DASH DIET COOKBOOK

The Complete Guide to Lower Blood Pressure with Flavorful Low-Sodium Recipes and 6 Weekly Plans to Improve your Health and Boost your Energy Level

Dorothy Brooks

Table of Contents

INTRODUCTION **10**

CHAPTER 1: WHY START A DASH DIET? **14**

WHO SHOULD FOLLOW THE DASH DIET? **14**
HOW TO LOSE WEIGHT QUICKLY & HEALTHILY
USING DASH **14**
DASH DIET PLAN BENEFITS **15**

CHAPTER 2: THE DASH DIET AT WORK **18**

DEFINITION & PRINCIPLES **18**
DASH DIET TYPES **18**
DASH-FRIENDLY FOODS **18**
DAIRY PRODUCTS **18**
FRUITS **19**
SUGGESTED SWEETENERS **20**
VEGETABLES **20**
FATS & OILS **21**
SEEDS - NUTS & LEGUMES **22**
WHOLE GRAINS **22**
LEAN PROTEIN **23**
LIMITED FOODS ALLOWED ON THE DASH PLAN **24**

CHAPTER 3: DASH RECIPES **26**

SMOOTHIES **27**
CANTALOUPE DASH SMOOTHIE **27**
CHOCOLATE BERRY DASH SMOOTHIE **27**
CHOCOLATE SMOOTHIE WITH BANANA & AVOCADO **27**
FRESH FRUIT SMOOTHIE **28**
GINGER CARROT & TURMERIC SMOOTHIE **28**
GREEN SMOOTHIES **28**
HIGH-PROTEIN STRAWBERRY SMOOTHIE **29**
ORANGE JUICE SMOOTHIE **29**
ORANGE- TOFU LOVER'S SMOOTHIES **29**
SPINACH & AVOCADO SMOOTHIE - GLUTEN-FREE **29**
BREAKFAST MUFFINS - TEA CAKES & SCONES **31**
APPLE CORN MUFFINS **31**
BLUEBERRY & LEMON SCONES **31**
BLUEBERRY MUFFINS - LOW-CARB **32**
CINNAMON ROLLS **32**
CRANBERRY ORANGE MUFFINS **33**
MIXED BERRY WHOLE-GRAIN COFFEE CAKE **33**

PECAN - RHUBARB MUFFINS **34**
PUMPKIN-HAZELNUT TEA CAKE **34**
RASPBERRY-CHOCOLATE SCONES **35**
3-GRAIN RASPBERRY MUFFINS **35**
BREAD OPTIONS **38**
CARROT & SPICE QUICK BREAD **38**
HONEY WHOLE-WHEAT BREAD **38**
IRISH BROWN BREAD **39**
LEMON BREAD **39**
WHOLE-GRAIN BANANA BREAD **40**
ZUCCHINI BREAD **40**
OTHER BREAKFAST OPTIONS **42**
ASPARAGUS OMELET TORTILLA WRAP **43**
BAKED BANANA-NUT OATMEAL CUPS **43**
BLUEBERRY LOW-SODIUM PANCAKES **43**
BREAKFAST SCRAMBLED EGG BURRITO **44**
BUCKWHEAT PANCAKES **44**
GERMAN APPLE PANCAKE **45**
GRILLED SPLIT BANANA BOWL **45**
MUESLI BREAKFAST BARS **46**
MUSHROOM HASH WITH POACHED EGGS - MEAL
PREP **46**
PEANUT BUTTER & CHIA BERRY JAM ENGLISH
MUFFIN DIABETIC-FRIENDLY **47**
POPOVERS **47**
RASPBERRY PEACH PUFF PANCAKE **47**
ROASTED PORTOBELLO MUSHROOMS FLORENTINE **48**
SPINACH & MUSHROOM QUICHE **48**
WHITE CHEDDAR - BLACK BEAN FRITTATA **49**
WHOLE-GRAIN BANANA BREAD **49**
WHOLE GRAIN BANANA PANCAKES **49**
ZUCCHINI & TOMATO PIE BREAKFAST PIE **50**
CEREAL FAVORITES **51**
BAKED OATMEAL **51**
BERRY MUESLI **51**
HERBED SAVORY WILD MUSHROOM OATMEAL **51**
OVERNIGHT OATS WITH FRUIT **52**
OVERNIGHT PEANUT BUTTER OATS - GLUTEN-FREE
- VEGAN **52**
QUICK-COOKING OATS - VEGAN **52**
SIX-GRAIN HOT CEREAL **53**
SOUP & CURRY OPTIONS **55**
ASPARAGUS SOUP **55**
BEEF STEW WITH FENNEL & SHALLOTS **55**
CHICKEN CHILI VERDE – DIABETIC-FRIENDLY **56**
CHICKPEA & POTATO CURRY **56**
CHILEAN LENTIL STEW WITH SALSA VERDE **57**
CREAM OF WILD RICE SOUP **57**
CURRIED CREAM OF TOMATO SOUP WITH APPLES **58**

Dijon Salmon with Green Bean Pilaf 100
Easy Low-Sodium Salmon with Lime & Herbs 100
Honey Mustard Salmon with Mango Quinoa
100
Lemon-Herb Salmon with Caponata & Spelt -
Diabetic-Approved 101
Roasted Salmon 102
Roasted Salmon with Olives - Garlic &
Tomatoes 102
Roasted Salmon with Maple Glaze 102
Roasted Salmon with Smoky Chickpeas &
Greens 103
Salmon & Asparagus with Lemon-Garlic
Butter Sauce 103
Salmon with Cilantro-Pineapple Salsa 104
Salmon & Edamame Cakes 104
Spicy Salmon 105
Poultry **107**
Balsamic Roasted Chicken 107
BBQ Basil Turkey Burgers 107
Cabbage Lo Mein - Heart Healthy 107
Chicken Cutlets & Sun-Dried Tomato Cream
Sauce 108
Chicken Fajitas - Party Pack 109
Chicken Souvlaki Kebabs & Mediterranean
Couscous 109
Chicken-Spaghetti Squash Bake 110
Chicken & Spinach Skillet Pasta with Lemon &
Parmesan 111
Chicken - Spring Pea & Farro Risotto with
Lemon 111
Chicken Stir-Fry with Basil - Eggplant &
Ginger 112
Chicken & Vegetable Penne with Parsley-
Walnut Pesto 113
Cinnamon Carrots & Chicken Sheet Pan
Favorite - Meal Prep 113
Creamy Chicken & Mushrooms 114
Easy Low-Sodium Chicken Breast 114
Greek Chicken with Roasted Spring
Vegetables & Lemon Vinaigrette 115
Greek Meatball Mezze Bowls - Meal Prep 115
Greek Turkey Burgers with Spinach - Feta &
Tzatziki 116
Harissa Chicken & Vegetables Sheet-Pan 116
Lemon-Thyme Roasted Chicken with
Fingerlings 117
Mediterranean Chicken Quinoa Bowls 117
Mushroom-Swiss Turkey Burgers 118
1-Pan Chicken & Asparagus Bake - Heart &
Diabetic Friendly 119
Orange Rosemary Roasted Chicken 119
Paella with Chicken Leeks & Tarragon 120
Pineapple Chicken Stir-Fry 120
Roasted Red Pepper Chicken Wrap 121
Roasted Turkey 121
Sesame Ginger Chicken Stir-Fry with
Cauliflower Rice 122
Skillet Lemon Chicken & Potatoes with Kale
123
Thai Chicken & Pasta Skillet 123
Zucchini Noodles & Quick Turkey Bolognese
- Meal Prep 123
The Quick & Delicious Turkey Meat Sauce 124
Meats **125**
Beef & Bean Sloppy Joes - Diabetic & Heart-
Friendly 125
Beef & Blue Cheese Penne with Pesto 125
Beef Stroganoff 126
Chinese Ginger Beef Stir-Fry with Baby Bok
Choy 126
Low-Sodium Dash Meatloaf 127
Philly Cheesesteak Stuffed Peppers 127
Sesame - Garlic Beef & Broccoli with Whole-
Wheat Noodles 127
Skillet Steak with Mushroom Sauce - Diabetic-
Friendly 128
Slow-Cooked Braised Beef with Carrots &
Turnips 129
Spaghetti & Quick Meat Sauce - Diabetic-
Friendly 129
Spicy Orange Beef & Broccoli Stir-Fry 130
Veggie-Filled Meat Sauce with Zucchini
Noodles 131
Pork Specialties **133**
Brown Sugar Pork Tenderloin Stir-Fry 133
Irish Pork Roast with Roasted Root
Vegetables 133
Pork Carnitas - Slow-Cooked 134
Pork & Cherry Tomatoes 134
Pork Chops with Tomato Curry - Diabetic-
Friendly 135
Pork Tenderloin with Apple-Thyme Sweet
Potatoes 135
Vegan Dishes **137**
Gnocchi Pomodoro 137
Lasagna - Vegan-Style - Diabetic-Friendly 137
Roasted Tofu & Peanut Noodle Salad 138
Spaghetti Squash with Tomato Basil Sauce -
Vegan-Friendly 138
Vegan Mushroom Bolognese 139
Sides - Veggies & Rice & Other Healthy
Dishes **140**
Acorn Squash with Apples 140
Black Bean & Sweet Potato Rice Bowls 140
Brown Rice Pilaf 140
Brussels Sprouts & Shallots 141
Bulgur & Quinoa Lunch Bowls - Meal Prep 141
Carrots - Honey-Sage-Flavored 142
Carrots with Mint 142

CURRIED SWEET POTATO & PEANUT SOUP	58
GARDEN VEGETABLE BEEF SOUP - DIABETIC-FRIENDLY	59
GINGER CHICKEN NOODLE SOUP	59
GREEN BEAN & TOMATO SOUP	60
MEDITERRANEAN CHICKEN & CHICKPEA SOUP - SLOW-COOKED	60
POTATO FENNEL SOUP	61
QUICK CREAMY TOMATO CUP-OF-SOUP	61
SALMON CHOWDER	61
SLOW-COOKED CHICKEN & WHITE BEAN STEW - DIABETIC-FRIENDLY	62
SOUTHWESTERN VEGETABLE CHOWDER	62
SPICY BEAN CHILI	63
TURKEY & BEAN SOUP	63
VEGETABLE & TOFU SOUP - VEGETARIAN-FRIENDLY	64
SALAD OPTIONS	**65**
APPLE SALAD WITH FIGS & ALMONDS	65
ASIAN VEGETABLE SALAD	65
BABY BEET & ORANGE SALAD	65
BALSAMIC BEAN SALAD WITH VINAIGRETTE	66
CHICKEN & SPRING VEGETABLE TORTELLINI SALAD	66
CHOPPED SUPERFOOD SALAD WITH SALMON & CREAMY GARLIC DRESSING	67
CITRUS SALAD	67
COBB SALAD THAI-STYLE	68
CREAMY PESTO CHICKEN SALAD WITH GREENS	68
CUCUMBER SALAD WITH TZATZIKI	68
LEAFY ROTISSERIE CHICKEN SALAD WITH CREAMY TARRAGON DRESSING	69
SALAD SKEWER WEDGES	69
SHRIMP & NECTARINE SALAD - DIABETIC-FRIENDLY	69
STRAWBERRY-BLUE CHEESE STEAK SALAD	70
TURKEY MEDALLIONS WITH TOMATO SALAD	71
WARM RICE & PINTOS SALAD - DIABETIC-FRIENDLY	71
WINTER KALE & QUINOA SALAD WITH AVOCADO	72
SALSA	**73**
AVOCADO SALSA	73
LOW-SODIUM RED SALSA	73
MEDITERRANEAN SALSA	73
VEGETABLE SALSA	73
SALAD DRESSINGS	**76**
BLUE CHEESE DRESSING	76
CARAMELIZED BALSAMIC VINAIGRETTE	76
CILANTRO LIME DRESSING	76
ORANGE BASIL VINAIGRETTE	76
SAUCES	**78**
BANANA-PECAN COMPOTE	78
BASIL BUTTER & SUN-DRIED TOMATO SAUCE	78
CITRUS REMOULADE	78
ORANGE-CRANBERRY GLAZE	78
SPAGHETTI SAUCE	79
TZATZIKI SAUCE	79
DIPS	**80**
ARTICHOKE DIP	80
ARTICHOKE - SPINACH & WHITE BEAN DIP	80
AVOCADO DIP	80
BABA GHANOUSH	80
BLACK BEAN & CORN RELISH	81
HUMMUS	81
MEDITERRANEAN LAYERED HUMMUS DIP	82
SKINNY QUINOA VEGETABLE DIP	82
SNACKS & APPETIZERS	**84**
ALMOND & APRICOT BISCOTTI	84
ASPARAGUS & HORSERADISH DIP	84
BAKED BRIE ENVELOPES	84
BASIL-PESTO STUFFED MUSHROOMS	85
CHICKPEA POLENTA WITH OLIVES	85
ROASTED ROOT VEGETABLES WITH GOAT CHEESE POLENTA	86
FISH & SEAFOOD	**87**
BAKED COD	87
BAKED PARCHMENT-PACKED TUNA STEAKS & VEGGIES WITH SAUCE	87
BROILED SEA BASS	87
CHARRED SHRIMP & PESTO BUDDHA BOWLS - DIABETIC-FRIENDLY	88
CHIMICHURRI MEAL-PREP NOODLE BOWLS - DIABETIC-FRIENDLY	88
COCONUT SHRIMP	89
CREAMY LEMON PASTA WITH SHRIMP	89
CRISPY OVEN-FRIED FISH TACOS	90
GARLIC SHRIMP & SPINACH - DIABETIC-FRIENDLY	90
GRILLED FISH WITH PEPERONATA - DIABETIC-FRIENDLY	91
GRITS & SHRIMP	91
PEPPERED SOLE	92
PEPPERY BARBECUE-GLAZED SHRIMP WITH VEGETABLES & ORZO	92
PROVENÇAL BAKED FISH WITH ROASTED POTATOES & MUSHROOMS	93
SEARED SCALLOPS & WHITE BEAN RAGU WITH CHARRED LEMON	93
SHRIMP ORZO & FETA	94
SHRIMP SCAMPI ZOODLES	94
SPICY JERK SHRIMP	95
SPINACH-STUFFED SOLE	96
STEAMED TROUT WITH MINT & DILL DRESSING	96
SWEET CHILI & PISTACHIO MAHI MAHI	96
SWORDFISH WITH ROASTED LEMONS	97
TILAPIA ON THE GRILL WITH SALSA	97
TURKISH SEARED TUNA WITH BULGUR & CHICKPEA SALAD	98
THE ULTIMATE FISH TACOS - DIABETIC-FRIENDLY	99
CHILI-LIME SALMON WITH PEPPERS & POTATOES IN A SHEET-PAN	99

CELERY ROOT 143
CREAMY LOW-SODIUM MACARONI & CHEESE 143
EASY BROWN RICE 143
EGGPLANT PARMESAN 144
FRIED RICE 144
GARLIC MASHED POTATOES 145
GINGER-MARINATED-GRILLED PORTOBELLO MUSHROOMS 145
GREEN BEANS WITH PEPPERS & GARLIC 145
GRILLED EGGPLANT & TOMATO PASTA - DIABETIC-FRIENDLY 146
LENTIL MEDLEY 146
MARINATED PORTOBELLO MUSHROOMS WITH PROVOLONE 147
MEDITERRANEAN CHICKPEA QUINOA BOWL - VEGETARIAN 147
MUSHROOM STROGANOFF 148
PEA & SPINACH CARBONARA - VEGETARIAN 148
POTATO SALAD 149
RICE NOODLES & SPRING VEGGIES 149
ROASTED CHICKPEA & SWEET POTATO PITAS 150
SHEET PAN ROASTED ROOT VEGGIES 150
SPICY ROASTED BROCCOLI 151
SPICY SNOW PEAS 151
STEAK FRIES 151
STUFFED POTATOES WITH SALSA & BEANS - DIABETIC APPROVED 152
WARM RICE & PINTOS 152
SNACKS **153**
AIR-FRIED CRISPY CHICKPEAS 153
ALMOND & APRICOT BISCOTTI 153
ALMOND CHAI GRANOLA 154
ALMOND - FRUIT BITES 154
ALMONDS WITH A SPICY KICK 154
AMBROSIA WITH COCONUT & TOASTED ALMONDS 155
APPLES & DIP 155
APRICOT & ALMOND CRISP 156
APRICOT & SOY NUT TRAIL MIX 156
ARTICHOKES ALLA ROMANA 156
BAKED APPLES WITH CHERRIES & ALMONDS 157
BERRIES MARINATED IN BALSAMIC VINEGAR 157
CINNAMON-RAISIN OATMEAL COOKIES 158
CRISPY POTATO SKINS 158
FRESH TOMATO CROSTINI 159
FRUIT COMPOTE & YOGURT ALA MODE 159
FRUIT KEBABS 159
FRUIT & NUT BAR 159
FRUIT SALSA & SWEET CHIPS 160
PEANUT BUTTER ENERGY BALLS - G.F. & DIABETIC-FRIENDLY 160
RAINBOW ICE POPS 160
SPICY-SWEET SNACK MIX 161
STRAWBERRY-CHOCOLATE GREEK YOGURT BARK 161
SANDWICHES **163**
BAKED FALAFEL SANDWICHES WITH YOGURT-TAHINI SAUCE 163
BUFFALO CHICKEN SALAD 163
CHICKEN & CHERRY LETTUCE WRAPS 164
SPINACH WRAP & TUNA SALAD 164
TURKEY WRAP 165
VEGGIE & HUMMUS SANDWICH - VEGAN & DIABETIC FRIENDLY 165
DELICIOUS DESSERTS **166**
APPLE DUMPLINGS 166
APPLE-BERRY COBBLER 166
APPLE & BLUEBERRY COBBLER 167
APPLE PIE 167
BANANA SPLITS 168
BLUEBERRY CHEESECAKE 168
CARROT & SPICE QUICK BREAD 168
CHOCOLATE CAKE 169
CHOCOLATE PEANUT BUTTER VEGETARIAN ENERGY BARS 170
CRAN-FRUIT COFFEE CAKE WITH CRUMB TOPPING 170
CREAMY FRUIT DESSERT 171
EASY PEACH COBBLER DUMP CAKE 171
FLOURLESS HONEY-ALMOND CAKE 171
FRUIT CAKE 172
GLAZED CHOCOLATE-PUMPKIN BUNDT CAKE 172
GRILLED PINEAPPLE WITH CHILI-LIME 173
GRAPEFRUIT- LIME & MINT YOGURT PARFAIT 173
LEMON PUDDING CAKES 174
MIXED BERRY PIE 174
PEACH TART 175
PEACHES & CREAM 175
POACHED CITRUSY PEARS 175
RHUBARB & ALMOND CRUMBLE TART 176
RICE - FRUITY PUDDING 176
RICE - MANGO PUDDING 177
DELICIOUS BEVERAGE OPTIONS **178**
BLUEBERRY-LAVENDER LEMONADE 178
CHOCOLATE-PEANUT BUTTER PROTEIN SHAKE 179
COOKIES & CREAM SHAKE 179
CRANBERRY SPRITZER 179
GINGER-CINNAMON & BLACKBERRY ICED TEA 179
ICED LATTE 180
ISLAND CHILLER 180
MINTY-LIME ICED TEA 180
MOCK CHAMPAGNE 181
NON-ALCOHOLIC MARGARITA 181
STRAWBERRY-BANANA MILKSHAKE 181
STRAWBERRY MOCKARITA 181
TROPICAL HURRICANE PUNCH 182
WATERMELON-CRANBERRY AGUA FRESCA 182

CHAPTER 4: SIX-WEEK MEAL PLAN **184**

HOW TO SAVE MONEY WITH SHOPPING LISTS &
MEAL PLANS   184
REMAIN FOCUSED   185
TWEAK YOUR COOKING HABITS   185
MEAL PLANS & SHOPPING LISTS - SIX WEEKS   186
BASIC FOOD ITEMS - SIX WEEKS   186
WEEK ONE - MEAL PLAN   188
WEEK ONE: INGREDIENT SHOPPING LIST   189
WEEK TWO - MEAL PLAN   191
WEEK TWO - INGREDIENT SHOPPING LIST   192
WEEK THREE - MEAL PLAN   194
WEEK THREE - INGREDIENT SHOPPING LIST   195
WEEK FOUR -MEAL PLAN   197
WEEK FOUR - INGREDIENT SHOPPING LIST   198
WEEK FIVE - MEAL PLAN   201
WEEK FIVE - INGREDIENT SHOPPING LIST   202
WEEK SIX - MEAL PLAN   204
WEEK SIX - INGREDIENT SHOPPING LIST   205

CHAPTER 5: DASH-APPROVED
RESTAURANT DINING   207

CHAPTER 6: BIG CHANGES TO YOUR DIET
BEGIN - ALWAYS FROM SMALL CHANGES212

HANDLE SNACK TIME   216
TIPS TO RESET YOUR DIET & LIFESTYLE   217

CONCLUSION   221

Dorothy Brooks

Introduction

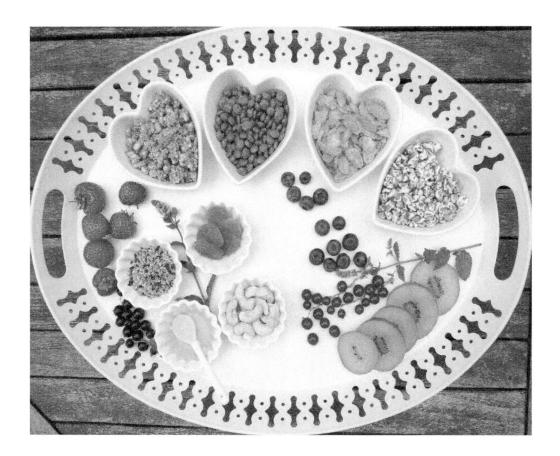

Congratulations on purchasing *Dash Diet Cookbook,* and thank you for doing so. Are you also seeking a diet where you will make healthier food choices? Has your physician told you that you need to find a healthier diet that matches your needs?

Your new cookbook contains a collection of healthy recipes without sacrificing taste, with a sample six-week meal plan to get you started. The Dietary Approaches to Stop Hypertension, or DASH for short, is a lifetime method to prevent and treat high blood pressure/hypertension. The following chapters will discuss its origins, leading benefits, and tons of new recipes for you to use in your new dieting way.

The DASH technique is based on the principle that you should eat various nutrient-rich foods while lowering sodium usage in your daily meal plan. DASH will reduce your blood pressure by using the elements of magnesium, potassium, and calcium.

The Worldwide Health Organization (WHO) noted the expansions in the processed food industry significantly impacted the amount of salt consumed worldwide. On top of that, stress can also raise your blood pressure. Keep in mind; underlying conditions can cause hypertension.

DASH diet trials were executed to test the effect of the diet on your blood pressure. One study originated in August of 1993 and did not end till July of 1997. Results indicated dietary patterns used with high intakes of specific fiber and minerals were linked with lower blood pressures.

The Mayo Clinic indicates hypertension is a common ailment after long-term forced blood has been pushed against the artery walls, resulting in heart disease issues. Normal blood pressure generally runs 120 over 80. If your blood pressures exceed 130 over 80, you have hypertension. Many instances of hypertension are caused by underlying conditions such as medication.

It's essential to understand the symptoms of high blood pressure so you can be aware. You may have blurred vision issues or a pounding feeling in your chest. You may also have bloody urine, which can be very discomforting. Chronic fatigue will probably be present, both mental and physical, since you may become confused - for no apparent reason. What's important is to test your blood pressure at a regular time daily to ensure you're getting an accurate reading. The testing should be done when you're not feeling any additional physical or mental stressors.

Consider the DASH diet methods as your new way of life. You will learn what the most common mistakes are when planning a meal plan. You will also better understand how to create a meal plan once you decide you are ready. Not everyone can do the DASH program, but you will also understand who cannot use the methods. The benefits are also extensive, as you will soon recognize.

Before we begin, let's review some of the abbreviations that are used in your new cookbook so you understand every step of the process:

Tablespoon = tbsp.
Teaspoon = tsp.
Gluten-Free = G.F.
All-Purpose = A.P.
Low-fat = l.f.
Reduced-Fat = r.f.
Reduced-sodium = r.s.

Fractions Included:

0.125 = 1/8
0.25 = 1/4
0.33 = 1/3
0.5 = 1/2
0.66 = 2/3
0.75 = 3/4

Most of the temperature settings and ingredients are shown with metric and US standards for your best cooking experience.
You may also see some of the recipes include "added sugars."

Two types of sugars exist in American diets.

✓ **Natural sugars:** are those found in whole, fresh and unprocessed foods, such as the fructose in bananas and other fruits or the lactose in a glass of milk. Foods with natural sugars tend to be low in calories and sodium and high in water and many important vitamins and minerals. In addition, the fiber in fruit slows down the rate at which the body digests it, so you don't get an excessive spike in blood sugar. The lactose in milk comes along with a good serving of protein, which provides long-term energy, so we feel full longer than when we drink a sugar-rich soda.

✓ ***Added sugars:*** those you need to worry about the most. Those nasty calories are also included as high fructose corn syrup, lurking in some ketchups and packaged breads, as well as honey, agave, molasses, fruit juice concentrates, maltose, dextrose, or similar products ending in "ose." that you could add to a cup of tea or smoothie.

Often, they are not found together with other nutrients such as proteins and fibers that can compensate for their effect, our body digests them more quickly, causing a rapid increase in blood sugar. And over time, having a consistently high blood sugar contributes to health problems like type 2 diabetes, obesity, and heart disease.

Be aware when the second ones type are found on the labels!

The DASH diet is rich in fruits and vegetables, nuts, with low fat and nonfat dairy, fish, lean meats, and poultry, mostly whole grains, and heart-healthy fats. You fill up on delicious fruits and vegetables paired up with protein-rich foods to quench your hunger.

This makes a plan that is so easy to follow.

Chapter 1:
Why Start a DASH Diet?

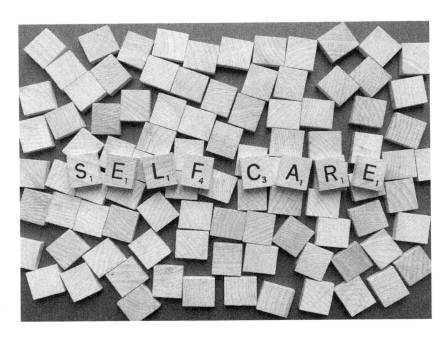

Who Should Follow the DASH Diet?

DASH can be safe for many people, but it's not for everyone. The following is a list of individuals who may need to reconsider the DASH diet plan:

- If you're unsure you're in good health
- A recorded family history of heart-related issues: Men before 55 or women before 65 years of age
- Overweight or obese
- You've had a heart attack
- A woman older than age 55 or men older than 45 years old
- You've got high blood pressure or high cholesterol issues
- If you have diabetes
- If you have a lingering health ailment - such as cardiovascular disease or lung disease
- Discomfort or pain, which is evident in your arms, chest, neck, or jaw during various forms of activity
- Not exercising regularly

How to Lose Weight Quickly & Healthily Using DASH

These are the basics:

- Switch refined grains for whole grains.
- Eat fruits and veggies daily.
- Shop low-fat or fat-free dairy products.
- Select lean proteins - beans, fish, or poultry.
- Eat limited portions of foods containing high counts of added sugars, including candy and soda pop.

DASH Diet Plan Benefits

Part of the reasoning of why so many people appreciate the DASH diet is because there is an abundance of documented research available on the topic about his benefits. Here we report the more important.

Blood Pressure is Lowered

Your blood pressure measures the force put on your organs and blood vessels as your blood is passed through them. The counts for your pressure include:

- Systolic pressure is the pressure in your blood vessels as your heart is beating.
- Diastolic pressure is the vessel pressure between heartbeats - your heart is at rest.

Blood pressure has been proven to be lower within two weeks of beginning the DASH Diet plan. The composition of magnesium, calcium, and potassium are the key elements. Too much sodium can cause fluid to build up, creating more pressure and strain on the heart, which increases your blood pressure.

Not only does the standard diet plan offer you options through an emphasis on fruits, vegetables, and low-dairy foods, you are also consuming fewer whole grains. The traditional diet plan allows you to consume 2,300 milligrams (mg) daily. On the other hand, the lower sodium dash diet plan allows only 1,500 mg daily.

On the plus side, both versions of the DASH choice will reduce sodium intake significantly compared to many of the 'normal' American diets, which can add up to 3,400 mg more of daily sodium.
According to the American Heart Association (AHA), all adults should be limited to no more than 1,500 mg daily. It is advisable to confer with your physician to be sure you are ingesting amounts within your limits. Many factors are considered, including your race, age, and past or current health issues. Remedy the intake of salt by removing the shakers from the dinner table. While cooking, choose no- or low-sodium condiments and foods. It is crucial to stay away from foods that are pickled, smoked, or cured.

Lowered Cholesterol

As you consume the whole grains, you provide a natural fiber source with oats, brown rice, and similar products. By receiving sufficient fiber, also research-proven, you will be reducing your cholesterol levels simultaneously. Women should consume about 25 grams daily versus men, who should aim for 38 grams every day.

Kidney Health

You can help prevent kidney stones, which can become very painful. The diet prevents the composition of the mineral deposits that lead to the generation of stones. Consuming high amounts of sodium can also lead to kidney failure. The National Kidney Foundation has praised DASH for its potential value to those who might be at risk of kidney failure. Once again, discuss this with your physician.

Avoid Diabetes

The DASH diet that is most useful against diabetes is its influence on the decrease in insulin resistance (type 2 diabetes, is also called insulin-independent), an effect intensified by constant physical exercise associated with compliance with the diet.
Without the starchy foods and empty carbohydrates, you can avoid the 'simple' sugars which your body easily absorbs and sends into your bloodstream. This intake can cause insulin levels and the body's glucose levels— via the chance of diabetes.

Weight Issues

You will learn how to get tuned in on important things to help you with healthier eating habits and become more physically active. You will notice the results if you make a plan you can follow.

You have to achieve a calorie deficit to accomplish weight loss. You can still substantially shed the unwanted pounds because the DASH diet pushes for nutrient-dense foods versus calorie-rich foods. High fiber also is a plus, as well as a plan filled with vital nutrients. Among the benefits, it is also aimed at decreasing water retention and increasing metabolism, useful for maintaining the results obtained and not regaining the lost pounds.

Osteoporosis

The high content of potassium, protein, and calcium is the DASH program's composition, helping slow the process or onset of osteoporosis.

The food in lean proteins, leafy vegetables, milk, grains, and fruits contribute to building strong bones.

Chapter 2:
The DASH Diet at Work

Definition & Principles

The DASH diet inspires you to lower your diet's sodium intake. Indulge in various nutrient-rich food to lower your blood pressure by increasing your calcium, magnesium, and potassium intake. At the end of two weeks, you *could* reduce your systolic (top number) pressure by about 14 points, making a compelling change to your health. Use Dash with conservative portions of nuts, whole grains, fish, and poultry.

Dash Diet Types

Choose the DASH plan version that will best suit your health demands:
- The standard DASH diet allows up to 2,300 milligrams (mg) of sodium daily.
- The lower-sodium DASH Diet is a phase of the DASH experience that restricts your daily sodium intake to 1,500 mg.

Both versions of the plan can help lower the sodium amounts in your diet. For example, you may not realize the usual American diet can tip the scales to 3,400 mg of sodium daily. If you're unsure which phase is appropriate for your case, it's advisable to discuss any changes with your physician.

Dash-Friendly Foods

Dairy Products

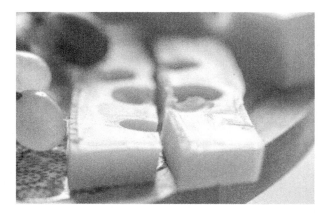

Aim for two to three dairy products daily to receive critical nutrients, including fat, protein, calcium, and Vitamin D. These are some of those choices with the suggested types and amounts that should be low-fat and fat-free or reduced-fat:

- Cheese - 1.5 oz. serving
- Skim or f.f. - 1% l.f. milk - skim or buttermilk - 1 cup
- Yogurt or frozen yogurt - 1 cup

Milk provides an array of high-quality milk proteins, which intensely help to increase calcium absorption. If lactose is your enemy, choose almond and coconut milk since neither one contains dairy properties. Limited research has discovered individuals can drop unwanted pounds by adding just one serving of yogurt daily. You will also achieve good intestinal bacteria, which may allow you to reach and maintain a healthier weight!

Fruits

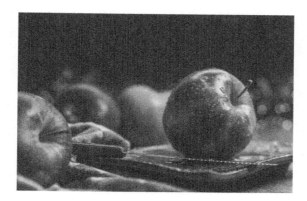

Dietitians recommend four to five servings of fruit daily to provide vital energy and necessary fiber content for the body to function correctly. Enjoy canned, frozen, dried, or fresh fruits. Be sure to carefully read each of the nutritional labels to avoid added sugar content. Most fruits contain large quantities of potassium, fiber, magnesium, and many are low in fat. Serving portions can include one of these:

- Fruit juice - .5 cup
- Canned, fresh, or frozen fruit - .5 cup
- Fruit - 1 medium or .25 cup of dried fruit

These are some of the examples of healthy fruit choices with approximate calorie content for your convenience:

- Bananas are one of America's favorite fruits. It provides approximately 13% of your daily needs for potassium. So, if you have leg cramps, have a banana. One medium banana is 105 calories.
- Apples are high in fiber and antioxidants. Two extra small apples are 105 calories.
- Pears are an excellent antioxidant and are also high in fiber content (102 calories for one medium or 178 grams).
- Apricots - 6 whole are 101 calories.
- Peaches - 2.5 medium peaches are 96 calories.
- Dates - 1.5 dates are 100 calories.
- Grapes - 30 grapes are 101 calories.
- Mangoes - 1 cup of sliced is 101 calories.
- Oranges - 2 small oranges are 90 calories.
- Cantaloupe Melons - 2 cups diced melon are 106 calories.
- Nectarines - 1.5 medium nectarines registers at 94 calories.
- Pineapples - 1.25 cups cut in chunks are 103 calories.
- Raisins - One small box or 1.5 oz. is 129 calories.
- Strawberries - 25 medium berries are 96 calories.
- Tangerines - 2 medium weigh about 100 calories.
- Raspberries - 1.5 cups or about 100 berries are 96 or 99 calories.
- Blueberries - 1.25 cups or about 125 berries are 103 or 97 calories.
- Blackberries - 100 berries or 1.5 cups are 100 or 93 calories.

Suggested Sweeteners

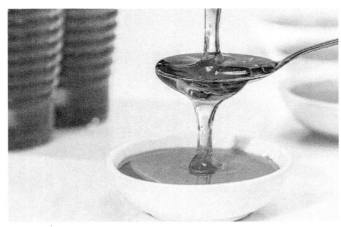

Weekly, you're allowed a maximum of five servings or less of sugar. The DASH plan doesn't require total abstinence from sweets, but you need to choose lower fat content options. Consider jelly beans, low-fat granola bars, or cookies. Maybe fruit ices if you are going to cheat. These are a few examples of one serving: One cup of lemonade - one tablespoon of sugar or one tablespoon of jam or jelly.

- *Sugar*: According to the American Heart Association, women are allowed 25 grams daily, whereby men are allowed 36 grams of sugar, which is about the same scale as considered by WHO. However, the average American will consume 82 grams of added sugar every single day. Consider this as a scale. One tablespoon of jam or jelly or 1/2 cup of sorbet will equal one tablespoon of sugar.

- *Raw Honey:* Honey has been used as a popular natural sweetener for many years. You can purchase raw honey as a comb, a whipped mixture (tubs like butter), and spreadable options.

- *Maple Syrup*: The natural sweetener is collected from sugar maple trees. It's available in dark, medium, or light in liquid form. It is also high in calcium content. Use caution because many of the grocery store items are not 100% natural maple syrup. Check at the health food store for natural syrup.

- *Agave Syrup*: This syrup is also sometimes called agave nectar and is a native of Mexico. The agave plant provides a natural nectar sweetener and is available in liquid form. It resembles honey - but it is even sweeter, fruitier, and has a much cleaner flavor. It can be in anything from BBQ sauce to catch it to baked goods or ice cream.

Vegetables

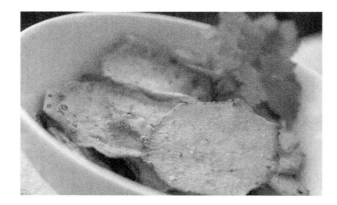

It is vital to consume four to five vegetable servings daily for fiber, potassium, vitamins, and magnesium. Be sure to check the nutrients and avoid sodium/salt. Enjoy some of these:

- *Beans*: Any beans are good choices, but white beans are the best. If you use canned options, just be sure to rinse the beans to reduce the sodium content.
- *Sweet Potatoes*: You will receive fiber and Vitamin A for boosts towards your blood vessel health.
- *Winter Squash*: Substitute spaghetti squash for pasta dishes to reduce the calorie intake.
- *Broccoli:* These delicious 'mini trees' provide you with tons of benefits, including decreasing your risk of overall mortality, diabetes, heart disease, and obesity. It's an excellent way to promote a healthy complexion and boost beautiful hair. You will also have increased energy and overall weight loss.

Other Vegetable Choices
- Arugula - About 2 cups - 40 grams are ten calories
- Cauliflower - 100 grams of boiled are 28 calories
- Kale - 100 grams of raw kale is 28 calories; boiled is 24 calories
- Carrots - 1 medium carrot is 25 calories
- Lima beans - 1 tbsp. of boiled limas are 13 calories
- Green beans - 100 grams are 23.5 calories
- Spinach - 23.18 calories per 100 grams
- Beets - 1 cup is 59 calories
- Garlic - 148.9 calories per 100 grams
- Onions - 1 scallion is five calories for 5 grams - 1 shallot is 43 grams or 31 calories
- Tomatoes - Fresh tomatoes are 17.69 calories per 100 grams

Fats & Oils

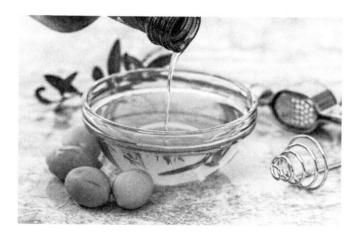

Dietitians recommend consuming a minimum of two to three servings of oils and fats daily. Your body needs them to strengthen your immune system and absorb nutrients. You must control the amount used because it's possible to lead to cardiovascular disease, obesity, or diabetes. You must know the difference. Consider a serving of 2 tablespoons of salad dressing or one teaspoon of mayonnaise, vegetable oil, or soft margarine. You can also choose from coconut, peanut, or extra-virgin olive oil (EVOO).

Seeds - Nuts & Legumes

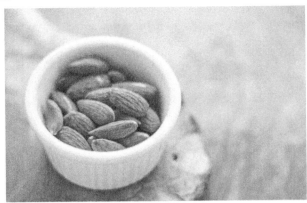

While you're making your plan for the week, be sure to include 5 to 6 servings of seeds, nuts, beans, and legumes. Healthy veggies will provide you with additional fiber, protein, magnesium, phytochemicals, and protein to your body. Some may have higher calorie counts. One serving could be .5 cup of cooked legumes, 1.5 ounces or .33 cup of nuts, two tablespoons of nut butter, or .5 ounces or two tablespoons of seeds. Consider some of these options:

- Kidney beans - 215 calories per one cup - 256 grams
- Peas - 125 calories per one cup - 160 grams
- Pistachios - 170 calories per .5 cup
- Almonds - 622 calories per 100 grams
- Cashews - 585 calories per 100 grams
- Peanuts - 427 calories per 73 grams or for each .5 cup

Whole Grains

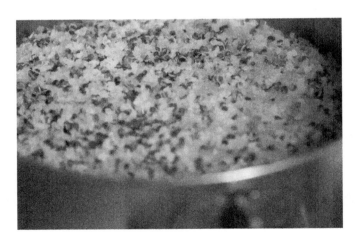

You should consume seven to eight servings of whole grains daily to receive an increased amount of fiber and nutrients versus consuming processed food products. Choose 100% whole wheat or grain. Select a variety of pasta, bread, and cereals. Avoid topping them off with butter, cheese, or cream. These are just a few:

- Quinoa - rinse thoroughly before cooking - 1 cup cooked is 222 calories.
- Brown rice - 218 calories per cooked cup
- Whole oats - ex. steel cut oats - 150 calories per .25 cup dry
- Popcorn - .25 cup for 248 calories - makes 10 cups

Lean Protein

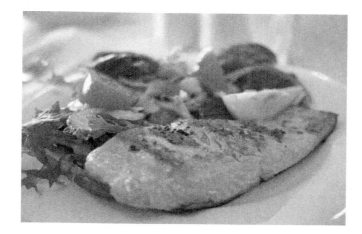

It's advisable to enjoy up to six servings of lean meat, fish, and poultry daily. Skinless and lean meat are good sources of B complex vitamins, zinc, iron, and protein. These are some of the choices:

- Eggs: 1 egg is one serving.
- Seafood & Fish: Get your Omega 3 fatty acids by eating herring, tuna, and salmon, which will help lower the cholesterol levels in your blood. Enjoy fresh - not canned - clams to reduce the preservatives and salt intake.
- Poultry is another lean option with its skin removed.

One ounce of cooked fish, seafood, and meat - roasted, baked, or grilled - is an appropriate amount, but you should avoid frying the options.

Limited Foods Allowed on the DASH Plan

You should limit your intake of foods in these categories:

- High Sodium Foods
- Dairy with high-fat content or whole milk or cream
- High sodium salad dressing
- High-fat snacks
- Added sugars and other sweets, including beverages composed of sugar
- Artificial sweeteners
- Saturated and trans fats
- Red meat - lean cuts only
- Salted Nuts or seeds
- Packaged Meals & Snacks
- Canned & Processed Meat
- Bread & Baked Goods
- Cheese
- Sauces
- Soup
- Salty Snacks
- Many Restaurant Foods

Chapter 3:
DASH Recipes

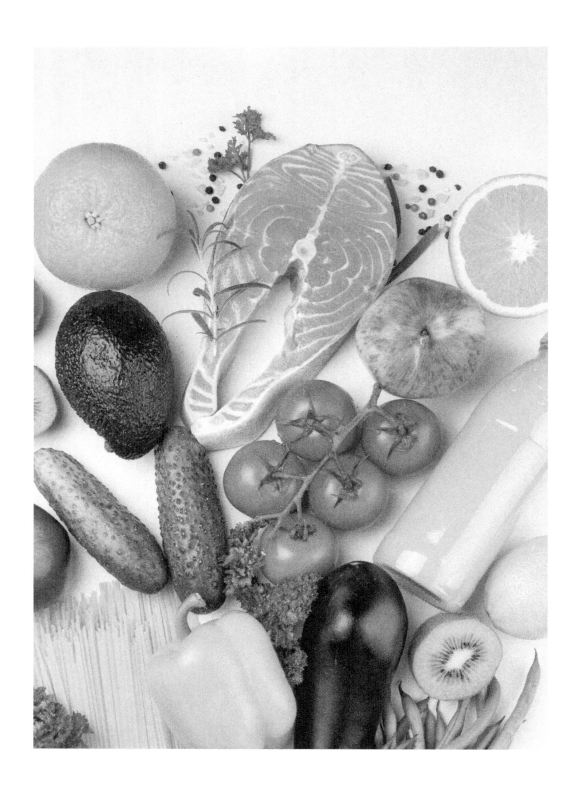

Smoothies

Cantaloupe Dash Smoothie

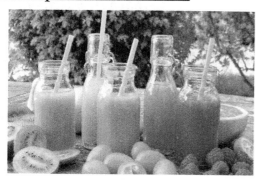

Portions Provided: 2 servings
Time Required: 5 minutes
Nutritional Statistics (Each Portion):
- Protein Counts: 11 grams
- Carbohydrates: 46 grams
- Fat Content: 1 gram
- Dietary Fiber: 3 grams
- Sodium: <trace mg
- Calories: 214

Essential Ingredients:
- Frozen cantaloupe (2.5 cups)
- Nonfat or low-fat milk (.5 cup)
- Frozen banana (1 sliced)
- Nonfat vanilla Greek yogurt (5.5 oz./160 g carton)
- Ice (.5 cup)
- Honey (1 tsp.)

Preparation Method:
1. Peel, cube, and freeze the cantaloupe.
2. Place the milk, banana, yogurt, ice, and honey in a blender.
3. Work and mix the fixings till incorporated and creamy.
4. Toss in the cantaloupe pieces - process until incorporated and creamy smooth.
5. Serve immediately.

Chocolate Berry Dash Smoothie

Portions Provided: 1 serving
Time Required: 5 minutes
Nutritional Statistics (Each Portion):
- Protein Counts: 6.4 grams
- Fat Content: 17.2 grams
- Sugars: 8 grams
- Dietary Fiber: 7.7 grams
- Sodium: 55 mg

- Calories: 250

Essential Ingredients:
- Cashews (2 tbsp.)
- Water - cold (340 g/12 oz.)
- Frozen blueberries (.25 cup)
- Avocado (half of 1)
- Organic cocoa powder (2 tbsp.)
- Vanilla extract (.5 tsp.)
- Agave nectar/sub honey (as desired)

Preparation Method:
1. Toss each of the fixings into a blender.
2. Set the function to high and mix for 40 to 60 seconds.
3. Pour and serve.

Chocolate Smoothie with Banana & Avocado

Portions Provided: 2 servings
Time Required: 5 minutes
Nutritional Statistics (Each Portion):
- Fat Content: 12 grams
- Carbohydrates: 33 grams
- Protein Counts: 11 grams
- Fiber: 8 grams
- Sugars: 8 grams
- Sodium: 102 mg
- Calories: 252

Essential Ingredients:
- Vanilla soy milk (2 cups)
- Medium banana (1)
- Avocado (half of 1)
- Splenda (2 individual packets)
- Unsweetened cocoa powder (.25 cup)

Preparation Method:
1. Peel the banana and remove the avocado peel and pit.
2. Toss each of the fixings into the blender - process them till they're creamy smooth.
3. Serve promptly and enjoy.

Fresh Fruit Smoothie

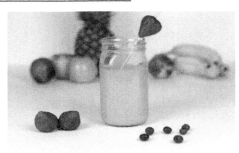

Portions Provided: 4 servings
Time Required: 10-15 minutes
Nutritional Statistics (Each Portion):
- Protein Counts: 1 gram
- Carbohydrates: 17 grams
- Fat Content: -0- grams
- Sugars: 13 grams
- Dietary Fiber: 1 gram
- Sodium: 7 mg
- Calories: 72

Essential Ingredients:
- Fresh pineapple chunks (1 cup)
- Cantaloupe or other melon chunks (.5 cup)
- Fresh strawberries (1 cup)
- Juice (from 2 oranges)
- Water (1 cup - cold)
- Agave nectar/sub honey (1 tbsp.)

Preparation Method:
1. Discard the rind from the pineapple and melon - slice them into pieces.
2. Remove the stems from strawberries. Toss each of the fixings into a blender. Mix them till they're incorporated and creamy smooth. Serve the smoothies cold.

Ginger Carrot & Turmeric Smoothie

Portions Provided: 2 servings
Time Required: 10 minutes
Nutritional Statistics (Each Portion):
- Protein Counts: 2.4 grams
- Carbohydrates: 32 grams
- Fat Content: 2.3 grams
- Sugars: 17.5 grams
- Dietary Fiber: 5 grams
- Sodium: 112 mg
- Calories: 144

Essential Ingredients:
The Juice:
- Carrots (2 cups)
- Filtered water (1.5 cups)

The Smoothie:
- Ripe banana (1 large + more for sweetness as desired)
- Frozen or fresh pineapple (1 cup or 140 g)
- Fresh ginger (.5 tbsp.)
- Carrot juice (.5 cup/120 ml.)
- Ground turmeric (.25 tsp.)
- Cinnamon (.5 tsp.)
- Lime juice (1 tbsp.)
- Unsweetened almond milk (1 cup or 240 ml.)
- Suggested: High-powered blender

Preparation Method:
1. Add the water and carrots to the blender. Mix till it's incorporated and smooth. Add more water as needed, scraping down its sides. Keep the juice in the refrigerator.
2. Toss the rest of the fixings into the blender for the smoothie and mix thoroughly.
3. Serve in two chilled glasses.

Green Smoothies

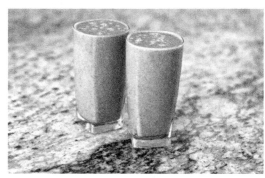

Portions Provided: 4 servings @ 6 oz./170 g each
Time Required: 6 minutes
Nutritional Statistics (Each Portion):
- Protein Counts: 1 gram
- Carbohydrates: 12 grams (Net: 10 grams)
- Fat Content: trace grams
- Dietary Fiber: 2 grams
- Sodium: 15 mg
- Calories: 64

Essential Ingredients:
- Banana (1)
- Juice (1 lemon/about 4 tbsp.)
- Strawberries (.5 cup)
- Berries - such as blueberries or blackberries (.5 cup)
- Baby spinach (2 oz./approx. 2 cups)
- Fresh mint (as desired)
- Ice or cold water (1 cup)

Preparation Method:
1. Toss each of the fixings into a blender or juicer.
2. Puree and serve in chilled mugs.

High-Protein Strawberry Smoothie

Portions Provided: 1 serving
Time Required: 10 minutes
Nutritional Statistics (Each Portion):
- Protein Counts: 22 grams
- Carbohydrates: 26 grams (Net: 2 grams)
- Fat Content: 2.8 grams
- Sugars: 21 grams
- Dietary Fiber: 3 grams
- Sodium: 141 mg
- Calories: 215

Essential Ingredients:
- Low-fat cottage cheese -low-salt (.5 cup)
- 1% milk (.75 cup)
- Fresh/frozen strawberries (1 cup) **

Preparation Method:
1. Toss each of the fixings into the mixing container dish (ex. Nutribullet cup).
2. Blend each of the fixings till creamy.
3. Pour it into a tall-chilled glass to serve.
4. *Note** You can substitute the berries for a banana, sliced mango, or a half cup of another favorite berry.*

Orange Juice Smoothie

Portions Provided: 2 servings @ 1 cup each
Time Required: 5 minutes
Nutritional Statistics (Each Portion):
- Protein Counts: 12 grams
- Carbohydrates: 41 grams
- Fat Content: trace grams
- Sugars: 26 grams
- Dietary Fiber: 5 grams
- Sodium: 177 mg
- Calories: 200

Essential Ingredients:
- Vanilla frozen yogurt - no sugar - f.f. (1 cup)
- Milk - fat-free (.75 cup)
- Frozen orange juice concentrate - no-sugar (.25 cup)

Preparation Method:
1. Toss each of the fixings into your blender - mixing till creamy.
2. Serve in a cold mug and enjoy them right away.

Orange- Tofu Lover's Smoothies

Portions Provided: 4 servings
Time Required: 6 minutes
Nutritional Statistics (Each Portion):
- Protein Counts: 3 grams
- Carbohydrates: 20 grams
- Fat Content: 1 gram
- Sugars: 4 grams
- Dietary Fiber: 1 gram
- Sodium: 40 mg
- Calories: 101

Essential Ingredients:
- Dark honey (1 tbsp.)
- Chilled light vanilla soy milk (1 cup)
- Vanilla extract (.5 tsp.)
- Chilled orange juice (1.5 cups)
- Soft/silken tofu (.33 cup)
- Orange zest (1 tsp.)

Preparation Method:
1. Grate the orange for zest and prepare the juice.
2. Pour the milk, orange juice, honey, vanilla, orange zest, tofu, and ice into a blender.
3. Mix till the smoothie is as desired (30 sec.).
4. Pour the smoothies into cold glasses. Garnish each glass with an orange segment.

Spinach & Avocado Smoothie - Gluten-Free

Portions Provided: 1 serving
Time Required: 5 minutes
Nutritional Statistics (Each Portion):
- Protein Counts: 17.7 grams
- Carbohydrates: 57.8 grams
- Fat Content: 8.2 grams
- Sugars: 39.3 grams
- Dietary Fiber: 7.8 grams
- Sodium: 237.9 mg
- Calories: 357

Essential Ingredients:
- Plain yogurt - nonfat (1 cup)
- Frozen banana (1)
- Avocado (¼ of 1)
- Fresh spinach (1 cup)
- Honey (1 tsp.)
- Water (2 tbsp.)

Preparation Method:
1. Toss the yogurt with avocado, honey, banana, water, and spinach in a blender.

2. Let the mixture work and puree till it's creamy smooth. Serve in a chilled mug.

Breakfast Muffins - Tea Cakes & Scones

Apple Corn Muffins

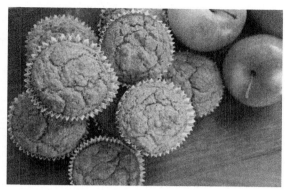

Portions Provided: 12 servings
Time Required: 40 minutes
Nutritional Statistics (Each Portion):
- Protein Counts: 4 grams
- Carbohydrates: 26 grams (Net: 18 grams)
- Fat Content: <1 gram
- Sugars: 7 grams
- Dietary Fiber: 1 gram
- Sodium: 127 mg
- Calories: 120

Essential Ingredients:
- Apple (1)
- Corn kernels (.5 cup)
- A. P. flour (2 cups)
- Yellow cornmeal (.5 cup)
- Brown sugar (.25 cup - packed tight)
- Salt (.25 tsp.)
- Baking powder (1 tbsp.)
- Egg whites (2)
- Fat-free milk (.75 cup)
- Also Needed: 12-count muffin tin

Preparation Method:
1. Line the containers with foil or paper liners.
2. Preheat the oven to reach 425° Fahrenheit/218° Celsius.
3. Peel and coarsely chop the apple.
4. Whisk the brown sugar with the cornmeal, salt, baking powder, and flour in a big mixing container.
5. Prepare another container and beat the eggs with the milk. Blend in the corn kernels and apple bits.
6. Whisk and combine all of the fixings till they are slightly moistened.

7. Scoop the batter into the cups (leaving ⅓ of the top open).
8. Set a timer to bake for ½ hour.
9. Test the muffins for doneness by gently pressing the center. They should spring back.

Blueberry & Lemon Scones

Portions Provided: 6 servings
Time Required: 50-55 minutes
Nutritional Statistics (Each Portion):
- Protein Counts: 45.1 grams
- Sodium: 35 mg
- Calories: 328

Essential Ingredients:
- A. P. flour (2 cups + more for dusting)
- Granulated sugar (.25 cup)
- No-sodium baking powder - your choice (1 tbsp.)
- Cold unsalted butter (6 tbsp.)
- Eggs (2 large)
- Lemon: Zest + juice (1 tbsp.)
- Half & Half (.5 cup)
- Fresh blueberries (1 cup)

Preparation Method:
1. Warm the oven temperature setting to reach 400° Fahrenheit/204° Celsius.
2. Cover a baking tray using a layer of parchment baking paper. Sprinkle it lightly using a tiny bit of flour.
3. Rinse, remove the stems, and dry the blueberries using a few paper towels. Prepare the lemon and set it aside for now.
4. Whisk the flour with butter, sugar, lemon zest, and baking powder into a big mixing container - mixing till it's crumbly.
5. Break and whisk two eggs into a smaller container. Whisk in the Half & Half and lemon juice - beating till it's thoroughly blended.
6. Toss the egg mix into the dry fixings - stir till blended.
7. Gently mix in the berries. Scoop the batter onto a floured surface - such as a chopping block.
8. Work the dough into a disc/ball - arrange it in the center of the parchment-lined baking

tray - as you flatten it into a one-inch circular disc. Use a floured knife to portion it into six wedges.

9. Put the baking tray in the fridge to chill and harden the dough's butter (15 min.).

10. When chilled, pop it into the oven to bake till it's nicely browned (20 min.).

11. Put the tray onto a wire rack to cool. Recut the scones while still warm.

12. Serve with a mix of honey and butter or plain unsalted butter.

Blueberry Muffins - Low-Carb

Portions Provided: 12 servings
Time Required: 60 minutes
Nutritional Statistics (Each Portion):
- Protein Counts: 5.8 grams
- Carbohydrates: 14.9 grams
- Fat Content: 14.6 grams
- Sugars: 9.9 grams
- Dietary Fiber: 2.9 grams
- Sodium: 230.1 mg
- Calories: 204

Essential Ingredients:
- Coconut flour (.25 cup)
- Bak. soda (.25 tsp.)
- Salt (.25 tsp.)
- Almond flour (1.75 cups)
- Bak. powder (1 tbsp.)
- Eggs (3 large)
- Light brown sugar (.33 cup + 2 tbsp.)
- Blueberries (1 cup)
- Vanilla extract (1.5 tsp.)
- Milk - reduced-fat (.5 cup)
- Avocado oil (.25 cup)

Preparation Method:
1. Warm the oven to reach 350° Fahrenheit/177° Celsius.
2. Use a generous portion of cooking oil spray to prepare the muffin tray wells.
3. Whisk both types of flour with salt, baking soda, and powder in a big mixing container. Fold in the berries - tossing to cover.
4. Whisk the eggs with the milk, vanilla, brown sugar, and oil in a separate mixing container. Stir in the dry fixings - stirring till it's thoroughly combined.
5. Portion the batter into the muffin cups (¼ cup each).
6. Bake the muffins till they're lightly browned around the edges (20-25 min.).

7. Leave them in the pan - place them onto a cooling rack (20 min.).

8. Transfer the muffins from the tin by using a butter knife to dislodge the edges if needed to serve.

Cinnamon Rolls

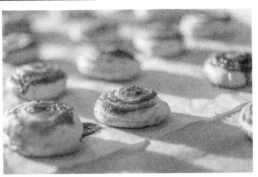

Portions Provided: 32 servings
Time Required: 4 hours (lots of waiting time)
Nutritional Statistics (Each Portion):
- Protein Counts: 3 grams
- Carbohydrates: 25 grams
- Fat Content: 2 grams
- Added Sugars: 8 grams
- Dietary Fiber: 2 grams
- Sodium: 30 mg
- Calories: 130

Essential Ingredients:
- Canola oil (.25 cup)
- Skim milk (1 cup)
- Salt (.25 tsp.)
- Sugar (.33 cup)
- Dry yeast (2 pkg. @ about 0.75 oz. each)
- Warm water (.25 cup)
- Eggs: Whole (1) + whites (2)
- A. P. flour (3 cups)
- Flour - whole-wheat (2.5 cups)
- Cooking spray (as needed)
- Brown sugar (.75 cup)
- Cinnamon (2 tbsp.)
- Raisins (.25 cup)
- Frozen juice concentrate - unsweetened apple (.5 cup)

Preparation Method:
1. Set the juice aside to thaw.
2. Use a small saucepan to warm the milk - do not boil. Mix in the salt, oil, and sugar. Set it aside to cool till it's tepid.
3. Whisk the water with the yeast, stir, and set aside for five minutes.
4. Whisk all of the eggs with the mixture after the waiting time.

5. Combine the flours, one cup at a time - to form a soft dough.

6. Lightly dust a working space with flour - knead gently till the dough is incorporated - yet elastic (5 min.).

7. Scoop the dough into the bowl - cover using a layer of plastic wrap. Wait for it to rise in a warm space until it has doubled in size (1.5 hrs.).

8. Portion the dough in half, shaping it into two dough balls. Put a plastic layer over the container and let it rest (10 min.).

9. Whisk the cinnamon and brown sugar with the raisins in a small mixing container.

10. Spray the baking pan with cooking oil spray.

11. Roll each dough ball into a rectangle using a rolling pin if you have one (noting -, a glass will also work) until it is about 16x8-inches. Lightly spritz the dough using a tiny bit of baking spray.

12. Sprinkle each of the rectangles using the cinnamon mixture. Roll and slice each rectangle into 16 portions - arrange them onto the baking tray. Wait for them to rise until their size is about doubled (1.5 hrs.)

13. Meanwhile, warm the apple juice using a medium-temperature setting - simmer until it is syrupy (5-7 min.) and set it to the side.

14. Warm the oven to reach 350° Fahrenheit/177° Celsius.

15. Brush the rolls with apple juice and bake until golden brown (15 min.) and serve warm.

Cranberry Orange Muffins

Portions Provided: 16 servings
Time Required: 30-35 minutes
Nutritional Statistics (Each Portion):
- Protein Counts: 4 grams
- Carbohydrates: 24 grams
- Fat Content: 5 grams
- Sugars: 10 grams
- Dietary Fiber: 1 gram
- Sodium: 148 mg
- Calories: 155

Essential Ingredients:
- Plain Greek yogurt - f.f. (230 g or 8 oz.)
- Eggs (2)
- Canola oil (.25 cup)
- Brown sugar (.25 cup)

- A. P. flour (1.75 cups)
- Flaxseed meal (.25 cup)
- Baking soda & powder (1 tsp. each)
- Salt (.125 or 1/8 tsp.)
- Granulated sugar (.5 cup)
- Cinnamon (.5 tsp.)
- Orange zest (2 tbsp.)
- Unsweetened concentrate - orange juice (2 tbsp.)
- Vanilla (2 tsp.)
- Fresh or frozen cranberries (1.5 cups)

Preparation Method:
1. Warm the oven to reach 350° Fahrenheit/177° Celsius.

2. Lightly spray the muffin tins or use muffin cup liners.

3. Whisk the yogurt with the eggs, oil, juice concentrate, sugars, vanilla, and orange zest.

4. Use a separate container to combine the baking soda and powder with the flaxseed, cinnamon, salt, and flour.

5. Use a mixer's low-speed setting to combine the dry and wet fixings - mixing till they're just combined (1-2 min.). Fold in cranberries. Scoop batter (¼ cup each) into the tin.

6. Set the timer to bake till the tops are golden brown (22-25 min.).

Mixed Berry Whole-Grain Coffee Cake

Portions Provided: 8 servings
Time Required: 45-50 minutes
Nutritional Statistics (Each Portion):
- Protein Counts: 4 grams
- Carbohydrates: 26 grams
- Fat Content: 5 grams
- Sugars: 13 grams
- Dietary Fiber: 3 grams
- Sodium: 153 mg
- Calories: 165

Essential Ingredients:
- Skim milk (.5 cup)
- Vinegar (1 tbsp.)
- Canola oil (2 tbsp.)
- Egg (1)
- Vanilla (1 tsp.)
- Brown sugar - tightly packed (.33 cup)
- Salt (.125 tsp.)
- Pastry flour - whole-wheat (1 cup)
- Baking soda (.5 tsp.)
- Cinnamon (.5 tsp.)

- Frozen mixed berries - ex. - raspberries, blueberries, or blackberries - *don't thaw* (1 cup)
- Granola - l.f. - slightly crushed (.25 cup)
- Suggested: 8-inch/20-cm round cake pan

Preparation Method:
1. Set the oven temperature setting at 350° Fahrenheit/177° Celsius.
2. Spray the cake pan using a spritz of cooking spray and dust with flour.
3. Whisk the milk with vinegar, vanilla, oil, brown sugar, and egg until creamy.
4. Stir in flour, cinnamon, baking soda, and salt till moistened. Gently fold in ½ of the berries and scoop the batter into the baking pan.
5. Decorate the top using the remainder of the berries and garnish with the granola.
6. Bake till it's a nice brown. The top should spring back when touched in its center (25-30 min.).
7. Allow it to cool in the pan on a cooling rack for ten minutes before serving.

Pecan - Rhubarb Muffins

Portions Provided: 12 servings
Time Required: 45 minutes
Nutritional Statistics (Each Portion):
- Protein Counts: 3 grams
- Carbohydrates: 26 grams
- Fat Content: 3 grams
- Sugars: 8 grams
- Dietary Fiber: 2 grams
- Sodium: 190 mg
- Calories: 143

Essential Ingredients:
- Canola oil (2 tbsp.)
- Egg whites (2)
- Applesauce - unsweetened (2 tbsp.)
- Orange juice - Calcium-fortified (.75 cup)
- Rhubarb (1.25 cups)
- Orange peel (2 tsp.)
- Chopped pecans (2 tbsp.)
- Salt (.5 tsp.)
- Sugar (.5 cup)
- Baking powder (1.5 tsp.)
- Flour - whole-wheat & all-purpose (1 cup of each)
- Baking soda (.5 tsp.)

Preparation Method:
1. Set the oven temperature at 350° Fahrenheit/177° Celsius.

2. Line a muffin tray using foil or paper liners.
3. In a big mixing container, sift each type of flour with salt, baking soda, sugar, and baking powder.
4. Grate the orange peel. Whisk the peels with the egg whites, juice, applesauce, and canola oil using an electric mixer until creamy in another container.
5. Mix the wet and dry fixings - blend till it's just moistened.
6. Finely chop and mix in the rhubarb.
7. Scoop the batter mix into the cups or about two-thirds full.
8. Sprinkle nuts (½ tsp.) over each muffin cup.
9. Bake till they "spring back" to the touch (25-30 min.).
10. Let them cool for five minutes in the pan - transfer them onto a cooling rack for thorough cooling before storing.

Pumpkin-Hazelnut Tea Cake

Portions Provided: 12 servings
Time Required: 1 hour 20 minutes
Nutritional Statistics (Each Portion):
- Protein Counts: 4 grams
- Carbohydrates: 28 grams
- Fat Content: 6 grams
- Sugars: 15 grams
- Dietary Fiber: 2.5 grams
- Sodium: 73 mg
- Calories: 166

Essential Ingredients:
- Canola oil (3 tbsp.)
- Unsweetened canned pumpkin puree (.75 cup)
- Honey (.5 cup)
- Brown sugar - firmly packed (3 tbsp.)
- Eggs (2)
- Flour - whole-wheat/meal (1 cup)
- A. P. flour (.5 cup)
- Baking powder (.5 tsp.)
- Flaxseed (2 tbsp.)
- Ground allspice (.5 tsp.)
- Salt (.25 tsp.)
- Ground cloves (.25 tsp.)
- Cinnamon (.5 tsp.)
- Ground nutmeg (.5 tsp.)
- Chopped hazelnuts (filberts) (2 tbsp.)
- Also Needed: 8x4-inch/20x10-cm loaf pan

Preparation Method:
1. Warm the oven to 350° Fahrenheit/177° Celsius.

2. Lightly coat the pan with a spritz cooking oil spray.
3. Using the low-speed setting of an electric mixer, mix the canola oil with the honey, pumpkin puree, eggs, and brown sugar until incorporated and thoroughly blended.
4. Whisk each type of flour with flaxseed, baking powder, cinnamon, allspice, nutmeg, salt, and cloves in a small mixing container.
5. Combine all of the fixings using the medium-speed setting till it's thoroughly mixed.
6. Dump the batter mix into the pan, sprinkling the hazelnuts over the top - gently pressing them into the mix.
7. Bake until they're nicely browned (50-55 min.).
8. Place the pan on a cooling rack (10 min.). Flip the cake from the pan and slice it into 12 portions to serve.

Raspberry-Chocolate Scones

Portions Provided: 12 servings
Time Required: 20-25 minutes
Nutritional Statistics (Each Portion):
- Protein Counts: 4 grams
- Carbs: 22 grams
- Fat Content: 5 grams
- Dietary Fiber: 2 grams
- Added Sugars: 3 grams
- Sodium: 143
- Calories: 149

Essential Ingredients:
- Pastry flour: A. P. & whole-wheat (1 cup each)
- Bak. soda (.25 tsp.)
- Bak. powder (1 tbsp.)
- Trans fat-free buttery spread (.33 cup)
- Raspberries 0 fresh/frozen (.5 cup)
- Chocolate chips - minis (.25 cup)
- Plain yogurt - f.f. (1 cup + 2 tbsp.)
- Honey (2 tbsp.)
- Sugar (.5 tsp.)
- Cinnamon (.25 tsp.)

Preparation Method:
1. Set the oven temperature at 400° Fahrenheit/204° Celsius.
2. Lightly grease a baking tray.
3. Mix each of the flours with baking soda and powder in a big mixing container. Use a pastry cutter to combine and mix in the butter spread until crumbly.

4. Gently fold in the mini chips and berries.
5. Whisk the yogurt with the honey in a small dish.
6. Combine the fixings until just blended.
7. Place a dough ball on the countertop - kneading a couple of times. Roll it into a ½-inch-thick circle and slice it into 12 wedges.
8. Arrange them on the baking tray.
9. Whisk the cinnamon and sugar to sprinkle over top of scones to bake (10-12 min.).
10. Serve as desired when they're ready.

3-Grain Raspberry Muffins

Portions Provided: 12 servings
Time Required: 30-35 minutes
Nutritional Statistics (Each Portion):
- Protein Counts: 3 grams
- Carbohydrates: 26 grams
- Fat Content: 5 grams
- Sugars: 13 grams
- Dietary Fiber: 2 grams
- Sodium: 126 mg
- Calories: 161

Essential Ingredients:
- Milk - 1 % or plain soy - l.f. (1 cup)
- A. P. flour (.75 cup)
- Rolled oats (.5 cup)
- Wheat bran (.25 cup)
- Cornmeal - coarse-ground (.5 cup)
- Salt (.25 tsp.)
- Baking powder (1 tbsp.)
- Honey (.5 cup)
- Canola oil (3.5 tbsp.)
- Lime zest - grated (2 tsp.)
- Egg (1)
- Raspberries (.66 or 2/3 cup)

Preparation Method:
1. Heat the oven to reach 400° Fahrenheit/204° Celsius.
2. Use foil or paper liners to line a 12-cup muffin pan.
3. Use a big microwave-safe mixing container to combine the milk and oats. Pop the container into the microwave using the high setting till the oats are tender and creamy (3 min.). Set aside.
4. Whisk the flour with the cornmeal, baking powder, bran, and salt till incorporated.
5. Whisk and mix in the canola oil, honey, oat mixture, lime zest, and egg - beating till the mixture is just moistened (slightly lumpy).
6. Lastly, take care and mix in the raspberries.

7. Scoop the batter into the prepared tin (2/3 full).
8. Bake till the muffins' tops are browned to your liking (16-18 min.).
9. Put the muffins on a cooling rack a few minutes before serving or freezing

Bread Options

Carrot & Spice Quick Bread

Portions Provided: 17 servings @ 0.5-inch slices
Time Required: 60-65 minutes
Nutritional Statistics (Each Portion):
- Protein Counts: 2 grams
- Carbohydrates: 15 grams
- Fat Content: grams
- Added Sugars: 6 grams
- Dietary Fiber: 1 gram
- Sodium: 82 mg
- Calories: 110

Essential Ingredients:
- Flour - whole-wheat (1 cup)
- Sifted a.p. flour (.5 cup)
- Bak. powder (2 tsp.)
- Bak. soda (.5 tsp.)
- Ground ginger (.25 tsp.)
- Cinnamon (.5 tsp.)
- Unchilled - trans-fat-free margarine (.33 cup)
- Brown sugar - firmly packed (.25 cup + 2 tbsp.)
- Skim milk (.33 cup)
- Orange juice - unsweetened (2 tbsp.)
- Egg whites (2)
- Vanilla extract (1 tsp.)
- Orange rind - grated (1 tsp.)
- Shredded carrots (1.5 cups)
- Golden raisins (2 tbsp.)
- Walnuts (1 tbsp.)
- Suggested: Two 0.5x-4.5x-8.5-inch loaf pans

Preparation Method:
1. Set the oven temperature at 375° Fahrenheit/191° Celsius.
2. Spray the loaf pans using a spritz of cooking oil spray.
3. Whisk or sift each type of flour with ginger, cinnamon, baking soda, and powder.
4. Use a separate container - by hand or with an electric mixer - cream the margarine with the sugar in a big mixing container. Mix in the egg, milk, vanilla, orange juice, and orange rind.
5. Finely chop the walnuts and toss them with the raisins and carrots.
6. Fold in the dry fixings - thoroughly mixing.
7. Dump the prepared batter into the pans. Bake till browned to your liking (45 min.).
8. Cool in the pan for about ten minutes. Transfer the bread to a cooling rack to thoroughly cool before storing.

Honey Whole-Wheat Bread

Portions Provided: 17 servings @ ½-inch slice
Time Required: 4.5-5 hrs. - lots of rising time
Nutritional Statistics (Each Portion):
- Protein Counts: 3 grams
- Carbohydrates: 15 grams
- Fat Content: 2 grams
- Added Sugars: 2 grams
- Dietary Fiber: 2 grams
- Sodium: 104 mg
- Calories: 90

Essential Ingredients:
- Rolled oats - dry (1 cup)
- Water (3 cups)
- Flour - whole-wheat (3 cups)
- Soy flour (.75 cup)
- Flaxseed (3 tbsp.)
- Ground flaxseed/flaxseed meal (.75 cup)
- Unbleached white flour (about 5 cups)
- Poppy & Sesame seeds (3 tbsp. each)
- Yeast (4.25 tbsp.)
- Sea salt (1 tbsp.)
- Applesauce - unsweetened (1 cup)
- Honey (.5 cup)
- Olive oil (.25 cup)
- Suggested pan size: 2 - 1 x 11 cm x 22 cm/0.5 x 4.5 x 8.5 inches

Preparation Method:
1. In a microwave-safe bowl, cook the oats mixed with water (about 120° Fahrenheit/ 49° Celsius to 130° Fahrenheit/54° Celsius).
2. In a heavy stand mixer with a dough hook, mix the whole-wheat and soy flour with the flaxseed/meal, yeast, and salt.
3. Mix the oil with the honey and applesauce by hand. Fold in the hot, rolled oats mixture.
4. When blended, start mixing with a dough hook to mix (3 min.).
5. Slowly mix in white flour until the dough comes away from the bowl's sides - it will become elastic and smooth.
6. Place a layer of plastic over the dough container and place it in a warm spot to rise till it's doubled in size (1.5-2 hrs.).
7. Punch dough down and scoop it onto the countertop. Divide evenly into four loaf pans - generously sprayed with cooking oil spray.

8. Cover and let them rise in a warm spot until nearly double in size (1.5-2 hrs.).

9. Warm the oven to reach 350° Fahrenheit/177° Celsius.

10. Bake until the loaf's tops are browned as desired (25 min.). Remove the bread from pans and cool on a wire rack. Slice the bread into half-inch-wide slices to serve.

Irish Brown Bread

Portions Provided: 24 servings
Time Required: 45 minutes + 2 hours cool time
Nutritional Statistics (Each Portion):
- Protein Counts: 4 grams
- Carbohydrates: 15 grams
- Fat Content: 1 gram
- Sugars: 1 gram
- Dietary Fiber: 1.5 grams
- Sodium: 170 mg
- Calories: 85

Essential Ingredients:
- Whole-wheat flour (2 cups)
- A. P. flour (1.5 cups + more for kneading & dusting)
- Wheat germ (.5 cup)
- Baking soda (2 tsp.)
- Salt (.25 tsp.)
- Buttermilk - l.f. (2 cups)
- Egg (1)

Preparation Method:
1. Set the oven temperature setting to 400° Fahrenheit/204° Celsius.
2. Prepare a nonstick baking tray.
3. Whisk all of the flour with baking soda, wheat germ, and salt. Whisk to blend.
4. Lightly whisk the egg with the buttermilk till moistened into a sticky dough.
5. Lightly flour a working surface. Turn the dough out and gently knead it eight to ten times, shaping it into a loose ball.
6. Shape it into a 7-inch round on the baking tray. Lightly dust the dough's top with a tiny bit of flour.
7. Slice a four-inch "X" into the dough's top (½-inch deep).
8. Bake till the bread splits open at the "X." It will make a hollow sound when tapped on its underside (25-30 min.).
9. When it's ready, place it onto a rack to cool for about two hours before slicing.

Lemon Bread

Portions Provided: 16 servings
Time Required: 1 hour 25 minutes
Nutritional Statistics (Each Portion):
- Protein Counts: 2.9 grams
- Carbohydrates: 21.4 grams
- Fat Content: 5 grams
- Sugars: 10.4 grams
- Dietary Fiber: 0.8 grams
- Sodium: 80.3 mg
- Calories: 140

Essential Ingredients:
- A. P. flour (1.75 cups)
- Baking powder (2 tsp.)
- Salt (.25 tsp.)
- Refrigerated/frozen egg product (.25 cup) or lightly whisked egg (1)
- Fat-free milk (1 cup)
- Butter - melted/cooking oil (.25 cup)
- Lemon peel (2 tsp.)
- Toasted almonds/walnuts (.5 cup)
  Optional:
- Sugar substitute blend equivalent to .75 cup sugar (.75 cup)
- Lemon juice - divided (1 tbsp. + 2 tbsp.)
- Sugar (1 tbsp.)
- Also Needed: 8x4x2-inch/20x10x5-cm loaf pan

Preparation Method:
1. Thaw the egg product if using. Set the oven temperature at 350° Fahrenheit/177° Celsius.
2. Generously grease the bottom and ½ -inch up the sides of the loaf pan.
3. Finely shred the lemon peel and juice it.
4. Using a medium mixing container, whisk/sift the flour, sugar (.75 cup), salt, and baking powder. Scoop a hole in the middle of the flour mixture - set to the side.
5. Use another mixing container to whisk the egg with the milk, oil, lemon peel, and lemon juice (1 tbsp.). Add the egg mixture all at once to the flour mix - stirring just until moistened (lumpy still). Chop and mix in the nuts. Scoop the batter into the greased pan.
6. Bake till it's a nice golden brown (45-55 min.).
7. Whisk lemon juice (2 tbsp.) with the sugar substitute (1 tbsp.). While the bread is still in the pan, brush the lemon-sugar mixture over its top.

8. Cool in the pan on a wire rack (10 min.) - move from the pan to thoroughly cool on a baking rack.
9. Wrap the bread as desired and store it overnight. Serve the next day.

Whole-Grain Banana Bread

Portions Provided: 14 servings
Time Required: 1 hour 20 minutes
Nutritional Statistics (Each Portion):
- Protein Counts: 4 grams
- Carbohydrates: 30 grams
- Sugars: 10 grams
- Fat Content: 3 grams
- Dietary Fiber: 2 grams
- Sodium: 146 mg
- Calories: 163

Essential Ingredients:
   Flour @ 0.5 cup each:
- Tapioca
- Amaranth
- Brown rice
- Quinoa
- Millet
   Rest of the Ingredients:
- Bak. soda (1 tsp.)
- Salt (.125 tsp.)
- Bak. powder (.5 tsp.)
- Egg substitute or use egg whites (.75 cup)
- Grapeseed oil (2 tbsp.)
- Raw sugar (.5 cup)
- Mashed banana (2 cups)
- Suggested: 5x9-inch/13x23-cm loaf pan

Preparation Method:
1. Warm the oven to 350° Fahrenheit/177° Celsius.
2. Prepare the pan using a light dusting of cooking oil spray. Dust with a tiny bit of flour - set aside.
3. Whisk each of the dry fixings except for the sugar in a big mixing container.
4. In another container, whisk the egg with the oil, sugar, and mashed banana.
5. Toss the wet mixture to dry fixings to combine thoroughly.
6. Dump the batter into the pan. Set a timer to bake (50 min.-1 hr.).
7. Transfer the pan of bread from the oven, cool, slice, and serve.

Zucchini Bread

Portions Provided: 18 servings or 2 loaves
Time Required: 1 hour 15 minutes
Nutritional Statistics (Each Portion):
- Protein Counts: 4 grams
- Carbohydrates: 22 grams
- Fat Content: 5 grams
- Added Sugars: 5 grams
- Dietary Fiber: 2 grams
- Sodium: 103 mg
- Calories: 141

Essential Ingredients:
- Egg whites (6)
- Canola oil (.25 cup)
- Unsweetened applesauce (.5 cup)
- Sugar (.5 cup)
- Vanilla extract (2 tsp.)
- Flour - A.P. & whole-wheat (1.25 cups of each)
- Baking soda and powder (1 tsp. each)
- Ground cinnamon (3 tsp.)
- Zucchini (2 cups)
- Walnuts - chopped (.5 cup)
- Crushed - unsweetened pineapple (1.5 cups)
- Suggested: Two 9-by-5-inch loaf pans

Preparation Method:
1. Warm the oven to reach 350° Fahrenheit/177° Celsius.
2. Lightly coat the pans with a tiny bit of cooking spray.
3. Whisk the egg whites with vanilla, canola oil, applesauce, and sugar (low-speed of an electric mixer) till it's thick and foamy.
4. Whisk each type of flour into a mixing container, set ½ cup to the side for now.
5. Mix in the baking soda and powder with the cinnamon into the container with the flour. Combine it with the egg white mixture. Use the electric mixer at the medium-speed setting to combine till the mixture is thoroughly blended.
6. Shred and mix in the walnuts with the pineapple and zucchini - stir till entirely combined. Modify the batter's consistency till it's thickened with the remaining half-cup of flour (add one tablespoon at a time).
7. Scoop half of the batter into each pan. Bake the bread for about 50 minutes - cool in the pans on a wire rack for ten minutes.
8. Dump the loaves onto the cooling rack to cool thoroughly.

9. Slice each bread loaf into nine (one-inch) slices to serve. You can also freeze one loaf for later.

Other Breakfast Options

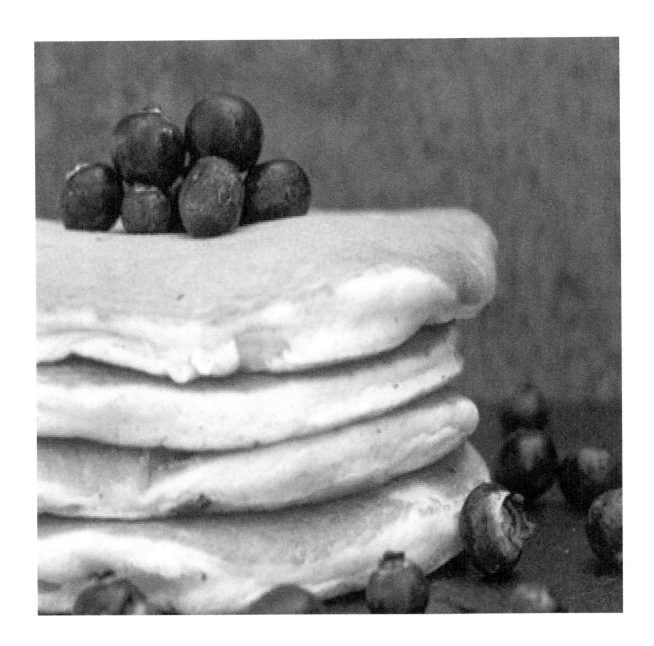

Asparagus Omelet Tortilla Wrap

Portions Provided: 1 serving
Time Required: 20 minutes
Nutritional Statistics (Each Portion):
- Protein Counts: 21 grams
- Carbohydrates: grams
- Fat Content: 13 grams
- Sugars: 4 grams Dietary Fiber: 3 grams
- Sodium: 444 mg Calories: 319

Essential Ingredients:
- Parmesan cheese - grated (2 tsp.)
- Black pepper (.125 or ⅛ tsp.)
- Fresh asparagus spears (4)
- Egg (1 whole large)
- Fat-free milk (1 tbsp.)
- Egg whites (2 large)
- Butter (1 tsp.)
- Green onion (1)
- Whole wheat tortilla (1 @ 8 inches - warmed)

Preparation Method:
1. Beat the eggs with the pepper, parmesan, and milk till it's incorporated.
2. Spritz a skillet using a tiny portion of cooking oil spray. Warm it using the medium temperature setting.
3. Add and sauté the asparagus (3-4 min.). Scoop the asparagus from the pan.
4. Use the same pan to warm the butter using med-high heat. Add and cook the eggs, pushing them to the center until it's one layer and thickened.
5. Trim and slice the asparagus and chop the onion.
6. When eggs are thickened, spoon the green onion and asparagus on one side. Fold the omelet in half and serve in a tortilla.

Baked Banana-Nut Oatmeal Cups

Portions Provided: 12 servings
Time Required: 50 minutes
Nutritional Statistics (Each Portion):
- Protein Counts: 5.2 grams
- Carbohydrates: 26.4 grams
- Fat Content: 6.2 grams
- Sugars: 10.5 grams
- Dietary Fiber: 3.1 grams
- Sodium: 165.6 mg
- Calories: 176
  Diabetic Exchanges:
- Other Carbohydrate: ½
- Fruit: ½
- Starch: 1
- Fat: 1

Essential Ingredients:
- Rolled oats (3 cups)
- Brown sugar - tightly packed (.33 cup)
- Milk - l.f. (1.5 cups)
- Ripe bananas (2 or about .75 cup)
- Large eggs (2)
- Salt (.5 tsp.)
- Baking powder (1 tsp.)
- Cinnamon (1 tsp.)
- Vanilla extract (1 tsp.)
- Toasted chopped pecans (.5 cup)

Preparation Steps:
1. Set the oven temperature to 375° Fahrenheit/191° Celsius.
2. Lightly spritz the cups of the muffin tin using a cooking oil spray.
3. Mash the bananas. Lightly whisk the eggs and mix with the oats, milk, bananas, baking powder, salt, brown sugar, cinnamon, and vanilla in a big mixing container.
4. Fold in pecans. Scoop the batter into the muffin cups (.33 or 1/3 cup).
5. Bake till they're nicely browned (25 min.). Allow cooling in the pan (10 min.).
6. Transfer the oatmeal cups onto a cooling rack to thoroughly cool before storing.
7. Serve as desired - either cooled or warm.
8. Meal Prep Tip: Wrap tightly in foil or place in a container in the refrigerator to enjoy for a day or two. They are a wonderful freezer option to prepare and save for up to three months.

Blueberry Low-Sodium Pancakes

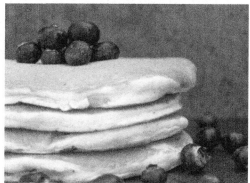

Portions Provided: 16 cakes
Time Required: 15 minutes
Nutritional Statistics (Each Portion):
- Protein Counts: 2 grams
- Carbohydrates: 16 grams

- Dietary Fiber: 4 grams
- Sodium: 113 mg
- Calories: 77

Essential Ingredients:
- A. P. flour (2 cups)
- Brown sugar (4 tbsp.)
- Reduced sodium baking powder (2 tbsp.)
- Vinegar - apple cider (1 tbsp.)
- Vanilla extract (1 tsp.)
- Oat milk (1 cup)

Preparation Method:
1. Toss all of the dry fixings (flour, brown sugar, baking powder & salt) into a mixing container. Whisk till it's all combined.
2. In another mixing container or liquid measuring cup, add the wet fixings (oat milk, apple cider vinegar & vanilla), whisking till incorporated.
3. Combine all of the components till creamy. Wait while it rests (5 min.).
4. Pour the batter (65 grams or ½ cup) into a griddle or skillet using a medium-temperature setting.
5. When the top begins to bubble, flip the pancake and continue cooking till they're nicely browned.
6. Serve warm with honey or syrup.

Breakfast Scrambled Egg Burrito

Portions Provided: 1 serving
Time Required: 25 minutes
Nutritional Statistics (Each Portion):
- Carbohydrates: 27.8 grams
- Dietary Fiber: 15 grams
- Sodium: 116 mg
- Calories: 273

Essential Ingredients:
- Tortilla (1 homemade - low or zero sodium - 1 @ 6-8 inch/15-20-cm tortilla)
- Small sweet pepper (1-2 tbsp. diced)
- Egg (1)
- Shredded Swiss & Gruyere cheese (1 tbsp.)
- Low/no sodium pasta sauce or salsa (1 tsp.)

Preparation Method:
1. Lightly spritz a skillet using a bit of cooking oil spray.
2. Whisk the egg and mix in the peppers and salsa.
3. Warm the skillet on the stovetop using a medium-temperature setting. When it's heated, stir in the egg mixture - folding the egg over itself until large curds begin to form. Move the skillet to a cool spot and set it aside.
4. Plate the tortilla flat and pop it into the microwave to heat for ten seconds.
5. Sprinkle a tablespoon of cheese down its center.
6. Add the scrambled egg and roll the tortilla - burrito-style.
7. Plate it again - seam side down and reheat it in the microwave to melt the cheese (5 sec.).
8. Cut the burrito on a diagonal across the middle and serve promptly with extra salsa as desired.

Buckwheat Pancakes

Portions Provided: 6 servings
Time Required: 15-20 minutes
Nutritional Statistics (Each Portion):
- Protein Counts: 5 grams
- Carbohydrates: 24 grams
- Fat Content: 3 grams
- Sugars: 6.5 grams
- Dietary Fiber: 3 grams
- Sodium: 150 mg
- Calories: 143

Essential Ingredients:
- Egg whites (2)
- Fat-free milk (.5 cup)
- Canola oil (1 tbsp.)
- Buckwheat flour (.5 cup)
- Sugar (1 tbsp.)
- A.P. flour (.5 cup)
- Baking powder (1 tbsp.)
- Sparkling water (.5 cup)
- Fresh sliced strawberries (3 cups)

Preparation Method:
1. Briskly whisk the eggs with the milk and oil in a mixing container.
2. Use another container to blend the sugar with the baking powder and each type of flour.
3. Blend in the egg white mixture and water until barely moist.
4. Use the medium-temperature setting to warm a nonstick griddle or frying pan— spoon the batter (½-cup each).
5. Continue cooking for about two minutes (bubbles over the top). Flip them over and proceed cooking till they're ready (1-2 min.).

6. Garnish each one with ½ cup of sliced berries and serve.

German Apple Pancake

Portions Provided: 4 servings
Time Required: 35 minutes
Nutritional Statistics (Each Portion):
Not included - counts for the powdered sugar or maple syrup:
- Carbohydrates: 39.7 grams
- Sodium: 71 mg
- Calories: 356

Essential Ingredients:
- Gala cooking apples (2 or minimum of 1.5 cups)
- Unsalted butter (5 tbsp.)
- Milk (1 cup)
- Eggs (2 large)
- A. P. flour (1 cup)
- Nutmeg - grated (.25 tsp.)
- Vanilla extract (1 tsp.)
  Optional Toppings:
- Powdered sugar
- Maple syrup
- Also Needed: 9-10-inch/23x25 cast-iron skillet

Preparation Method:
1. Set the oven temperature to heat at 475° Fahrenheit/246° Celsius.
2. Peel, remove the cores, and slice the apples.
3. Add unsalted butter (3 tbsp.) to a skillet to heat using a med-low temperature setting.
4. Once it's melted, add the apple slices - sauté them till they're just tender. OR, put them in a small-sized casserole dish and soften them in the microwave (6 min.), stirring every two minutes or so.
5. Whisk in the eggs, flour, milk, nutmeg, and vanilla in a mixing container till all of the fixings are incorporated, and the batter is smooth (no lumps).
6. Put the skillet into the oven to heat for at least five minutes - till it's scorching hot. Add butter (2 tbsp.) and pop it back into the oven to melt - not brown.
7. Transfer it to the stovetop and swirl the butter to cover the skillet's entire bottom and sides. Scoop the apple slices in the pan and add the batter over the slices.
8. Bake the mixture for about six minutes. Adjust the temperature setting to 425°

Fahrenheit/218° Celsius to bake (12-14 min.).
9. Remove the skillet and carefully tip the pancake upside down onto a prepared platter. Garnish as desired and slice it into four pieces.
10. Serve with maple syrup.
11. Delightful Note: You can also make this a dessert with a portion of custard or ice cream.

Grilled Split Banana Bowl

Portions Provided: 1 serving
Time Required: 20 minutes
Nutritional Statistics (Each Portion):
- Protein Counts: 23 grams
- Fat Content: 14 grams
- Carbohydrates: 108 grams
- Sugars: 75 grams
- Dietary Fiber: 8 grams
- Sodium: 59 mg
- Calories: 653

Essential Ingredients:
- Greek yogurt - l.f. & plain (.75 cup)
- Jam - Pure-red raspberry (2 tbsp.)
- Pure vanilla extract (.5 tsp.)
- Medium banana (2)
- Grapeseed oil (.5 tsp.)
- Fresh pineapple (.33 or 1/3 cup)
- Premium-quality almonds -sliced (1 tbsp.)
- Fresh strawberries (.33 cup)
- Chocolate morsels - semi-sweet (1 tbsp.)

Preparation Method:
1. Warm a grill pan or grill.
2. Whisk the yogurt with the fruit spread and vanilla extract till it's combined, and set it to the side for now.
3. Brush/rub the cut side of the banana halves with the oil.
4. Grill the banana halves - sliced side downward - over direct medium heat till they're caramelized (6-7 min.).
5. Next, grill the peeled side of the banana halves till heated (1 min.). Gently remove the peels.
6. Arrange the banana halves in a pasta dish and garnish using the yogurt mixture, almonds, pineapple, strawberries, and chips of chocolate.

Muesli Breakfast Bars

Portions Provided: 24 servings
Time Required: 40 minutes
Nutritional Statistics (Each Portion):
- Protein Counts: 5 grams
- Carbohydrates: 26 grams
- Fat Content: 5 grams
- Sugars: 17 grams
- Dietary Fiber: 2 grams
- Sodium: 81 mg
- Calories: 169

Essential Ingredients:
- Soy flour (.5 cup)
- Rolled oats - Old-fashioned (2.5 cups)
- Dry milk - f.f. (.5 cup)
- Toasted almonds (sliced) or pecans (chopped) (.5 cup)
- Dried apples - chopped (.5 cup)
- Wheat germ - toasted (.5 cup)
- Raisins (.5 cup)
- Salt (.5 cup)
- Dark honey (1 cup)
- Olive oil (1 tbsp.)
- Organic - unsalted peanut butter (.5 cup)
- Vanilla extract (2 tsp.)
- Suggested: 9x13-inch/23x33-cm baking pan

Preparation Method:
1. Warm the oven to 325° Fahrenheit/163° Celsius.
2. Spritz the baking tray using a tiny bit of cooking oil spray.
3. Whisk the oats with flour, wheat germ, dry milk, apples, raisins, almonds, and salt. Thoroughly mix and put it to the side for now.
4. Use a small saucepan to combine the peanut butter, honey, and olive oil using a med-low temperature setting till it's thoroughly blended (not boiling).
5. Whisk in the vanilla, adding the honey mixture to the dry fixings - quickly stir till it's thoroughly combined (sticky but not wet).
6. Firmly press the mixture into the baking pan.
7. Bake just until the edges begin to brown (25 min.).
8. Cool in the pan on a wire rack for ten minutes before slicing it into 24 bars.
9. Transfer the bars from the pan - set them aside onto a cooling rack till they're thoroughly cooled.
10. Keep them in the fridge for freshness.

Mushroom Hash with Poached Eggs - Meal Prep

Portions Provided: 4 servings
Time Required: 27 minutes
Nutritional Statistics (Each Portion):
- Protein Counts: 15 grams
- Carbohydrates: 15 grams
- Fat Content: 17 grams
- Sugars: 11 grams
- Dietary Fiber: 6 grams
- Sodium: 0.2 mg
- Calories: 283

Essential Ingredients:
- Rapeseed oil (1.5 tbsp.)
- Onions (2 large)
- Closed cup mushrooms (17.6 oz./500 g)
- Fresh thyme leaves (1 tbsp. + more for sprinkling)
- Fresh tomatoes (17.6 oz./500 g)
- Omega seed mix** (3 tsp.)
- Smoked paprika (1 tsp.)
- Large eggs (4)

Preparation Method:
1. Slice the onions into halves and thinly slice. Quarter the mushrooms and chop the tomatoes and thyme leaves.
2. Warm oil in a big frying pan to sauté the onions for a few minutes. Put a top on the pan to steam the onions (5 additional min.). Mix in the mushrooms with the thyme and continue sautéing till softened (5 min.).
3. Mix in the paprika and tomatoes - put the top on the pan - simmer till it is pulpy (5 min.). Thoroughly stir in the seed mix.
4. Poach eggs (2) in lightly simmering water till they are ready as desired.
5. Serve over half of the hash with a sprinkling of pepper and thyme.

Meal Prep Tip: Store the rest of the hash in a container for another meal.

*Note: **Make yourself the omega mix. Combine three tablespoons each of sunflower, sesame, and pumpkin seeds. Keep them in a closed container to use as desired.*

Peanut Butter & Chia Berry Jam English Muffin Diabetic-Friendly

Portions Provided: 1 serving
Time Required: 10 minutes
Nutritional Statistics (Each Portion):
- Protein Counts: 9.8 grams
- Carbohydrates: 40.5 grams
- Fat Content: 9.3 grams
- Sugars: 12 grams
- Dietary Fiber: 9.4 grams
- Sodium: 286.8 mg
- Calories: 262
  Diabetic Exchanges:
- Fat: 1 ½
- Fruit: ½
- Starch: 2

Essential Ingredients:
- Chia seeds (2 tsp.)
- Mixed frozen berries - unsweetened (.5 cup)
- Natural - organic peanut butter (2 tsp.)
- English muffin - Whole-wheat suggested (1 toasted)

Preparation Method:
1. Rinse and toss the berries into a microwave-safe container.
2. Cook them for ½ minute.
3. Stir and cook for another ½ minute. Mix in the seeds.
4. Prepare the muffin with peanut butter and a garnish of the berry mix to serve.

Popovers

Portions Provided: 6 servings
Time Required: 40 minutes
Nutritional Statistics (Each Portion):
- Protein Counts: 6 grams
- Carbohydrates: 18 grams
- Fat Content: trace grams
- Sugars: 2 grams
- Dietary Fiber: 0.5 grams
- Sodium: 156 mg
- Calories: 96

Essential Ingredients:
- Skim milk (1 cup)
- Salt (.25 tsp.)
- A.P. flour (1 cup)
- Egg whites (4)
- Also Needed: 6 large metal or glass muffin molds

Preparation Method:
1. Set the oven temperature setting to 425° Fahrenheit/218° Celsius.
2. Generously coat the muffin molds with cooking oil spray and warm them in the oven for two minutes.
3. Combine the milk with the salt, flour, and egg whites using an electric mixer till incorporated. Dump the batter into the cups (2/3 full).
4. Bake it in the uppermost part of the oven till they're nicely browned and puffy (½ hour). Serve promptly.

Raspberry Peach Puff Pancake

Portions Provided: 4 servings
Time Required: 35 minutes
Nutritional Statistics (Each Portion):
- Protein Counts: 9 grams
- Carbohydrates: 25 grams (Net: 11 grams)
- Fat Content: 7 grams
- Sugars: 11 grams
- Dietary Fiber: 3 grams
- Sodium: 173 mg
- Calories: 199

Essential Ingredients:
- Medium peaches (2)
- Sugar (.5 tsp.)
- Fresh raspberries (.5 cup)
- Butter (1 tbsp.)
- Unchilled large eggs (3)
- Fat-free milk (.5 cup)
- Salt (.125 or 1/8 tsp.)
- A. P. flour (.5 cup)
- Vanilla yogurt (.25 cup)
- Also Needed: 9-inch/23-cm pie plate

Preparation Method:
1. Warm the oven to 400° Fahrenheit/204° Celsius.
2. Peel, slice, and toss the peaches with sugar. Gently mix in raspberries.
3. Place butter on the pie plate. Warm it in the oven until the butter melts (2-3 min.).
4. Meanwhile, beat the milk, salt, and eggs till they're blended. Gradually whisk in the flour.
5. Transfer the pie plate to the countertop/stovetop and tilt it carefully to cover the sides and bottom with butter. Promptly stir in the egg mixture.

6. Bake until the pancake is puffed and browned (18-22 min.).
7. Remove it from the oven and serve immediately with fruit and yogurt.

Roasted Portobello Mushrooms Florentine

Portions Provided: 2 servings
Time Required: 25 minutes
Nutritional Statistics (Each Portion):
- Protein Counts: 11 grams
- Carbohydrates: 10 grams (Net: 3 grams)
- Fat Content: 5 grams
- Sugars: 4 grams
- Dietary Fiber: 3 grams
- Sodium: 472 mg
- Calories: 126

Essential Ingredients:
- Portobello mushrooms (2 large)
- Black pepper and salt (.125 or ⅛ tsp. each)
- Garlic salt (.125 or ⅛ tsp.)
- Olive oil (.5 tsp.)
- Large eggs (2)
- Crumbled goat or feta cheese (.25 cup)
- Small onion (1)
- Fresh baby spinach (1 cup)
- Optional: Freshly minced basil
- Cooking oil spray (as needed)
- Suggested: 15x10x1-inch or 38x25x3-cm pan

Preparation Method:
1. Set the oven temperature to 425° Fahrenheit/218° Celsius.
2. Remove the stems from the mushrooms.
3. Spritz mushrooms with cooking oil spray and arrange them in the baking tray, stem side up. Sprinkle them with pepper and garlic salt.
4. Roast them uncovered till tender (10 min.).
5. Meanwhile, warm the oil in a skillet using the med-high temperature setting.
6. Chop and sauté the onion till it's tender.
7. Fold in the spinach till it's wilted.
8. Whisk the eggs with the salt - cook until the eggs are thickened. Scoop them over the mushrooms. Sprinkle with cheese and basil to serve.

Spinach & Mushroom Quiche

Portions Provided: 6 servings
Time Required: 1 hour 5 minutes
Nutritional Statistics (Each Portion):
- Protein Counts: 17.1 grams
- Carbohydrates: 6.8 grams (Net: 2.1 grams)
- Fat Content: 20 grams
- Sugars: 3.2 grams
- Dietary Fiber: 1.5 grams
- Sodium: 442.5 mg
- Calories: 277

Essential Ingredients:
- Large eggs (6)
- Half-and-Half cream (.25 cup)
- Dijon mustard (1 tbsp.)
- Whole milk (.25 cup)
- Olive oil (2 tbsp.)
- Fresh mixed wild mushrooms - ex. -button - shiitake - crimini or oyster mushrooms (8 oz./230 g)
- Sweet onion (1.5 cups)
- Garlic (1 tbsp.)
- Fresh baby spinach (5 oz./about 8 cups)
- Fresh thyme leaves (1 tbsp. + garnishes)
- Salt & Black pepper (.25 tsp. each)
- Gruyère cheese - shredded (1.5 cups)

Preparation Method:
1. Warm the oven to reach 375° Fahrenheit/191° Celsius.
2. Cover a nine-inch pie pan with a spritz of cooking oil spray and put it to the side.
3. Thinly slice the onion and mushroom. Coarsely chop the spinach.
4. Warm oil in a big skillet using a med-high temperature setting - tilting the pan to thoroughly cover.
5. Toss in the mushrooms and sauté them till tender and lightly browned (8 min.).
6. Mince and toss in the garlic and sliced onion, cooking as you often stir it till it's softened and tender (5 min.). Fold in the spinach - continuously tossing till it's wilted (1-2 min.). Transfer the pan to a cool burner.
7. Vigorously whisk the milk with the cream, pepper, salt, thyme, and mustard in a mixing container. Fold in the cheese and mushroom mixture.
8. Scoop the quiche fixings into the prepared pie pan.

9. Set a timer to bake till it is a golden brown and set (½ hour). Wait for about ten minutes or so before slicing. Serve with a thyme garnish.

White Cheddar - Black Bean Frittata

Portions Provided: 6 servings
Time Required: 35-38 minutes
Nutritional Statistics (Each Portion):
- Carbohydrates: 9 grams (Net: 5 grams)
- Protein Counts: 13 grams
- Fat Content: 10 grams
- Sugars: 2 grams
- Dietary Fiber: 2 grams
- Sodium: 378 mg
- Calories: 183
- *Note: Toppings not included in counts*

Essential Ingredients:
- Canned black beans (1 cup)
- Large eggs (6 whole + 3 whites)
- Olive oil (1 tbsp.)
- Salsa (.25 cup)
- Fresh parsley (1 tbsp.)
- Black pepper & salt (.25 tsp. of each)
- Sweet green and red bell peppers (.33 cup of each)
- Green onions (3)
- Garlic cloves (2)
- Shredded white cheddar cheese (.5 cup)
  Optional Toppings:
- Fresh cilantro
- Sliced ripe olives
- Additional salsa
- Suggested: 10-inch ovenproof skillet

Preparation Method:
1. Rinse and drain the beans. Mince the parsley and cilantro, and set them aside for now. Preheat broiler.
2. Whisk the eggs with the salsa, pepper, and salt till they're thoroughly combined.
3. Warm the oil in the skillet using the med-high temperature setting.
4. Finely chop and add the peppers and green onions. Sauté them for three to four minutes. Adjust the temperature setting to medium - fold in the egg mixture.
5. Sauté them further with the lid off until nearly set (4-6 min.). Sprinkle it with cheese.
6. Broil three to four inches from the heating source until light golden brown and eggs are completely set (3-4 min.).

7. Let them stand for five minutes. Slice them into wedges.
8. Serve with the desired toppings.

Whole-Grain Banana Bread

Portions Provided: 14 servings
Time Required: 1 hour 10 minutes
Nutritional Statistics (Each Portion):
- Protein Counts: 4 grams
- Carbohydrates: 30 grams
- Fat Content: 3 grams
- Sugar Content: 10 grams
- Dietary Fiber: 2 grams
- Sodium: 150 mg
- Calories: 150

Essential Ingredients:
- Egg whites/egg substitute (.75 cup)
- Flour: 0.5 cups of each:
  - Quinoa
  - Millet
  - Rice
  - Tapioca
  - Amaranth - brown
- Baking powder (.5 tsp.)
- Salt (.125 or ⅛ tsp.)
- Bak. soda (1 tsp.)
- Grapeseed oil (2 tbsp.)
- Banana (2 cups)
- Raw sugar (.5 cup)
- Also Needed: 5x9 inches/13x23-cm loaf pan

Preparation Method:
1. Prepare the pan with a spritz of cooking oil spray. Sprinkle it using some flour and set it to the side.
2. Warm the oven to reach 350° Fahrenheit/177° Celsius.
3. Combine each of the dry fixings—omitting the sugar—in a large mixing container.
4. In another container, whisk the egg with the oil, mashed banana, and sugar.
5. Blend the ingredients and thoroughly mix - adding them to the loaf pan.
6. Bake for 50 minutes to one hour. Cool, slice, and serve.

Whole Grain Banana Pancakes

Portions Provided: 14 servings
Time Required: 1 hour 10 minutes
Nutritional Statistics (Each Portion):
- Protein Counts: 4 grams
- Carbohydrates: 30 grams
- Sugars: 7 grams

- Fat Content: 3 grams
- Dietary Fiber: 2 grams
- Sodium: 146 mg
- Calories: 163

Essential Ingredients:
- Brown rice - flour (.5 cup)
- Baking powder (.5 tsp.)
  Flour: 0.5 cup each:
- Amaranth flour
- Tapioca flour
- Millet flour
- Quinoa flour
- Baking soda (1 tsp)
- Salt (.125 or ⅛ tsp.)
- Egg substitute or egg whites (.75 cup)
- Mashed banana (2 cups)
- Grapeseed oil (2 tbsp.)
- Raw sugar (.5 cup)
- Suggested: 5-by-9-inch or 13-by-23-cm loaf pan

Preparation Method:
1. Set the oven temperature at 350° Fahrenheit/177° Celsius.
2. Lightly mist the pan using a spritz of cooking oil spray and dust using a tiny bit of flour and place it to the side for now.
3. Combine each of the dry fixings - omit the sugar.
4. In another container, whisk the egg with oil, mashed banana, and sugar.
5. Combine the wet mixture to dry ingredients and thoroughly incorporate.
6. Scoop the mix into the pan and set a timer to bake it (50 min to 1 hr.).
7. Check for doneness with a toothpick: it's ready when the toothpick is removed from the center and is clean when it's removed.
8. When it's ready, set it aside to cool before slicing it to serve.

Zucchini & Tomato Pie Breakfast Pie

Portions Provided: 6 servings
Time Required: 60 minutes
Nutritional Statistics (Each Portion):
- Carbohydrates: 18.7 grams
- Sodium: 223 mg
- Calories: 176

Essential Ingredients:
- Zucchini (1 cup)
- Onion (.5 cup)
- Tomato (1 cup)
- Shredded Swiss cheese (.33 or 1/3 cup)

- Low-sodium baking mix (.66 or 2/3 cup)
- 1% milk (.75 cup)
- Eggs (2 large)
- Black pepper (.25 tsp.)
- Herb & Garlic seasoning salt (.5 tsp.)
- Also Needed: 9-inch pie plate

Preparation Method:
1. Warm the oven setting to reach 400° Fahrenheit/204° Celsius.
2. Lightly spritz the bottom and sides of the pie plate using cooking oil spray.
3. Chop and scatter the zucchini, onion, tomato, and cheese evenly on the pie plate.
4. Whisk the remainder of the fixings using a fork and stir until blended.
5. Dump it over the veggies and cheese. Put the pie plate on a baking tray to catch any boil overs.
6. Bake till the pie is done. A knife inserted in the center should come out clean (35 min.).
7. Place the plate onto a wire rack for cooling - a minimum of ten minutes before slicing.
8. Slice the pie into six wedges.
9. Serve with a side salad as desired.

Cereal Favorites

Baked Oatmeal

Portions Provided: 8 servings
Time Required: 40 minutes
Nutritional Statistics (Each Portion):
- Protein Counts: 7 grams
- Carbohydrates: 33 grams
- Fat Content: 4 grams
- Sugars: 8.5 grams
- Dietary Fiber: 3 grams
- Sodium: 105 mg
- Calories: 196

Essential Ingredients:
- Egg substitute (equal to 4 egg whites/2 whole eggs)
- Unsweetened applesauce (.5 cup)
- Canola oil (1 tbsp.)
- Cinnamon (1 tsp.)
- Brown sugar (.33 cup)
- Baking powder (2 tsp.)
- Uncooked rolled oats (3 cups)
- Skim milk (1 cup)
- Suggested: 9x13 or 23x33-cm baking pan

Preparation Method:
1. Beat the eggs with oil, applesauce, and sugar. Mix in the dry fixings.
2. Spritz the pan generously with a cooking oil spray.
3. Scoop the oatmeal mixture into the pan.
4. Bake without a top at 350° Fahrenheit/177° Celsius for 30 minutes.

Berry Muesli

Portions Provided: 4 servings
Time Required: 5 minutes - overnight
Nutritional Statistics (Each Portion) varies:
- Protein Counts: 6 grams
- Carbohydrates: 27 grams
- Fat Content: 5 grams
- Dietary Fiber: 3 grams
- Sodium: 45 mg
- Calories: 170

Essential Ingredients:
- 1% milk (.5 cup)
- Fruit yogurt (1 cup)
- Apple (.5 cup)
- Dried fruit: Apricots - raisins or dates (.5 cup)
- Frozen blueberries (.5 cup)
- Rolled oats - raw - old-fashioned (1 cup)
- Toasted walnuts (.25 cup)

Preparation Method:
1. Whisk the yogurt with the oat milk and salt in a mixing container.
2. Place a lid or layer of foil over the container and pop it in the refrigerator to chill (6-12 hrs.).
3. Chop the apple and nuts.
4. Gently mix in the fresh and dried fruit.
5. Scoop the muesli in small serving dishes with a portion of nuts.
6. Pop any leftovers in the fridge to use within two to three hours.

Herbed Savory Wild Mushroom Oatmeal

Portions Provided: 4 servings
Time Required: 25 minutes
Nutritional Statistics (Each Portion):
- Protein Counts: 11 grams
- Carbohydrates: 30 grams
- Fat Content: 9 grams
- Sugars: 1 gram
- Dietary Fiber: 5 grams
- Sodium: 493 mg
- Calories: 247

Essential Ingredients:
- Olive oil (2 tsp.)
- Scallion (2 stalks)
- Sliced mushrooms (340 g/12 oz.)
- 100% Lemon juice (2 tsp.)
- Water (4 cups)
- Fresh rosemary (1 tsp.)
- Black pepper (.75 tsp.)
- Sea salt (1 tsp.)
- Old-fashioned dry oats (2 cups)
- Eggs (4)

Preparation Method:
1. Warm oil in a big saucepan using a med-high temperature setting.
2. Toss in the white part of the scallions, mushrooms, lemon juice, and pepper - sauté till the mushrooms are just cooked through (5 min.).
3. While the mushrooms are cooking, fry the eggs in a nonstick skillet using cooking spray.

4. Pour in the water, salt, and rosemary - boil using the high-temperature setting. Stir in the oats and green part of the scallions - adjust the heat to medium.
5. Simmer the mixture, occasionally stirring till the oats are thoroughly cooked (6 min.).
6. Sprinkle each serving with the cheese or top with an egg to serve. Garnish the dish with a few more scallions and serve.

Overnight Oats with Fruit

Portions Provided: 1 serving
Time Required: 10 minutes + chilling time
Nutritional Statistics (Each Portion):
- Protein Counts: 11 grams
- Carbohydrates: 53 grams
- Fat Content: 13 grams
- Sugars: 31 grams
- Dietary Fiber: 5 grams
- Sodium: 53 mg
- Calories: 345

Essential Ingredients:
- Old-fashioned oats (.33 cup)
- Plain yogurt - reduced-fat (3 tbsp.)
- Honey (1 tbsp.)
- Milk - fat-free (3 tbsp.)
- Assorted fresh fruit (.5 cup)
- Walnuts (2 tbsp.)
- Needed: Mason jar/similar freezer container

Preparation Method:
1. Toast and chop the nuts.
2. Load the jar with the oats, milk, yogurt, and honey.
3. Add the oats with nuts and fruit - lastly.
4. Close the top and pop it into the fridge overnight.
5. Wake up, stir, and serve cold or hot.

Overnight Peanut Butter Oats - Gluten-Free - Vegan

Portions Provided: 1 serving
Time Required: 6 hours 5 minutes
Nutritional Statistics (Each Portion):
- Protein Counts: 15 grams
- Carbohydrates: 52 grams (Net: 13 grams)
- Fat Content: 23 grams
- Sugars: 16 grams

- Dietary Fiber: 8 grams
- Sodium: 229 mg
- Calories: 452

Essential Ingredients:
- Unsweetened plain almond/coconut/soy/hemp milk (.5 cup)
- Chia seeds (.75 tbsp.)
- Natural salted peanut or almond butter - crunchy or creamy (2 tbsp.)
- Maple syrup/organic brown sugar/coconut sugar/stevia (1 tbsp. or as desired)
- Rolled oats - gluten-free (.5 cup)
  Optional Toppings:
- Strawberries/raspberries/sliced banana
- Granola
- More chia seeds or flaxseed meal
- Also Needed: Mason jar or small bowl with a lid.

Preparation Method:
1. Pour the milk, peanut butter, chia seeds, and maple syrup into the chosen container. Mix it using a wooden spoon.
2. Mix in the oats and stir a few more times. Pack the mixture tightly.
3. Cover securely with a top or foil. Pop it into the fridge overnight (at least 6 hrs.) to set. Open to serve.[1]

Quick-Cooking Oats - Vegan

Portions Provided: 1 serving
Time Required: 5 minutes
Nutritional Statistics (Each Portion):
- Protein Counts: 5 grams
- Carbohydrates: 27 grams
- Fat Content: 3 grams
- Sugars: 1 gram
- Dietary Fiber: 4 grams
- Sodium: 152.4 mg
- Calories: 150

Essential Ingredients:
- Water/low-fat milk (1 cup)
- Salt (1 pinch)
- Quick-cooking oats (.5 cup)
  To Serve:
- Low-fat milk (1 fl. oz./2 tbsp./as desired)
- Cinnamon (1-2 pinches)
- Honey or cane or brown sugar (1-2 tsp.)

Preparation Method:
Stovetop Steps: Prepare a saucepan to combine water/milk and salt. Wait for it to boil.

---

[1] *Optional Warming Tips*: Warm the oats in the microwave for 45 seconds to one minute. You can also scoop the oats into a saucepan to warm using the medium-temperature. It's not freezer-friendly.

1. Measure and toss in the oats - lowering the heat setting to medium to cook (1 min.).
2. Transfer the pan to a cold burner, place a lid on it, and wait two to three minutes before eating.
3. *Microwave Steps*: Combine water (or milk), salt, and oats in a two-cup microwave-safe bowl - cook using the high setting (1.5-2 min.). Stir before serving.
4. Serve with your favorite toppings, including milk, sweetener, dried fruits, cinnamon, and nuts.

Six-Grain Hot Cereal

Portions Provided: 14 servings @ ½ cup each
Time Required: 45-50 minutes
Nutritional Statistics (Each Portion):
- Protein Counts: 4 grams
- Carbohydrates: 21 grams
- Fat Content: 1 gram
- Sugars: -0- grams
- Dietary Fiber: 3 grams
- Sodium: 74 mg
- Calories: 114

Essential Ingredients:
- Uncooked red wheat berries (.5 cup)
- Uncooked quinoa (3 tbsp.)
- Uncooked brown rice (.5 cup)
- Uncooked steel-cut oats (.25 cup)
- Kosher salt (.5 tsp.)
- Uncooked pearl barley (.5 cup)
- Flaxseed (2 tbsp.)
- Water (1.5 quarts)

Preparation Method:
1. Toss each of the fixings in a big saucepan by pouring water over each cereal. Set the temperature on medium.
2. Stir and wait for them to boil.
3. Adjust the temperature setting to low. Simmer and occasionally stir the cereal for 45 minutes. Serve as desired.

Soup & Curry Options

Asparagus Soup

Portions Provided: 12 servings or ¾ cup each
Time Required: 1 hour 15 minutes
Nutritional Statistics (Each Portion):

- Protein Counts: 4 grams
- Carbohydrates: 11 grams (Net: 7 grams)
- Fat Content: 3 grams
- Sugars: 2 grams
- Dietary Fiber: 2 grams
- Sodium: 401 mg
- Calories: 79

Essential Ingredients:

- Carrot (1 medium)
- Fresh asparagus (2 lb. or 910 g)
- Medium onion (1)
- Olive oil (1 tbsp.)
- Butter (1 tbsp.)
- Pepper (.25 tsp.)
- Salt (.5 tsp.)
- Dried thyme (.25 tsp.)
- Uncooked - long-grain brown rice (.66 or 2/3 cup)
- Chicken broth - reduced-sodium (6 cups)
  Optional - Count & Add the Carbs:
- Sour cream - reduced fat
- Salad croutons
- Suggested: Immersion blender

Preparation Method:

1. Trim the asparagus into one-inch pieces. Chop the onion and thinly slice the carrot.
2. In a six-quart stockpot, warm the oil and butter using the medium-temperature setting.
3. Stir in the seasonings and veggies - cook till vegetables are tender - occasionally stirring (8-10 min.).
4. Stir in the broth and rice - wait for it to boil.
5. Lower the temperature setting and simmer with a lid on the pot till the rice is nice and tender - occasionally stirring (40-45 min.).
6. Puree the soup with the blender. (Alternately, lightly cool it and prepare it in batches using a regular blender.
7. Mix the blended soup into the pot and heat through. Serve with sour cream and croutons to your liking.
8. *Freezer Option*: Freeze the cool soup in freezer containers.
9. *Serving Time*: Partially thaw the soup in the refrigerator overnight. Warm it till it's boiling, whisking until blended.

Beef Stew with Fennel & Shallots

Portions Provided: 6 servings @ 1 cup each
Time Required: 2 hours - varies
Nutritional Statistics (Each Portion):

- Protein Counts: 21 grams
- Carbohydrates: 22 grams
- Fat Content: 8 grams
- Sugars: 8 grams
- Dietary Fiber: 4.5 grams
- Sodium: 185 mg
- Calories: 244

Essential Ingredients:

- Plain A. P. flour (3 tbsp.)
- Lean beef stew meat (1 lb./450 g)
- Olive/canola oil (2 tbsp.)
- Fennel bulb (half of 1)
- Shallots (3 large/about 3 tbsp.)
- Black pepper (.75 tsp. - divided)
- Bay leaf (1)
- Fresh thyme sprigs (2)
- Vegetable stock/broth - no-salt (3 cups)
- Carrots (4 large)
- Red-skinned or white potatoes (4 large)
- Boiling onions (18 small/about 10 oz./280 g total weight)
- Portobello mushrooms (3)
- Fresh Italian parsley - flat-leaf (.33 cup)
- Optional: Red wine (.5 cup/not included in the analysis)

Preparation Method:

1. Trim away the fat from the meat- cut it into cubes (1.5-inches).
2. Prep the veggies. Peel and slice the potatoes and carrots into one-inch cubes. Slice the onions into halves. Brush clean the mushrooms and chop them into one-inch chunks.
3. Add flour to a shallow dish and dip in the cubed beef. Use a big saucepan or dutch oven to warm the oil using a medium-temperature setting.
4. Place the beef in the pan to cook till it's browned (5 min.). Transfer the meat to a holding container for now.

5. Trim and thinly slice the fennel and chop the shallots - toss them into the pan using a medium-temperature setting. Sauté them till they're lightly browned and softened (6-8 min.). Mix in pepper (¼ tsp.), bay leaf, and thyme sprigs. Sauté them for about one minute.

6. Add the vegetable stock, beef, and wine to the dutch oven or chosen pan. Wait for it to boil, adjust the temperature setting to low. Put a top on the pan and let the mixture simmer till the meat is tender (40-45 min.). Toss in the potatoes, carrots, onions, and mushrooms. Simmer the stew gently till the veggies are fork-tender (another ½ hr.).

7. Discard the thyme sprigs and bay leaf. Finely chop and stir in the remainder of the pepper (½ tsp.) and parsley.

8. Scoop the delicious stew into warmed serving dishes to serve immediately.

Chicken Chili Verde – Diabetic-Friendly

Portions Provided: 6 servings @ 1.5 cups each
Time Required: 30 minutes
Nutritional Statistics (Each Portion):
- Protein Counts: 31.6 grams
- Carbohydrates: 40.5 grams
- Fat Content: 9.8 grams
- Sugars: 8.6 grams
- Dietary Fiber: 8.6 grams
- Sodium: 569.6 mg
- Calories: 408
  Diabetic Exchanges:
- Starch: 3
- Lean Protein: 1
- Vegetable 1 ½
- Fat: 2

Essential Ingredients:
- No-salt-added pinto beans - divided (2 - 430 g/15 oz. cans)
- Canola oil (1 tbsp.)
- Chicken thighs (1.5 lb.)
- Yellow onion (1 medium/2 cups)
- Poblano peppers (2 cups/2 large)
- Garlic cloves (5/about 1.5 tbsp.)
- Unsalted chicken stock (4 cups)
- Prepared salsa verde (1.5 cups)
- Salt (.5 tsp.)
- Frozen corn kernels (about 12 oz./2 cups)
- Fresh cilantro (1.5 cups)
- Spinach (2 cups/about 2 oz.)
- Sour cream (6 tbsp.)

Preparation Method:
1. Dump the beans into a colander, rinse them, and let them drain.
2. Trim the chicken to remove the bones and fat. Chop it into bite-sized chunks.
3. Chop the onions, peppers, garlic, spinach, and cilantro.
4. Mash one cup of beans in a mixing container using a potato masher or whisk.
5. Warm oil in a big heavy-duty pot using the high-temperature setting.
6. Add chicken and fry it till it's brown - occasionally turning (4-5 min.).
7. Toss in the prepared onion, poblanos, and garlic. Sauté the mixture till the onion is translucent and tender (4-5 more min.).
8. Mix in the rest of the whole beans, mashed beans, salsa, salt, and stock.
9. Wait for it to boil, lower the temperature setting to medium, and cook it till the chicken is thoroughly cooked (3 min.).
10. Fold in spinach, corn, and cilantro. Cook till the spinach is wilted (1 min.).
11. Serve topped with sour cream as desired to serve.

Chickpea & Potato Curry

Portions Provided: 4 servings @ 1¼ cups each
Time Required: 35 minutes
Nutritional Statistics (Each Portion):
- Protein Counts: 8.9 grams
- Carbohydrates: 46.5 grams
- Fat Content: 11.6 grams
- Fiber Counts: 8.8 grams
- Sugars: 6.6 grams
- Sodium: 532.8 mg
- Calories: 321

Essential Ingredients:
- Yukon Gold potatoes (450 g/1 lb.)
- Canola/grapeseed oil (3 tbsp.)
- Garlic cloves (3)
- Onion (1 large)
- Curry powder (2 tsp.)
- Salt (.75 tsp.)
- Cayenne pepper (.25 tsp.)
- No-salt-added diced tomatoes (400 g/14 oz. can)
- Water (.75 cup - divided)

- Low-sodium chickpeas (430 g/15 oz. can)
- Frozen peas (1 cup)
- Garam masala (.5 tsp.)

Preparation Method:

1. Pour one inch of water into a big pot fitted with a steamer basket.
2. Peel and slice the potatoes into one-inch chunks. Mince or dice the onions and garlic. Dump the chickpeas into a colander and thoroughly rinse; let them drain.
3. Toss the potatoes into the pot. Put a top on it to simmer/steam until tender (6-8 min.). Set the potatoes aside. Dry the pot.
4. Warm oil in the fresh pot using the med-high temperature setting. Chop/dice the onion and toss it into the pot. Stir often - until it's softened and translucent (3-5 min.).
5. Mince and add the garlic, salt, cayenne, and curry powder - let it simmer - stirring continuously for one minute. Mix in the tomatoes and juices - cook for another two minutes - adding the mixture into a food processor.
6. Pour in water (½ cup) and pulse till it's creamy smooth. Return the puree to the pot.
7. Pulse the rest of the water (¼ cup) in the food processor to rinse the sauce residue.
8. Pour it into the pot with the reserved potatoes, peas, chickpeas, and garam masala.
9. Simmer and stir till it's hot (5 min.) and serve.

Chilean Lentil Stew with Salsa Verde

Portions Provided: 4 servings **Time Required:** 40 minutes

Nutritional Statistics (Each Portion):

1 ¼ cups lentils + 2 tbsp. Salsa Verde:

- Protein Counts: 18.8 grams
- Carbohydrates: 53.1 grams
- Fat Content: 5.2 grams Sugars: 6.1 grams Dietary Fiber: 13.6 grams
- Sodium: 454.7 mg Calories: 322

Essential Ingredients:

- Olive oil (1 tbsp.)
- Fennel (1 bulb)/Celery (4-6 stalks) = (1.25 cups total)
- Carrots (.5 cup/3 small)
- Red bell pepper (.5 cup)
- Shallot (5 tbsp./1 large divided)

- Garlic (2 large cloves)
- Tomato paste (2 tbsp.)
- French green lentils (1.5 cups)
- Vegetable/chicken broth - l.s. - or water (4 cups)
- Ground pepper - divided (.75 tsp.)
- Salt - divided (.5 tsp.)
- Italian parsley (.75 cup/1 small bunch)
- Vinegar - white wine suggested (2 tbsp.)
- Lime juice (2 tbsp./1 large)
- Suggested: 4-6-qt. pot

Preparation Method:

1. Warm oil in a soup pot using a med-high temperature setting.
2. Sort and rinse the lentils.
3. Peel and mince or chop the fixings as desired.
4. Meanwhile, chop and add the parsley with the remaining shallots (2 tbsp.), vinegar, pepper, salt (¼ tsp. each), and lime juice in a mixing container.
5. Scoop the stew into four serving bowls - topping each one with a scoop of the salsa verde. Serve the rest of the salsa in another dish.

Cream of Wild Rice Soup

Portions Provided: 4 servings
Time Required: 45 minutes
Nutritional Statistics (Each Portion):

- Protein Counts: 12 grams
- Carbohydrates: 38 grams (Net: 14 grams)
- Fat Content: 4 grams
- Sugars: 12 grams
- Dietary Fiber: 7 grams
- Sodium: 180 mg
- Calories: 236

Essential Ingredients:

- Canola oil (.5 tbsp.)
- Unsalted prepared white beans (1 cup) or White beans (½ of a 15.5 oz. can) 1 % milk (2 cups)
- Yellow onion (1.5 cups)
- Carrot (1 cup)
- Kale (1.5 cups)
- Celery (1 cup)
- Minced parsley (1 tbsp.)
- Garlic (2 cloves)
- Low-sodium vegetable stock (2 cups)
- Fennel seeds - crushed (1 tsp.)
- Wild rice - cooked (.5 cup)
- Black pepper (1 tsp.)

Preparation Method:
1. Warm a saucepan or soup pot using a medium temperature setting - pour in canola oil to get hot.
2. Rinse and drain the beans.
3. Dice/chop and sauté the carrot, celery, garlic, and onions until lightly browned.
4. Chop and fold in the kale, parsley, stock, and other spices. Wait for it to boil.
5. Use a blender to puree the beans with milk. Mix the bean mixture into the soup. Simmer and add rice (½ hour).
6. Serve in heated bowls.

Curried Cream of Tomato Soup with Apples

Portions Provided: 8 servings
Time Required: 45 minutes
Nutritional Statistics (Each Portion):
- Protein Counts: 8 grams
- Carbohydrates: 32 grams
- Fat Content: 5 grams
- Dietary Fiber: 3 grams
- Sodium: 89 mg
- Calories: 205

Essential Ingredients:
- Olive oil (2 tbsp.)
- Garlic (1 tsp.)
- Onion (1.5 cups)
- Celery (1 cup)
- Curry powder (1 tbsp./as desired)
- Tomatoes - canned - no-salt - drained (3 cups)
- Ground black pepper (as desired)
- Long-grain brown rice (1 cup)
- Vegetable/chicken broth - l.s. (6 cups)
- Milk - Fat-free (1 cup)
- Apple cubes (1.5 cups)
- Thyme (.5 tsp.)
- Bay leaf (1)

Preparation Method:
1. Warm oil using the medium-temperature setting in a big saucepan or dutch oven.
2. Finely chop and toss in the garlic, onion, and celery. Sauté them till tender (4 min.).
3. Mix in the curry powder, thyme, tomatoes, bay leaf, rice, and black pepper while heating it.
4. Mix in the broth and wait for it to begin boiling. Cook it for about ½ hour. The rice should be tender. Trash the bay leaf.

5. Dump the soup into a food processor. Close the lid - mix it till it's creamy smooth.
6. Empty the smooth and creamy soup in the dutch oven. Fold in the apple cubes and milk, stirring until it's thoroughly heated.
7. Promptly serve the soup in warmed bowls while piping hot.

Curried Sweet Potato & Peanut Soup

Portions Provided: 6 servings @ 1 cup each
Time Required: 40 minutes
Nutritional Statistics (Each Portion):
- Protein Counts: 12.6 grams
- Carbohydrates: 37.4 grams
- Fat Content: 9.7 grams
- Fiber Counts: 8.4 grams
- Sugars: 6.8 grams
- Sodium: 593.7 mg
- Calories: 345

Essential Ingredients:
- Yellow onion (1.5 cups)
- Garlic (1 tbsp.)
- Fresh ginger (1 tbsp.)
- Red curry paste (4 tsp.)
- Serrano chili (1 rib & seeds removed, minced)
- Sweet potatoes (1 lb. @ ½-inch pieces)
- Canola oil (2 tbsp.)
- Water (3 cups)
- Coconut milk - lite (1 cup)
- White beans (430 g/15 oz. can)
- Salt (.75 tsp.)
- Ground pepper (.25 tsp.)
- Fresh cilantro (.25 cup)
- Roasted pumpkin seeds - unsalted (.25 cup)
- Dry-roasted peanuts - unsalted (.75 cup)
- Lime: Juice (2 tbsp.) + wedges

Preparation Method:
1. Thoroughly rinse the beans in a colander. Chop the cilantro.
2. Warm oil in a dutch oven using a med-high temperature setting.
3. Dice and mix in the onion to sauté till they're translucent and softened (4 min.).
4. Mince the garlic and ginger - sautéing them with the serrano and curry paste (1 min.).
5. Peel and cube the potatoes. Stir in water and wait for them to boil.
6. Adjust the temperature setting to med-low and simmer with the lid slightly ajar till the potatoes are softened (10-12 min.).

7. Pour about ½ of the soup into a blender - mix with the peanuts and coconut milk to puree (be careful while pureeing).

8. Dump the mixture back into the pot - adding in the pepper, salt, and beans - thoroughly heat and transfer it to a cool burner.

9. Stir in cilantro, lime juice, and pumpkin seeds. Serve with lime wedges.

Garden Vegetable Beef Soup - Diabetic-Friendly

Portions Provided: 8 servings or 3.5 quarts (1¾ cup portions)
Time Required: 1 hour 15 minutes
Nutritional Statistics (Each Portion - No Cheese):
- Protein Counts: 21 grams
- Carbohydrates: 14 grams (Net: 4 grams)
- Fat Content: 7 grams
- Sugars: 7 grams
- Dietary Fiber: 3 grams
- Sodium: 621 mg
- Calories: 207
  Diabetic Exchanges:
- Lean meat: 3
- Vegetables: 2

Essential Ingredients:
- 90% lean ground beef (680 g/1.5 lb.)
- Medium onion (1)
- Garlic cloves (2)
- Julienned carrots (280 g/10 oz. pkg.)
- Celery (2 ribs)
- Tomato paste (.25 cup)
- Diced tomatoes - undrained (410 g/14.5 oz. can)
- Shredded cabbage (1.5 cups)
- Medium zucchini (1)
- Red potato (about 140 g/5 oz./1 medium)
- Fresh or frozen cut green beans (.5 cup)
- Dried oregano (.5 tsp.)
- Black pepper and salt (.25 tsp. each)
- Dried basil (1 tsp.)
- Reduced-sodium beef broth (4 cans @ 410 g/14.5 oz. each)
- Optional: Grated Parmesan cheese
- Suggested: 6-qt./5.7-L. stockpot

Preparation Method:
1. Chop/mince the onion and garlic. Cover a platter using a few paper towels.
2. Prepare the stockpot to cook the beef with the onion and garlic using the medium-temperature setting till the beef is thoroughly done (not pink), breaking up the beef into crumbles (5-8 min.). Scoop the crumbles onto the prepared platter to drain the fats.
3. Julienne or dice the carrots.
4. Fold in carrots and celery to the pot, cook, and stir till tender (6-7 min.). Stir in tomato paste - cook for one more minute. Coarsely chop the zucchini and finely chop the cabbage and potato. Add tomatoes, cabbage, potatoes, zucchini, green beans, seasonings, cooked meat, and broth.
5. Once it's boiling, lower the temperature setting and simmer with a lid on the cooker until vegetables are tender (35-45 min.).
6. Garnish each portion with cheese to your liking - making sure to add the counts to your daily totals.

Ginger Chicken Noodle Soup

Portions Provided: 8 servings
Time Required: 20-25 minutes
Nutritional Statistics (Each Portion):
- Protein Counts: 19 grams
- Carbohydrates: 16 grams (Net: 10 grams)
- Fat Content: 5 grams
- Sugars: 4 grams
- Dietary Fiber: 2 grams
- Sodium: 267 mg
- Calories: 185

Essential Ingredients:
- Olive oil (1 tbsp.)
- Dried soba noodles (3 oz./85 g)
- Yellow onion (1 large)
- Carrot (1)
- Fresh ginger (1 tbsp.)
- Chicken broth or stock (4 cups)
- Garlic (1 clove)
- Soy sauce - reduced-sodium (2 tbsp.)
- Shelled edamame (1 cup)
- Chicken breasts (1 lb./450 g)
- Freshly chopped cilantro/coriander (.25 cup)
- Plain soya/soy milk (1 cup)

Preparation Method:
1. Toss the noodles in a prepared saucepan ¾ full of boiling water (5 min.).
2. Use the stovetop and set the burner using the medium-temperature setting. Use a big pan to heat the oil. Dice and sauté the onion (4 min.).

3. Peel, chop and toss in the carrot and ginger and sauté one more minute. Mince and toss the garlic into the pan - sautéing for another thirty seconds (don't brown the garlic).

4. Pour the soy sauce and add the garlic, bringing it to a boil.

5. Trim the bones and fat from the chicken and chop it into chunks.

6. Add the edamame and chicken and wait for them to boil.

7. Adjust the temperature setting to med-low; simmer another four minutes.

8. Pour in the soy milk and noodles, cooking until completely heated.

9. Take the pan from the burner to add the cilantro.

10. Serve the soup as desired.

Green Bean & Tomato Soup

Portions Provided: 9 servings
Time Required: 45 minutes
Nutritional Statistics (Each Portion):
- Protein Counts: 4 grams
- Carbs: 10 grams (Net: 2 grams)
- Fat Content: 1 gram
- Sugars: 5 grams
- Dietary Fiber: 3 grams
- Sodium: 535 mg
- Calories: 58

Essential Ingredients:
- Carrots (1 cup)
- Butter (2 tsp.)
- Onion (1 cup)
- Chicken/vegetable broth - reduced-sodium (6 cups)
- Fresh green beans (1 lb.)
- Garlic (1 clove)
- Diced fresh tomatoes (3 cups)
- Freshly minced basil (.25 cup) or Dried basil (1 tbsp.)
- Salt (.5 tsp.)
- Pepper (.25 tsp.)

Preparation Method:
1. Warm a big pan and melt the butter.
2. Chop and sauté the carrots with the onions (5 min.).
3. Cut the beans into one-inch pieces and mince the garlic. Stir in the beans, broth, and garlic. Wait for it to boil.

4. Lower the temperature setting and put a top on the saucepan to cook until the veggies are tender (20 min.).

5. Mix in the tomatoes, salt, basil, and pepper.

6. Put a top on the pan - simmer the soup for five more minutes.

Mediterranean Chicken & Chickpea Soup - Slow-Cooked

Portions Provided: servings **Time Required**: 4 hours 20 minutes
Nutritional Statistics (Each Portion):
- Protein Counts: 33.6 grams
- Carbohydrates: 43 grams
- Fat Content: 15.3 grams
- Sugars: 8.5 grams
- Dietary Fiber: 11.6 grams
- Sodium: 761.8 mg
- Calories: 447
  Diabetic Exchanges:
- Fat: ½
- Vegetable: 2
- Starch: 2
- Lean Protein: 4 ½

Essential Ingredients:
- Dried chickpeas (1.5 cups)
- Water (4 cups)
- Yellow onion (1 large)
- Tomato paste (2 tbsp.)
- Fire-roasted diced tomatoes - no-salt (430 g/15 oz can)
- Garlic (4 cloves)
- Paprika (4 tsp.)
- Bay leaf (1)
- Cayenne pepper (.25 tsp.)
- Black pepper (.25 tsp.)
- Ground cumin (4 tsp.)
- Chicken thighs - bone-in (910 g/2 lb.)
- Artichoke hearts 400 g/ (14 oz. can)
- Pitted oil-cured olives (.25 cup)
- Salt (.5 tsp.)
- Fresh parsley or cilantro (.25 cup)
- Suggested: Slow Cooker (6-qt. or larger)

Preparation Method:
1. Soak the chickpeas overnight. Drain the artichokes and cut them into quarters.
2. Finely chop the garlic and onions. Slice the olives into halves. Chop the parsley.
3. Drain chickpeas and place them into the cooker. Add four cups of water, tomato paste, onions, tomatoes with juices, bay leaf,

garlic, cumin, paprika, cayenne, and ground pepper; stir to combine. Trim the chicken and remove the fat; toss it into the cooker.

4. Cover and cook for eight hours (low setting) or four hours (high setting).
5. Transfer the chicken to a chopping block and let cool slightly. Discard bay leaf.
6. Add in the artichokes, olives, and salt - stir to combine.
7. Shred the chicken, discarding bones. Stir the chicken into the soup.
8. Serve the soup topped with parsley or cilantro as desired.

Potato Fennel Soup

Portions Provided: 8 servings
Time Required: 35-40 minutes
Nutritional Statistics (Each Portion):
- Protein Counts: 6 grams
- Carbohydrates: 28 grams
- Fat Content: 1.5 grams
- Sugars: 7 grams
- Dietary Fiber: 3 grams
- Sodium: 104 mg
- Calories: 149

Essential Ingredients:
- Fennel bulb (1 large/910 g/about 2 lb.)
- Red onion (1 cup)
- Russet potatoes (2 large)
- Milk - fat-free (1 cup)
- Olive oil (1 tsp.)
- Chicken broth - reduced sodium (3 cups)
- Lemon juice (2 tsp.)
- Toasted fennel seeds (2 tsp.)

Preparation Method:
1. Warm the oil using the medium-temperature setting in a big dutch oven or similar pot.
2. Chop and toss in the fennel and onions. Sauté until softened (5 min.).
3. Peel and slice the potatoes. Toss them into the pot with lemon juice, milk, and chicken broth.
4. Put a lid on the pot and adjust the temperature setting to a simmer until the potatoes are done (15 min.).
5. Pour the soup into a food processor - preparing in batches if needed and mix till it's smooth. (Carefully fill - no more than 1/3 full to avoid burns.)

6. Add it back to the pot and heat it to serve. Garnish the soup with fennel seeds to serve.

Quick Creamy Tomato Cup-of-Soup

Portions Provided: 1 serving
Time Required: 5 minutes
Nutritional Statistics (Each Portion):
- Protein Counts: 5.1 grams
- Carbohydrates: 18.3 grams (Net: 4.6 grams)
- Fat Content: 2.7 grams
- Fiber Counts: 3.6 grams
- Sugar: 10.1 grams
- Sodium: 244.9 mg
- Calories: 105

Essential Ingredients:
- No-salt-added canned tomato puree (.75 cup)
- Chicken broth - l.s. (.25 cup)
- Reduced-fat cream cheese (1 tbsp.)

Preparation Method:
1. Whisk the puree with the broth and cream cheese in a big heat-proof mug.
2. Microwave using the high setting, occasionally stirring till it's thoroughly heated and creamy (2 min.).

Salmon Chowder

Portions Provided: 8 servings
Time Required: 35 minutes
Nutritional Statistics (Each Portion):
- Protein Counts: 11 grams
- Carbohydrates: 26 grams
- Fat Content: 2.5 grams
- Dietary Fiber: 2 grams
- Sodium: 207 mg
- Calories: 166

Essential Ingredients:
- Olive oil (1 tsp.)
- Celery (.5 cup)
- Garlic (1 clove)
- Chicken broth - l.s. (430 g/15 oz. can)
- Frozen country-style hash browns with green peppers & onions (2.5 cups)
- Frozen peas and carrots (1 cup)
- Pink salmon - deboned (170 g/6 oz. can/pouch)
- Evaporated skim milk (340 g/12 oz. can)
- Dill (.5 tsp.)
- Black pepper (.5 tsp.)
- No-salt-added cream-style corn (420 g/14.75 oz. can)

Preparation Method:

1. Heat the oil using the medium-temperature setting in a big saucepan.
2. Chop and add the celery to sauté for ten minutes.
3. Mince and toss in the garlic to sauté (1 min.).
4. Add in the broth and mix it with pepper, dill, hash browns, and carrots. Wait for it to boil and adjust the temperature setting. Cook it until the vegetables are done but not overcooked (10 min.).
5. Separate and mix in the salmon. Pour in the corn and milk. Serve when it's piping hot.

Slow-Cooked Chicken & White Bean Stew - Diabetic-Friendly

Portions Provided: 6 servings @ 1¼ cups each
Time Required: 7 hours 35 minutes
Nutritional Statistics (Each Portion):

- Protein Counts: 44.2 grams
- Carbohydrates: 53.8 grams
- Fat Content: 10.9 grams
- Sugars: 4.5 grams
- Dietary Fiber: 27.4 grams
- Sodium: 518.4mg
- Calories: 493
  Diabetic Exchanges:
- High-fat Protein: ½
- Vegetable: 1
- Fat: 1
- Starch: 2
- Lean Protein: 4 1/2

Essential Ingredients:

- Olive oil (2 tbsp.)
- Dried cannellini beans - soaked overnight & drained (1 lb.**)
- Unsalted chicken broth (6 cups)
- Carrots (1 cup)
- Yellow onion (1 cup)
- Parmesan cheese rind (110 g/4 oz.) + grated parmesan (.66 or 2/3 cup) divided
- Chicken breasts (2 bone-in/1 lb. each)
- Kale (4 cups)
- Fresh rosemary (1 tsp.)
- Kosher salt & black pepper (.5 tsp. each)
- Flat-leaf parsley leaves (.25 cup)
- Lemon juice (1 tbsp.)
- Suggested: Six-quart slow cooker

Preparation Method:

1. Chop the onion, carrots, rosemary, kale, and parsley.
2. Load the cooker with the rind of parmesan, rosemary, carrots, onion, broth, and beans. Add the chicken last and securely close the lid.
3. Set the timer for seven or eight hours using the low-temperature setting - the veggies should be fork-tender. Transfer the chicken to the chopping block - waiting till it's cool enough to handle (10 min.). Trim the chicken of all its fat and bones while you shred it into the cooker. Stir in the lemon juice, pepper, salt, and kale. Put the lid back on the slow cooker and simmer till the kale is also fork-tender (20-30 min.).
4. Trash the parmesan rind and serve the stew with a spritz of oil. Lightly dust it using a sprinkle of parsley and parmesan.
5. Meal Prep Tip: **You can substitute four (15 oz.) cans of rinsed - no-salt-added cannellini beans to replace the soaked dried beans.

Southwestern Vegetable Chowder

Portions Provided: 6 servings @ 1½ cups each
Time Required: 45 minutes
Nutritional Statistics (Each Portion):

- Protein Counts: 11.2 grams
- Carbohydrates: 43.4 grams
- Fat Content: 10 grams
- Sugars: 7 grams
- Dietary Fiber: 10 grams
- Sodium: 310.3 mg
- Calories: 307

Essential Ingredients:

- Olive oil (3 tbsp.)
- Celery (1 cup)
- Dried oregano (1 tsp.)
- Onion (1 cup)
- Salt (.25 tsp.)
- A.P. flour (.5 cup)
- Chili powder (1 tbsp.)
- Vegetable broth - Reduced-sodium (4 cups)
- Whole milk (1 cup)
- Medium poblanos or red/green bell peppers (2)
- Diced sweet potato (2 cups)
- Black beans (2 cans @ 15 oz./430 g each)
- Ground cumin (1.5 tsp.)
  To Garnish:
- Toasted pepitas
- Cilantro
- Lime wedges

Preparation Method:

1. Rinse the beans in a colander.
2. Dice the onion, peeled potatoes, peppers, and celery.
3. Warm oil in a big pot using the medium temperature setting. Toss in the celery and onion - cook the veggies while often stirring till they're softened (3-6 min.).
4. Sprinkle the mixture using flour, salt, chili powder, cumin, and oregano over the veggies and simmer for another minute. Mix in the vegetable broth and milk - stirring till it reaches a gentle boil.
5. Fold in the peppers and sweet potatoes - bring just to a simmer.
6. Continue heating, occasionally stirring till the veggies are tender (12-15 min.).
7. Mix in the black beans and cook till they're thoroughly heated (2-4 min.).
8. Enjoy them with a portion of pepitas, cilantro, and lime wedges.

Spicy Bean Chili

Portions Provided: 4 servings @ 1 cup each
Time Required: 35 minutes
Nutritional Statistics (Each Portion):

- Protein Counts: 17 grams
- Carbohydrates: 45 grams
- Fat Content: 2 grams
- Dietary Fiber: 17 grams
- Sodium: 643 mg
- Calories: 270

Essential Ingredients:

- Grapeseed oil (2 tsp.)
- Medium red onion (1)
- Jalapeno pepper (1)
- Garlic (2 cloves)
- Red kidney beans - l.s. (30 oz./850 g)
- Vegetable broth - l.s. (1.25 cups)
- Crushed tomatoes - canned (1 cup)
- Chili powder (1.5 tsp.)
- Sea salt (.5 tsp.)
- Cinnamon (.25 tsp.)
  Optional Garnishes:
- Fresh cilantro
- Organic sour cream - l.f.

Preparation Method:

1. Warm the oil in a big saucepan using a med-high temperature setting.

2. Chop and toss in the onion and jalapeño. Sauté till the onion is lightly caramelized (5 min.).
3. Mince and toss in the garlic - sauté until fragrant (½ minute).
4. Stir in the rest of the fixings and wait for it to boil. Simmer for one minute.
5. Put a lid on the pan and adjust the temperature setting to low. Simmer till the flavors are meld (10 min.) or using the med-low setting without a top.
6. Garnish as desired using sour cream and cilantro.

Turkey & Bean Soup

Portions Provided: 6 servings
Time Required: 40 minutes
Nutritional Statistics (Each Portion):

- Protein Counts: 26 grams
- Carbohydrates: 30 grams
- Fat Content: 2 grams
- Dietary Fiber: 10 grams
- Sodium: 204 mg
- Calories: 242

Essential Ingredients:

- Ground turkey breast (450 g/1 lb.)
- Unsalted cannellini beans (430 g/15 oz. can)
- Onions (2 medium)
- Celery (2 stalks)
- Garlic (1 clove)
- Ketchup (.25 cup)
- Unsalted tomatoes - diced (410 g/14.5 oz. can)
- Chicken bouillon - l.s. (3 cubes)
- Water (7 cups)
- Dried basil (1.5 tsp.)
- Freshly cracked black pepper (.25 tsp.)
- Cabbage (2 cups)

Preparation Method:

1. Cook the turkey in a big saucepan.
2. Add the beans to a colander to thoroughly rinse and drain.
3. Chop/mince and toss in the garlic, onions, and celery. Sauté them until the veggies are softened. The turkey should be done.
4. Shred the cabbage.
5. Add the tomatoes, ketchup, water, pepper, bouillon, basil, beans, and cabbage.
6. Once boiling, lower the temperature setting.
7. Put a top on the saucepan - cook for ½ hour and serve.

Vegetable & Tofu Soup - Vegetarian-Friendly

Portions Provided: 4 servings @ 1¾ cups each
Time Required: 2 hours 35 minutes
Nutritional Statistics (Each Portion):
- Protein Counts: 15.6 grams
- Carbohydrates: 19.2 grams
- Fat Content: 14.9 grams
- Sugars: 10.7 grams
- Dietary Fiber: 9.8 grams
- Sodium: 574 mg
- Calories: 259
  Diabetic Exchanges:
- Starch: ½
- Lean Protein: 1 ½
- Vegetable: 2 ½
- Fat: 2 ½

Essential Ingredients:
- Tofu - extra-firm - bean curd (340 g/12 oz. tub)
- Olive oil (2 tbsp.)
- Cooking oil spray (as needed)
- Chicken broth - l.s. (2 cups)
- Dried Italian seasoning (1 tsp.)
- Tomatoes - diced with garlic - basil & oregano - no-salt - undrained (14.5 oz. can)
- Fresh button mushrooms (3 cups/8 oz.)
- Fresh/frozen-thawed peas (.5 cup)
- Asparagus (.5 cup - 1-inch pieces)
- Chopped roasted red sweet pepper (.5 cup)
- Green olives (.25 cup)
- Dried tomatoes - oil-packed - drained & finely diced (.33 cup)
- Parmesan cheese (1 pinch - finely grated)
- Suggested: Dutch oven (5-6-quart)

Preparation Method:
1. Drain and slice the tofu into ¾-inch cubes. Toss them into a zipper-type plastic bag. Mix in the Italian seasoning and oil.
2. Close the bag while flipping it to coat the tofu. Pop it in the fridge to marinate for two to four hours.
3. Coat the dutch oven with a spritz of cooking oil spray and warm it using a med-high temperature setting.
4. Mix in the undrained tofu - cook until the tofu is browned, turning once (5-8 min.).
5. Add in the canned tomatoes and broth. Wait for it to boil.
6. Slice and toss in the mushrooms, peas, and asparagus. Lower the temperature and simmer just until the veggies are tender (5-7 min.).
7. Fold in the dried tomatoes, sweet pepper, and diced olives.
8. Warm thoroughly and garnish with a portion of cheese.

Salad Options

Apple Salad with Figs & Almonds

Portions Provided: 6 servings
Time Required: 5-7 minutes
Nutritional Statistics (Each Portion):
- Protein Counts: 2 grams
- Carbohydrates: 19 grams
- Fiber Count: 3 grams
- Fat Content: 1 gram
- Sodium: 33 mg
- Calories: 93

Essential Ingredients:
- Carrots (2 or about .75 cup)
- Celery (2 ribs/about 2 cups)
- Red apples (2 large/about 4 cups)
- Dried figs (6/about 1 cup)
- Lemon yogurt - f.f. (.5 cup)
- Almonds - slivered (2 tbsp.)

Preparation Method:
1. Peel and grate the carrots.
2. Remove the core and dice the apples.
3. Chop the figs and dice the celery.
4. Toss the celery with the figs, apples, and carrots.
5. Mix in the yogurt. Top with slivered almonds and serve.

Asian Vegetable Salad

Portions Provided: 4 servings
Time Required: 10 minutes
Nutritional Statistics (Each Portion):
- Calories: 113
- Protein Counts: 3 grams
- Fat Content: 4 grams
- Total Carbs: 14 grams (Net: 4 grams)
- Dietary Fiber: 4 grams
- Sugars: 6 grams
- Sodium: 168 mg

Essential Ingredients:
- Julienned red bell pepper (.5 cup)
- Spinach (1.5 cups)
- Yellow onion (.5 cup)
- Bok choy (1.5 cups)
- Garlic (1 tbsp.)
- Carrot (1.5 cups)
- Red cabbage (1 cup)
- Snow peas (1.5 cups)
- Cilantro (1 tbsp.)
- Cashews (1.5 tbsp.)
- Soy sauce - l.s. (2 tsp.)
- Toasted sesame oil (2 tsp.)

Preparation Method:
1. Thoroughly wash the veggies using cold running tap water - tossing them in a colander to drain.
2. Julienne (like matchsticks) the pepper, carrot, onion, and red cabbage. Chiffonade (cut across the grain - narrow strips) the spinach, cabbage, and cilantro. Mince the garlic.
3. Toss the cut veggies with garlic, chopped cashews, and snow peas in a large mixing container.
4. Spritz using the oil and a portion of soy sauce over the salad.
5. Toss thoroughly and serve.

Baby Beet & Orange Salad

Portions Provided: 4 servings
Time Required: 55 minutes
Nutritional Statistics (Each Portion):
- Calories: 118
- Protein Counts: 3 grams
- Carbohydrates: 22 grams
- Fat Content: 2 grams
- Dietary Fiber: 6 grams
- Sodium: 135 mg

Essential Ingredients:
- Olive oil (.5 tbsp.)
- Celery (2 ribs or .5 cup)
- Baby beets with greens (2 bunches/about 1 cup greens + 4 cups of beets)
- Napa cabbage (1.5 cups or ¼ of 1 head)
- Yellow onion (1 small/.5 cup)
- Orange - Juice & zest (1)
- Orange - peeled into segments (1)
- Black pepper (as desired)

Preparation Method:
1. Warm the oven in advance to 400° Fahrenheit/204° Celsius.
2. Cut the greens from the beets and wash them thoroughly using cold tap water, placing them in a colander to drain.
3. Rinse the beets and grease with oil. Use a sheet of foil to wrap the beets. Place them in the oven to bake till they're tender (45 min.). Cool to remove the outer skin and slice. Set to the side.

4. Slice the beet greens into strips and toss them into a mixing container.

5. Chop the onion, cabbage, and celery, and toss into the bowl.

6. Zest and juice one orange into a bowl. Peel the other orange - slice it into segments. Add to a mixing container.

7. Drizzle oil (½ tbsp.) and black pepper over the salad.

8. Serve the salad on chilled plates topped with sliced beets.

Balsamic Bean Salad with Vinaigrette

Portions Provided: 6 servings
Time Required: 15-20 minutes
Nutritional Statistics (Each Portion):
- Calories: 206
- Protein Counts: 7 grams
- Carbohydrates: 22 grams (Net: 4 grams)
- Fat Content: 10 grams
- Sugars: 4 grams
- Dietary Fiber: 8 grams
- Sodium: 174mg

Essential Ingredients:
The Vinaigrette:
- Balsamic vinegar (2 tbsp.)
- Ground black pepper (as desired)
- Olive oil (.25 cup)
- Fresh parsley (.33 cup)
- Garlic cloves (4)
The Salad:
- Medium red onion (1)
- Lettuce leaves (6)
- Celery (.5 cup)
- Black beans - low-sodium (15 oz. or 430 g can)
- Garbanzo beans - l.s. (15 oz. can)

Preparation Method:
1. Finely chop the cloves, celery, onion, and parsley. Rinse and drain the beans.

2. Prepare the vinaigrette by whisking the vinegar with garlic, parsley, pepper, and oil.

3. Toss the onion with the beans and mix in the vinaigrette. Place a lid or foil over the dish and pop it into the refrigerator to chill for now.

4. Arrange one lettuce leaf on each plate with a portion of the salad - garnishing them using a bit of celery to serve.

Chicken & Spring Vegetable Tortellini Salad

Portions Provided: 6 servings @ 1.5 cups
Time Required: 30 minutes
Nutritional Statistics (Each Portion):
- Protein Counts: 23.6 grams
- Carbohydrates: 35.5 grams
- Fat Content: 12.7 grams
- Sugars: 2.9 grams
- Dietary Fiber: 3.8 grams
- Sodium: 452.1 mg
- Calories: 357
  Diabetic Exchanges:
- Fat: 1 ½
- Lean Protein: 2
- Vegetable: ½
- Starch: 2

Essential Ingredients:
- Chicken breast (450 g/1 lb.)
- Bay leaves (2)
- Water (6 cups)
- Fresh cheese tortellini (570 g/20 oz. pkg.)
- Peas - fresh/frozen (.5 cup)
- Creamy salad dressing - ex. - peppercorn/ranch (.25 cup)
- Red-wine vinegar (2 tbsp.)
- Fresh herbs - ex. - chives - dill or basil - divided (5 tbsp.)
- Marinated artichokes (.5 cup + 2 tbsp. marinade - divided)
- Pea shoots/baby arugula (1 cup)
- Radishes (.5 cup)
- Sunflower seeds (2 tbsp.)

Preparation Method:
1. Trim the chicken, removing all bones and skin. Chop the herbs and set them to the side. Chop the artichokes and julienne the radishes.

2. Toss the chicken in with the bay leaves and water in a big saucepan. Wait for it to boil using a high-temperature setting.

3. Adjust the temperature to low, once boiling, and simmer till it reaches an internal temp of 165° Fahrenheit/74° Celsius (10-12 min.). Move the chicken to a chopping block - wait for it to slightly cool.

4. Discard the bay leaves. Add tortellini to the pot and wait for it to boil.

5. Simmer till the tortellini is tender (3 min.).

6. Add peas and simmer for an additional minute. Dump them into a colander and rinse using cool water.

7. Make the dressing with vinegar, herbs (3 tbsp.), and artichoke marinade in a large bowl.

8. Shred the chicken and add to the dressing, peas, tortellini, artichokes, radishes, and pea shoots/arugula). Thoroughly toss and serve the salad topped with the rest of the sunflower seeds and herbs (2 tbsp.).

Chopped Superfood Salad with Salmon & Creamy Garlic Dressing

Portions Provided: 4 servings
Time Required: 30 minutes
Nutritional Statistics (Each Portion):
3-4 oz. salmon + 3 cups salad:
- Calories: 409
- Protein Counts: 31.9 grams
- Carbohydrates: 18.7 grams (Net: 5.5 grams)
- Fat Content: 24.2 grams
- Sugars: 7.4 grams
- Dietary Fiber: 5.8 grams
- Sodium: 356.4 mg

Essential Ingredients:
- Salmon fillet (1 lb.)
- Mayonnaise (.25 cup)
- Lemon juice (2 tbsp.)
- Plain yogurt - l.f. (.5 cup)
- Fresh parsley & chives (1 tbsp. each)
- Tamari/soy sauce - reduced sodium (2 tsp.)
- Garlic (1 medium clove)
- Ground pepper (.25 tsp.)
- Carrots (2 cups)
- Broccoli (2 cups)
- Curly kale (8 cups)
- Red cabbage (2 cups)
- Sunflower seeds - toasted (.5 cup)
- Parmesan cheese (2 tbsp.)

Preparation Method:
1. Grate the parmesan and snip the chives. Finely dice/chop the carrots, parsley, and garlic.
2. Chop the broccoli, kale, and cabbage. Dice the carrots.
3. Arrange the oven rack in the uppermost oven section. Warm the broiler using the high-temperature setting. Cover a baking tray using a layer of aluminum foil.

4. Arrange the salmon on the tray with the skin-side down.
5. Broil, rotating the pan - once till the salmon is opaque in the center (8-12 min.). Cut the salmon into four portions.
6. Meanwhile, whisk the yogurt with mayonnaise, garlic, parmesan, lemon juice, chives, parsley, tamari/soy sauce, and pepper in a mixing container.
7. Toss the kale with the broccoli, carrots, cabbage, and sunflower seeds in a big mixing container. Add the dressing (¾ of a cup) while tossing to thoroughly cover.
8. Portion the salad into four dinner plates with a portion of salmon and dressing (1 tbsp. each).
9. This recipe will also provide a heart-healthy and diabetic-appropriate option.

Citrus Salad

Portions Provided: 4 servings
Time Required: 20 minutes
Nutritional Statistics (Each Portion):
- Calories: 166
- Protein Counts: 2 grams
- Carbohydrates: 17 grams
- Fat Content: 10 grams
- Sugars: -0- grams
- Dietary Fiber: 3 grams
- Sodium: 11 mg

Essential Ingredients:
- Oranges (2)
- Olive oil (2 tbsp.)
- Red grapefruit (1)
- Orange juice (2 tbsp.)
- Pine nuts (2 tbsp.)
- Spring greens (4 cups)
- Balsamic vinegar (1 tbsp.)
- Optional for Garnish: Chopped mint (2 tbsp.)

Preparation Method:
1. For each orange and grapefruit: Remove the bottoms and tops to expose the flesh.
2. Remove the peelings, membrane, and white pith. Over a small bowl, slice along each side to remove the membrane and seeds - reserving the sections and juices.
3. Using a separate container, combine the vinegar with the orange juice and oil. Gently empty it over the segments of fruit to evenly coat each surface.

4. Serve with a layer of spring greens, fruit, and dressing. Garnish it with ½ of a tablespoon of the pine nuts or mint if desired.

Cobb Salad Thai-Style

Portions Provided: 6 servings
Time Required: 15 minutes
Nutritional Statistics (Each Portion):
- Calories: 382
- Protein Counts: 23 grams
- Carbohydrates: 18 grams (Net: 3 grams)
- Fat Content: 25 grams
- Sugars: 10 grams
- Dietary Fiber: 5 grams
- Sodium: 472 mg

Essential Ingredients:
- Medium ripe avocado (1)
- Fresh snow peas - halved (1 cup)
- Medium carrot (1)
- Sweet red pepper (1 medium)
- Romaine - torn (1 bunch)
- Shredded rotisserie chicken (2 cups)
- Hard-boiled large eggs (3)
- Unsalted peanuts (.5 cup)
- Fresh cilantro leaves (.25 cup)
- Asian toasted sesame salad dressing (.75 cup)
- Creamy peanut butter (2 tbsp.)

Preparation Method:
1. Peel and thinly slice the avocado, shred the carrot, and julienne the red pepper.
2. Place romaine on a large serving platter.
3. Coarsely chop the eggs.
4. Arrange chicken, eggs, avocado, vegetables, and peanuts over romaine; sprinkle with cilantro.
5. Whisk the peanut butter with the salad dressing until it's creamy smooth. Serve with salad.

Creamy Pesto Chicken Salad with Greens

Portions Provided: 4 servings
Time Required: 30 min.
Nutritional Statistics (Each Portion):
0.5 cup of salad + 2 cups of greens:
- Protein Counts: 27.1 grams
- Carbohydrates: 9.2 grams
- Fat Content: 19.7 grams
- Sugars: 3.2 grams
- Dietary Fiber: 2.3 grams
- Sodium: 453.9 mg
- Calories: 324

Essential Ingredients:
- Chicken breast (1 lb.)
- Olive oil (2 tbsp.)
- Pesto (.25 cup)
- Mayo - low-fat (.25 cup)
- Red-wine vinegar (2 tbsp.)
- Salt & black pepper (.25 tsp. each)
- Red onion (3 tbsp.)
- Mixed salad greens (5 oz. pkg./approx. 8 cups)
- Cherry/grape tomatoes (1 pint)

Preparation Method:
1. Trim the chicken and remove all bones and fat. Slice the tomatoes into halves. Finely chop the onion.
2. Put the prepared chicken into a saucepan or skillet, pouring in enough water to cover the chicken by about one inch, and wait for it to boil.
3. Put a lid on the pot and adjust the temperature setting to low to simmer till done - not pink in the center (10-15 min.). Place it on a chopping block to cool slightly - shred into bite-size pieces.
4. Combine the mayo with the pesto and onion in a mixing container and toss in the chicken to coat.
5. Whisk oil with vinegar, pepper, and salt in a big mixing container - stir in the tomatoes and greens - tossing to cover.
6. Serve the salad greens topped with the chicken salad.

Cucumber Salad with Tzatziki

Portions Provided: 4 servings
Time Required: 20 minutes
Nutritional Statistics (Each Portion):
- Protein Counts: 2.2 grams
- Carbohydrates: 4.2 grams
- Fat Content: 0.6 grams
- Sugars: 3.1 grams
- Dietary Fiber: 0.7 grams
- Sodium: 169.2 mg
- Calories: 30

Essential Ingredients:
- Cucumbers (1 large or 2 small)
- Clove of garlic (1)
- Salt (.25 tsp.)
- Plain yogurt - l.f. (.5 cup)
- Fresh mint (2 tbsp.) or Dried (2 tsp.)
- Black pepper (as desired)

Preparation Method:

1. Chop the fresh mint. Peel and slice the cucumbers in halves, removing the seeds. Coarsely shred the cucumber - gently squeezing it to remove excess liquid.
2. Mince the garlic and dust using some of the salt. Work the salted garlic into a paste.
3. Work the garlic paste with yogurt and mint in a medium-sized mixing container.
4. Fold in the cucumber - adding pepper and salt to serve.

Leafy Rotisserie Chicken Salad with Creamy Tarragon Dressing

Portions Provided: 4 servings
Time Required: 20 minutes
Nutritional Statistics (Each Portion):

- Protein Counts: 26 grams
- Carbohydrates: 39 grams
- Fat Content: 11 grams
- Sugars: 9 grams
- Dietary Fiber: 8 grams
- Sodium: 65 mg
- Calories: 357

Essential Ingredients:

- White beans (430 g/15 oz. can)
- White balsamic vinegar (.33 cup)
- Olive oil (1 tbsp.)
- Garlic clove (1)
- Fresh tarragon (2 tbsp.)
- Mesclun Salad Mix (6 cups)
- Medium red onion (half of 1)
- Chicken breast - cooked (1.33 cup)
- Grapes (12 red or green)
- English Cucumber (1 cup)
- Pine nuts (3 tbsp.)
- Black pepper (.75 tsp.)

Preparation Method:

1. Add the beans (½ cup), the vinegar, oil, garlic, and tarragon (1 tbsp.) to a blender. Cover and puree.
2. Toss the greens onto a large platter. Top with the rest of the beans, cucumber, chicken, onion, grapes, nuts, pepper, and remaining tarragon (1 tbsp.).
3. Serve the dressing on the side to your liking.

Salad Skewer Wedges

Portions Provided: 8 servings
Time Required: 10 minutes
Nutritional Statistics (Each Portion):

- Calories: 238
- Protein Counts: 8 grams
- Dietary Fiber: 5 grams
- Carbohydrates: 10 grams (Net: 2 grams)
- Fat Content: 19 grams
- Sugars: 3 grams
- Sodium: 401 mg

Essential Ingredients:

- Red onion (1)
- Avocados (2)
- Iceberg lettuce (1 head)
- Cucumber (sliced - peeled or unpeeled (1)
- Roma tomatoes (4)
- Cooked bacon (5 slices)
- Wooden skewers (8)
  To Garnish:
- Green onions (diced)
- Blue cheese crumbles (140 g/5 oz. container)
- Blue cheese dressing (approx. 1 small 12 oz./340 g bottle/as desired)

Preparation Method:

1. Rinse the veggies. Slice the lettuce into wedges.
2. Slice the tomatoes into halves and the bacon into thirds.
3. Slice the avocados and red onion into one-inch pieces.
4. Dice the green onions.
5. Prepare one skewer at a time. Add an iceberg wedge, tomato, onion, avocado, two bacon pieces, another iceberg wedge, and the cucumber.
6. Continue until all skewers have been made. Garnish with crumbled blue cheese, blue cheese dressing, and diced green onions to serve.

Shrimp & Nectarine Salad - Diabetic-Friendly

Portions Provided: 4 servings
Time Required: 30 minutes
Nutritional Statistics (Each Portion):

- Protein Counts: 23 grams
- Carbohydrates: 27 grams (Net: 8 grams)
- Fat Content: 7 grams
- Sugars: 14 grams

- Dietary Fiber: 5 grams
- Sodium: 448 mg
- Calories: 252
  Diabetic Exchanges:
- Lean meat: 3
- Vegetable: 2
- Fat: 1
- Starch: ½
- Fruit: ½

Essential Ingredients:
- Orange juice (.33 cup)
- Honey (1.5 tsp.)
- Dijon mustard (1.5 tsp.)
- Cider vinegar (3 tbsp.)
- Tarragon - fresh (1 tbsp.)
  The Salad:
- Canola oil (4 tsp. - divided)
- Fresh/frozen corn (1 cup)
- Salt (.25 tsp.)
- Lemon-pepper seasoning (.5 tsp.)
- Uncooked shrimp - 26-30 per pound (1 lb.)
- Mixed salad greens (8 cups - torn)
- Medium nectarines (2)
- Red onion (.5 cup)
- Grape tomatoes (1 cup)

Preparation Method:
1. Finely chop the onion and slice the tomatoes into halves. Mince the tarragon.
2. Whisk the orange juice with the vinegar, mustard, and honey till blended. Mix in tarragon.
3. Prepare a big skillet to warm the oil (1 tsp.) using the med-high temperature setting.
4. Pour in the corn to simmer till it's crispy-tender (1-2 min.). Scoop it into a holding container for now.
5. Peel and devein the shrimp - sprinkle them with lemon pepper and salt.
6. Use the same skillet to warm the rest of the oil using the med-high temperature setting. Stir in the prepared shrimp - sauté till the shrimp turn pink (3-4 mi.). Stir in the corn.
7. Slice the nectarines into one-inch pieces.
8. Toss the rest of the fixings in a big mixing container. Drizzle with dressing (⅓ cup) and toss to coat.
9. Portion the mixture among four serving plates and add the shrimp mixture with the rest of the dressing. Serve right away.

Strawberry-Blue Cheese Steak Salad

Portions Provided: 4 servings
Time Required: 30 minutes
Nutritional Statistics (Each Portion):
- Protein Counts: 29 grams
- Carbohydrates: 12 grams (Net: 3 grams)
- Fat Content: 15 grams
- Sugars: 5 grams
- Dietary Fiber: 4 grams
- Sodium: 452 mg
- Calories: 289
  Diabetic Exchanges:
- Vegetable: 2
- Lean meat: 4
- Fruit: ½
- Fat: 2

Essential Ingredients:
- Beef - top sirloin steak (1 lb. @ ¾-inch thickness)
- Olive oil (2 tsp.)
- Pepper (.25 tsp.)
- Salt (.5 tsp.)
- Lime juice (2 tbsp.)
  For the Salad:
- Romaine (1 bunch/about 10 cups)
- Fresh strawberries (2 cups)
- Red onion (.25 cup)
- Blue cheese (.25 cup)
- Walnuts - toasted & chopped (.25 cup)
- Reduced-fat balsamic vinaigrette

Preparation Method:
1. Lightly sprinkle the steak with pepper and salt - as desired.
2. Warm a big skillet and warm the oil using the medium-temperature setting.
3. Place the steak in the pan - cook till it's as desired (5-7 min. per side). Use a meat thermometer to test the meat for doneness (med-rare ~ 135° F or 57° C or medium ~ 140° F or 60° C or med-well ~ 145° F or 63° C).
4. Place the steak on a plate to rest briefly (5 min.).
5. Slice the meat into small strips and toss them using lime juice.
6. Tear the romaine as desired. Thinly slice the onion and slice the berries into halves.
7. Prepare a plate. Toss the lettuce with the onion and berries.
8. Toss the steak over the top with a sprinkle of nuts and crumbled cheese.

9. Serve with a drizzle of vinaigrette to your liking.

Turkey Medallions with Tomato Salad

Portions Provided: 6 servings
Time Required: 45 minutes
Nutritional Statistics (Each Portion):
- Protein Counts: 29 grams
- Carbohydrates: 13 grams (Net: 7 grams)
- Fat Content: 21 grams
- Sugars: 4 grams
- Dietary Fiber: 2 grams
- Sodium: 458 mg
- Calories: 351

Essential Ingredients:
- Olive oil (2 tbsp.)
- Salt (.25 tsp.)
- Sugar (.5 tsp.)
- Medium green pepper (1)
- Celery (1 rib)
- Red onion (.25 cup)
- Fresh basil (1 tbsp.)
- Dried oregano (.25 tsp.)
- Medium tomatoes (3)
  For the Turkey:
- Egg (1 large)
- Lemon juice (2 tbsp.)
- Panko breadcrumbs (1 cup)
- Parmesan cheese - grated (.5 cup)
- Walnuts (.5 cup)
- Lemon-pepper seasoning (1 tsp.)
- Turkey breast tenderloins (20 oz./570 g pkg.)
- Black pepper & salt (.25 tsp. each)
- Olive oil (3 tbsp.)
- To Garnish: Additional fresh basil

Preparation Method:
1. Whisk the first five ingredients (oil, vinegar, sugar, salt, and oregano) in a mixing container.
2. Coarsely chop and add in the green pepper, celery, onion, and basil.
3. Slice the tomatoes into wedges - cut wedges in half. Stir into the pepper mixture.
4. Whisk the egg with the lemon juice in a shallow mixing dish.
5. Chop the walnuts. In another shallow container, toss the breadcrumbs with cheese, walnuts, and lemon pepper.
6. Cut the tenderloins crosswise into one-inch slices - flattening the slices using a meat mallet (½-inch thickness). Dust them using a bit of pepper and salt.
7. First, dip them in the egg mix and through the crumb mix while patting to adhere.
8. Use a big frying pan to warm one tablespoon oil using a med-high temperature setting.
9. Add 1/3 of the turkey and cook until it is a nice brown (2-3 min. each side).
10. Repeat twice with the rest of the oil and turkey.
11. Serve with tomato mixture and a sprinkle of thinly sliced basil.

Warm Rice & Pintos Salad - Diabetic-Friendly

Portions Provided: 4 servings
Time Required: 30 minutes
Nutritional Statistics (Each Portion):
- Protein Counts: 12 grams
- Carbohydrates: 50 grams
- Fat Content: 8 grams
- Sugars: 5 grams
- Dietary Fiber: 9 grams
- Sodium: 465 mg
- Calories: 331

Essential Ingredients:
- Frozen corn (1 cup)
- Small onion (1)
- Garlic cloves (2)
- Chili powder (1.5 tsp.)
- Pinto beans (15 oz./430 g can)
- Olive oil (1 tbsp.)
- Ready-to-serve brown rice (8.8 oz./250 g pkg.)
- Chopped green chilies (4 oz./110 g can)
- Salsa (.5 cup)
- Ground cumin (1.5 tsp.)
- Fresh cilantro (.25 cup)
- Romaine (1 bunch)
- Finely shredded cheddar cheese (.25 cup)

Preparation Method:
1. Rinse and drain the beans in a colander. Prepare a big skillet to warm the oil using the med-high temperature setting.
2. In the meantime, chop the cilantro and onion.
3. Add corn and onion - sauté them till the onion is tender (4-5 min.).
4. Mince the garlic - combine with cumin and chili powder - add it to the skillet.

5. Simmer as you continue to stir one more minute.
6. Add beans, rice, green chilies, salsa, and cilantro; heat through, stirring occasionally. Slice the romaine lengthwise into wedges. Serve the mixture over the fresh romaine wedges. Sprinkle it with cheese.

Winter Kale & Quinoa Salad with Avocado

Portions Provided: 2 servings
Time Required: 35 minutes
Nutritional Statistics (Each Portion):
1 ¼ cups salad + 3 tbsp. dressing:
- Protein Counts: 14.6 grams
- Carbohydrates: 54.4 grams
- Fat Content: 19.7 grams
- Sugars: 4.6 grams
- Dietary Fiber: 13.8 grams
- Sodium: 252.6 mg
- Calories: 439

Essential Ingredients:
- Sweet potato (1 small/1.5 cups)
- Olive oil (2.5 tsp. divided)
- Avocado (half of 1)
- Lime juice (1 tbsp.)
- Garlic (1 clove)
- Black pepper and salt (.125 or ⅛ tsp. each)
- Ground cumin (.5 tsp.)
- Water (1-2 tbsp.)
- Cooked quinoa (1 cup)
- Canned black beans - No-salt-added (.75 cup)
- Baby kale (1.5 cups)
- Pepitas (2 tbsp.)
- Scallion (1 chopped)

Preparation Method:
1. Set the oven temperature at 400° Fahrenheit/204° Celsius.
2. Peel the garlic. Rinse the beans and chop the kale. Peel and slice the potato into ½-inch pieces.
3. Toss the potato with the oil (1 tsp.) in a big rimmed baking sheet. Roast until it's tender - stirring once halfway through the cycle (25 min.).
4. Meanwhile, combine the rest of the oil (1,5 tsp.), avocado, garlic, cumin, lime juice, pepper, salt, and water (1 tbsp.) in a food processor - mixing till it's creamy smooth.
5. Add water (1 tbsp.) as needed.
6. Combine the quinoa with the potato, kale, and black beans in a mixing container. Drizzle it using avocado dressing - tossing to thoroughly cover.
7. Top with pepitas and scallion to serve.
8. Meal Prep Tip: Prepare the potato (Steps one and two) and dressing (step three). Refrigerate the fixings individually for up to two days.

Salsa

Avocado Salsa

Portions Provided: 20 servings @ 2 tbsp. each
Time Required: 8-10 minutes
Nutritional Statistics (Each Portion):
- Protein Counts: 1 gram
- Sugar: 1 gram
- Total Carbs: 3 grams
- Fiber Counts: 2 grams
- Fat Content: 3 grams
- Sodium: 62 mg
- Calories: 41

Essential Ingredients:
- Roma tomatoes (5)
- Avocados (3)
- Red onion (half of 1)
- Cilantro (2 tbsp.)
- Garlic (2 cloves)
- Juiced lime (half of 1)
- Salt (.25 tsp.)
- Freshly cracked black pepper (to your liking)

Preparation Method:
1. Chop the tomatoes, onion, and cilantro.
2. Cube the avocados and mince the garlic.
3. Juice the lime.
4. Load a mixing container with tomatoes, avocados, red onion, cilantro, and garlic. Toss and add lime juice and pepper with salt as desired.
5. Mix well and serve.

Low-Sodium Red Salsa

Portions Provided: 4 cups
Time Required: 25 minutes
Nutritional Statistics (Each Portion):
- ½ cup = 5 mg. sodium
- Calories: 35

Essential Ingredients:
- Diced tomatoes - no salt (410 g/14.5 oz. can)
- Sweet onion (half of 1)
- Fresh jalapeno (1)
- Chopped cilantro (.25 to .5 cup)
- Minced garlic (2 cloves)
- Cumin (.5 tsp.)
- Mexican oregano (.25 tsp.)

Preparation Method:
1. Place diced tomatoes in a microwave-proof bowl.
2. Cut jalapeno in half and onion into quarters - add to a mixing container with garlic, cilantro, cumin, and oregano. Microwave for five minutes.
3. Once veggies have cooled a bit, place in a food processor to blend - adding a tiny bit of water for a thinner sauce.

Mediterranean Salsa

Portions Provided: 6 servings @ ½ cup each
Time Required: 20 minutes
Nutritional Statistics (Each Portion):
- Protein Counts: 0.8 grams
- Fiber: 1.3 grams
- Fat Content: 1.7 grams
- Carbs: 4.4 grams
- Sodium: 124 mg
- Calories: 33

Essential Ingredients:
- Lemon juice (2 tsp.)
- Tomato (1.5 cups)
- Zucchini (1 cup)
- Roasted bell peppers (.5 cup)
- Red onion (2 tbsp.)
- Fresh parsley - flat-leaf (1 tbsp.)
- Capers (1.5 tsp.)
- Salt (.25 tsp.)
- Fresh basil (1 tbsp.)
- Black pepper (.125 tsp.)
- Olive oil (2 tsp.)
- Garlic (1 clove)

Preparation Method:
1. Squeeze the lemon for juice. Chop and deseed the tomato. Mince the clove.
2. Finely chop the roasted peppers, red onion, zucchini, basil, and parsley.
3. Toss all of the fixings into a big mixing container.
4. Store the delicious salsa in the fridge for no more than two days.

Vegetable Salsa

Portions Provided: 16 servings @ ½ cup each
Time Required: 40 minutes
Nutritional Statistics (Each Portion):
- Protein Counts: 1 gram
- Carbohydrates: 5 grams (Net: 2 grams)
- Fat Content: -0- grams
- Sugars: 2 grams

- Dietary Fiber: 1 gram
- Sodium: 77 mg
- Calories: 24

Essential Ingredients:

- Red & green bell peppers (2/about 2 cups *each*)
- Zucchini (1 cup)
- Tomatoes (4/approx. 2 cups)
- Fresh cilantro (.5 cup)
- Red onion (1 cup)
- Black pepper (1 tsp.)
- Garlic (2 cloves)
- Sugar (2 tsp.)
- Salt (.5 tsp.)
- Lime juice (.25 cup)

Preparation Method:

1. Prepare all of the vegetables by washing them thoroughly.
2. Seed and dice the peppers and tomatoes.
3. Chop the zucchini, red onion, and cilantro. Mince the garlic.
4. Toss each of the fixings into a big mixing container, cover, and refrigerate for the ingredients to marinate (½ hour) and serve.

Salad Dressings

Blue Cheese Dressing

Portions Provided: 16 servings @ 2 tbsp. each
Time Required: 5-6 minutes
Nutritional Statistics (Each Portion):
- Protein Counts: 1 gram
- Carbohydrates: 2.5 grams
- Fat Content: 2 grams
- Sugars: 1.5 grams
- Dietary Fiber: trace grams
- Sodium: 172 mg
- Calories: 32

Essential Ingredients:
- Blue cheese (.5 cup)
- Garlic (1 tbsp.)
- Mayonnaise - f.f. (1 cup)
- Horseradish (1 tbsp.)
- Worcestershire sauce (1 tsp.)
- Buttermilk - l.f. (.5 cup)
- Cayenne pepper (.5 tsp.)

Preparation Method:
1. Mince the garlic and crumble the cheese.
2. Toss each of the fixings into a food processor, mixing till fully incorporated.
3. Chill till you are ready to use the delicious dressing.

Caramelized Balsamic Vinaigrette

Portions Provided: 8 servings @ 1 tbsp. each
Time Required: 15 minutes
Nutritional Statistics (Each Portion):
- Protein Counts: -0- grams
- Carbohydrates: 14 grams
- Fat Content: 3 grams
- Sugars: 14 grams
- Dietary Fiber: -0- grams
- Sodium: 62 mg
- Calories: 89

Essential Ingredients:
- Water (.5 cup)
- Sugar (6 tbsp.)
- Dark balsamic vinegar (.5 cup)
- Olive oil (2 tbsp.)
- Garlic cloves (4)
- Kosher salt & black pepper (.25 tsp. each)

Preparation Method:
1. Warm a saucepan using a med-low temperature setting.
2. Pour in water and sugar - simmering till the sugar begins to caramelize.
3. Mince the garlic. Add the vinegar, oil, garlic, salt, and pepper to the sugar mixture.
4. Place the pan on a cool burner - whisk - set aside to cool.
5. Remove the garlic with a strainer and discard.
6. Serve the prepared dressing right away or store it for another time.

Cilantro Lime Dressing

Portions Provided: 16 servings @ 2 tbsp. each
Time Required: 5 minutes
Nutritional Statistics (Each Portion):
- Protein Counts: 4 grams
- Fat Content: 4 grams
- Carbs: 2 grams
- Sugars: 1 gram
- Sodium: 188 mg
- Calories: 54

Essential Ingredients:
- Olive oil (.25 cup)
- 1% cottage cheese (2 cups)
- Garlic (1 clove)
- Whole limes (2)
- Salt (.5 tsp.)
- Cilantro (.5 cup)
- Sugar (.5 tsp.)
- Black pepper (.25 tsp.)

Preparation Method:
1. Juice the limes and roughly chop the cilantro. Dice the garlic.
2. Toss each of the fixings into a blender or food processor.
3. Mix till it's all creamy smooth to serve.

Orange Basil Vinaigrette

Portions Provided: 8 servings @ 1/3 cup each
Time Required: varies - 30 minutes
Nutritional Statistics (Each Portion):
- Protein Counts: trace grams
- Carbohydrates: 9 grams (Net: 4 grams)
- Fat Content: 1 gram
- Sugars: 5 grams
- Dietary Fiber: trace grams
- Sodium: 33 mg
- Calories: 45

Essential Ingredients:
- Cornstarch (2 tbsp.)

- White wine vinegar (.33 cup)
- Olive oil (2 tsp.)
- Orange juice (2 cups)
- Mustard - Dijon-style (2 tsp.)
- Fresh basil (1 tbsp.) or Dried (2 tsp.)

Preparation Method:

1. Using a small pan, mix the cornstarch with the orange juice—bringing it to a boil.
2. Continuously stir - allowing it to simmer for approximately one minute.

Empty the dressing mix into a jar and pop it in the fridge till it's chilled.

3. Once it's dinner, whisk the vinegar with the oil, basil, and mustard - whisking until it's thoroughly mixed.
4. Serve as desired.

Sauces

Banana-Pecan Compote

Portions Provided: 6 servings @ 1/3 cup each
Time Required: 10 minutes
Nutritional Statistics (Each Portion):
- Protein Counts: 1 gram
- Fat Content: 2 grams
- Carbohydrates: 24 grams
- Sugars: 14 grams
- Dietary Fiber: 2 grams
- Sodium: 2 mg
- Calories: 109

Essential Ingredients:
- Very ripe medium bananas (4)
- Brown sugar (2 tbsp.)
- Orange juice (.5 cup)
- Vanilla (1 tsp.)
- Cinnamon (.5 tsp.)
- Pecans (2 tbsp.)

Preparation Method:
1. Slice the bananas and chop the pecans.
2. Warm a saucepan using a medium-temperature setting.
3. Stir in the sugar with the bananas - sautéing till the sugar is liquified (1-2 min.).
4. Stir in the cinnamon, vanilla, and orange juice.
5. Simmer till the juice is reduced (2 min.), stirring occasionally.
6. Top with pecans before serving.

Basil Butter & Sun-Dried Tomato Sauce

Portions Provided: 4 servings @ 1/3 cup each
Time Required: 15 minutes
Nutritional Statistics (Each Portion):
- Protein Counts: 1 gram
- Carbohydrates: 3 grams
- Fat Content: 3 grams
- Sugars: -0- grams
- Dietary Fiber: 0.5 grams
- Sodium: 111 mg
- Calories: 43

Essential Ingredients:
- Butter (1 tbsp.)
- A.P. flour (1 tbsp.)
- Chicken broth - no-salt (1 cup)
- Fresh basil (1 tbsp.) or dry (1 tsp.)
- Sun-dried tomato paste (1 tbsp.)

Preparation Method:
1. Use a heavy-duty saucepan to melt the butter using a low-temperature setting.
2. Sift in the flour - simmer till the mixture is lightly browned (2 min.). Stir the mixture continuously.
3. Pour in the chicken broth. Raise the temperature setting to medium, stirring till it's thickened (5 min.).
4. Finely chop and mix in the basil and tomato paste.
5. Adjust the temperature setting to low - simmer (2 min.). Serve warm.

Citrus Remoulade

Portions Provided: 16 servings @ 1 tbsp. each
Time Required: 5-6 minutes
Nutritional Statistics (Each Portion):
- Protein Counts: -0- grams
- Carbohydrates: 2 grams
- Fat Content: 4 grams
- Sugars: 1 gram
- Sodium: 95 mg
- Calories: 45

Essential Ingredients:
- Orange juice (1 tbsp.)
- Salt (1 pinch/as desired)
- Light mayonnaise (1 cup)
- Orange zest (1 tsp.)

Preparation Method:
1. Toss each of the fixings into a mixing bowl.
2. Whisk till they're thoroughly incorporated.
3. Serve as desired and store the leftovers for another time.

Orange-Cranberry Glaze

Portions Provided: 4 servings @ ¼ cup each
Time Required: 10 minutes
Nutritional Statistics (Each Portion):
- Protein Counts: trace grams
- Fiber Content: 1 gram
- Carbohydrates: 9 grams
- Sodium: 1 mg
- Calories: 36

Essential Ingredients:
- Fresh cranberries (1 cup)

- Unsweetened orange juice (.66 or 2/3 cup)
- Cornstarch (1 tbsp.)
- Sugar substitute (as desired)

Preparation Method:

1. Chop the berries. Use a microwavable bowl to add the orange juice, cranberries, and cornstarch. Thoroughly mix.
2. Microwave using the high setting till the mixture thickens (3-4 min.). Stir several times while it's cooking and set aside to cool.
3. Add the sugar substitute. The glaze should be tart to serve over turkey, pork, or chicken.
4. The sauce is excellent for roasting, grilling, or using as a marinade.

Spaghetti Sauce

Portions Provided: 8 servings @ ½ cup each
Time Required: 40 minutes
Nutritional Statistics (Each Portion):

- Protein Counts: 1 gram
- Carbohydrates: 8 grams
- Fat Content: -0- grams
- Sugars: 5 grams
- Dietary Fiber: 1 gram
- Sodium: 26 mg
- Calories: 35

Essential Ingredients:

- Chopped onions (.25 cup)
- Tomato sauce (430 g/15 oz. can)
- Tomato paste - no-salt (8 tbsp.)
- Sugar (1.5 tbsp.)
- Garlic (3 tsp.)
- Ground oregano (1.5 tsp.)
- Dried leaves of basil (2 tbsp.)
- Red pepper flakes - crushed (.125 tsp.)
- Water (1.5 cups)

Preparation Method:

1. Mist a pan using a cooking oil spray.
2. Chop and sauté the onions till they're translucent. Mince and add the garlic.
3. Mix in tomato sauce, tomato paste, and water.

4. Stir in all the spices, and let the sauce simmer using the low setting (½ hr.).
5. Ground beef is optional.

Tzatziki Sauce

Portions Provided: 3.5 cups @ ¼ cup each
Time Required: varies - 2-3 hours
Nutritional Statistics (Each Portion):

- Protein Counts: 3 grams
- Carbohydrates: 4 grams
- Fat Content: -0- grams
- Sugars: 1 gram
- Dietary Fiber: -0- grams
- Sodium: 38 mg
- Calories: 37

Essential Ingredients:

- Plain low-fat yogurt (3 cups)
- Lemon juice (3 tbsp.)
- Medium cucumbers (2)
- Garlic (1 clove)
- Salt (.5 tsp.)
- Fresh dill (1 tbsp.)
- Freshly cracked black pepper (.25 tsp.)

Preparation Method:

1. Peel and deseed the cucumbers. Mince the garlic clove.
2. Use a bowl to strain the yogurt using a paper-lined strainer. Put the container into the refrigerator for two hours, so the yogurt can drain and seep through the straining filter.
3. Transfer the strained yogurt into a big mixing container.
4. Grate the cucumber into a mixing dish and sprinkle it with salt. Wrap the cucumber in towels to remove the liquid and add it to the yogurt.
5. Blend in the garlic, chopped dill, lemon juice, pepper, and the rest of the salt.
6. Let the sauce blend in the fridge for a few hours until it's cold.
7. Serve at room temperature or chilled.

Dips

Artichoke Dip

Portions Provided: 8 servings
Time Required: 40 minutes
Nutritional Statistics (Each Portion):
- Carbohydrates: 10 grams
- Protein Counts: 5 grams
- Fat Content: 2 grams
- Sugars: 1.5 grams Dietary Fiber: 6 grams
- Sodium: 130 mg Calories: 78

Essential Ingredients:
- Artichoke hearts in water (440 g/15.5 oz. can)
- Raw spinach (4 cups)
- Fresh thyme (1 tsp.) or dried (.33 tsp.)
- Garlic (2 cloves)
- Fresh parsley (1 tbsp.) or dried (1 tsp.)
- Unsalted white beans (1 cup or ½ of a 15.5-oz. can)
- Grated parmesan cheese (2 tbsp.)
- Sour cream - low-fat (.5 cup)
- Black pepper (1 tsp.)

Preparation Method:
1. Preheat the oven to reach 350° Fahrenheit/177° Celsius. Rinse and drain the beans and artichokes into a colander. Chop the spinach. Mince the garlic, thyme, and parsley.
2. Add each of the fixings into a big mixing container. Scoop it into an oven-safe glass/ceramic dish to bake for ½ hour. Serve it promptly while it's nice and warm.

Artichoke - Spinach & White Bean Dip

Portions Provided: 8 servings
Time Required: 35 minutes
Nutritional Statistics (Each Portion):
- Protein Counts: 8 grams
- Carbohydrates: 16 grams
- Fat Content: 3 grams
- Sugars: -0- grams
- Dietary Fiber: 7.5 grams
- Sodium: 114 mg
- Calories: 123

Essential Ingredients:
- Artichoke hearts (2 cups)
- Black pepper (1 tbsp.)
- Spinach (4 cups)
- Dried thyme (1 tsp.)
- Garlic (2 cloves)
- Fresh parsley (1 tbsp.)
- Cooked white beans (1 cup)
- Parmesan cheese - grated (2 tbsp.)
- Sour cream - l.f. (.5 cup)

Preparation Method:
1. Warm the oven to 350° Fahrenheit/177° Celsius.
2. Chop the artichoke, parsley, thyme, spinach, and garlic.
3. Toss all of the fixings in a baking dish to bake for ½ hour.
4. Serve with your favorite veggies.

Avocado Dip

Portions Provided: 4 servings
Time Required: 5-6 minutes
Nutritional Statistics (Each Portion):
- Protein Counts: 2 grams
- Carbohydrates: 8 grams
- Fat Content: 5 grams
- Sugars: trace grams
- Dietary Fiber: 2.5 grams
- Sodium: 57 mg
- Calories: 85

Essential Ingredients:
- Sour cream - fat-free (.5 cup)
- Hot sauce (.125 or 1/8 tsp.)
- Onion (2 tsp.)
- Ripe avocado (1 peeled - pitted & mashed/about ½ cup)

Preparation Method:
1. Chop the onion.
2. Combine sour cream, onion, hot sauce, and avocado in a small mixing container.
3. Mix to evenly blend all of the fixings.
4. Serve with sliced veggies or baked tortilla chips.

Baba Ghanoush

Portions Provided: 4 servings
Time Required: 35-40 minutes
Nutritional Statistics (Each Portion):
- Protein Counts: 7 grams
- Carbohydrates: 40 grams
- Fat Content: 5 grams
- Sugars: 11 grams
- Dietary Fiber: 12 grams
- Sodium: 150 mg
- Calories: 233

Essential Ingredients:
- Fresh lemon juice (4 tbsp.)
- Garlic (8 cloves/1 bulb)
- Eggplants (2)
- Bell pepper (1 red)
- Fresh basil (1 tbsp.)
- Black pepper (1 tsp./as desired)
- Whole-wheat pita or other flatbread (2 rounds)
- Olive oil (1 tbsp.)

Preparation Method:
1. Spray cold grill using a cooking oil spray.
2. Warm one side of the grill using the high-temperature setting (Or move coals to one side of the grill.)
3. Slice the top off the garlic bulb and wrap it in foil, and put it on the coolest part of the grill.
4. Roast for 20 minutes to ½ hour.
5. Slice the pepper in half and deseed it.
6. Slice the eggplants lengthwise with the skin removed.
7. On the hot part of the grill, place the bell pepper and eggplant slices - grilling for two to three minutes per side.
8. Squeeze the roasted garlic from the bulb and place it in the food processor.
9. Also, toss in the grilled peppers and eggplant.
10. Chop and add basil, olive oil, lemon juice, and pepper.
11. Pulse until it's creamy.
12. Place the dip in a serving bowl.
13. Warm bread on the grill for a few seconds on each side.
14. Serve with dip.

Black Bean & Corn Relish

Portions Provided: 8 servings @ 1 cup each
Time Required: 40 minutes
Nutritional Statistics (Each Portion):
- Protein Counts: 6 grams
- Carbohydrates: 22 grams
- Fat Content: 0.5 grams
- Sugars: 3 grams
- Dietary Fiber: 6 grams
- Sodium: 93 mg
- Calories: 112

Essential Ingredients:
- Black beans (15.5 oz. can/about 2 cups)
- Frozen corn kernels (1 cup)
- Tomatoes (4 or about 3 cups)

- Garlic cloves (2)
- Medium red onion (half of 1)
- Parsley (.5 cup)
- Bell pepper: Yellow/Green or red (1 or about 1 cup)
- Sugar (2 tsp.)
- Juice (from 1 lemon)

Preparation Method:
1. Thaw the corn till it's at room temperature.
2. Remove the seeds and dice the tomatoes and bell pepper.
3. Mince/dice the garlic, onions, and parsley.
4. Rinse and drain the beans in a colander.
5. Toss all of the fixings in a big mixing container with a lid - tossing gently to combine.
6. Put a lid or layer of foil over the container. Place it in the fridge for a minimum of 30 minutes for the flavors to blend.

Hummus

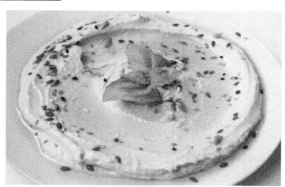

Portions Provided: 14 @1.5 cups
Time Required: 1 hour 15 minutes
Nutritional Statistics (Each Portion):
- Protein Counts: 1 gram
- Carbohydrates: 4 grams
- Fat Content: 0.2 grams
- Fiber: 0.7 grams
- Sugars: 0.2 grams
- Sodium: 47 mg
- Calories: 39

Essential Ingredients:
- Tahini (.25 cup) or toasted sesame seeds (.33 cup)
- Garbanzo beans (15-oz. can/2 cups cooked)
- Crushed red chilies (.125 or ⅛ tsp.)
- Orange/lemon or lime juice (⅛ cup)
- Salt (.5 tsp.)

- Olive oil (2 tbsp.)
- Garlic (.5 tsp.)

Preparation Method:

1. Rinse and drain the beans.
2. Set the oven temperature to 350° Fahrenheit/177° Celsius to toast the sesame seeds. Scatter them over a cookie tray to toast (8-12 min.). Stir the seeds often till they're browned.
3. Load a food processor and blend the chilies with the tahini/sesame seeds and beans. Mince and toss in the garlic, salt, and juice of choice. Puree till the mixture is creamy smooth.
4. Pour in the oil - continue to process until you reach the desired consistency.
5. Wait for the hummus to rest and meld the flavors for an hour before serving.

Mediterranean Layered Hummus Dip

Portions Provided: 12 servings
Time Required: 15 minutes
Nutritional Statistics (Each Portion):

- Protein Counts: 4 grams
- Carbohydrates: 6 grams (Net: 3 grams)
- Fat Content: 5 grams
- Sugars: 1 gram
- Fiber: 2 grams
- Sodium: 275 mg
- Calories: 88

Essential Ingredients:

- Red onion (.25 cup)
- Greek olives (.5 cup)
- Medium tomatoes (2)
- Large English cucumber (1)
- Hummus (10 oz. carton)
- Crumbled feta cheese (1 cup)
- Baked pita chips

Preparation Method:

1. Finely chop the olives and onion. Discard the seeds and chop the tomatoes and cucumber.
2. Spread the hummus into a shallow ten-inch round dish.
3. Begin with a layer of the onion, olives, tomatoes, cucumber, and cheese.
4. Pop the dish into the fridge until serving.
5. Serve with pita chips.

Skinny Quinoa Vegetable Dip

Portions Provided: 32 servings @ ¼ each
Time Required: 35 minutes
Nutritional Statistics (Each Portion):

- Protein Counts: 2 grams
- Carbohydrates: 8 grams (Net: 5 grams)
- Fat Content: 3 grams
- Sugar: 1 gram
- Sodium: 54 mg
- Fiber Count: 2 grams
- Calories: 65
- Note: Does not count the cucumber slices
  Diabetic Exchanges:
- Fat: ½
- Starch: 1/2

Essential Ingredients:

- Black beans (2 cans @ 430 g/15 oz.)
- Ground cumin (1.5 tsp.)
- Cayenne pepper (.5 tsp.)
- Water - divided (1.66 or 1-2/3 cups)
- Salt & black pepper (as desired)
- Paprika (1.5 tsp.)
- Quinoa (.66 or 2/3 cups)
- Lime juice (5 tbsp. - divided)
- Ripe avocados (2 medium)
- Sour cream (2 tbsp. + ¾ cup - divided)
- Fresh cilantro (.25 cup)
- Plum tomatoes (3)
- Cucumber (.75 cup)
- Zucchini (.75 cup)
- Red onion (.25 cup)
- Cucumber slices
- Suggested: Food processor

Preparation Method:

1. Rinse the quinoa in a colander.
2. Rinse, drain and pulse the beans and cumin, paprika, cayenne, and 1/3 cup water in the processor until smooth. Add pepper and salt to your liking.
3. Cook the quinoa in a saucepan with the rest of the water (1.33 cups) according to package instructions. Use a fork to fluff it, and drizzle using lime juice (2 tbsp.). Set aside.
4. Chop the cilantro. Peel and quarter the avocado. Mash the avocados with two tablespoons of sour cream, cilantro, and remaining lime juice.
5. Deseed and chop the tomatoes.
6. Peel, deseed, and chop the cucumber, onion, and zucchini.

7. Use a 2.5-quart baking dish and layer the quinoa, bean mixture, avocado mixture, tomatoes, zucchini, onion, cucumber, and sour cream.

8. Serve promptly with a few cucumber slices for dipping, or pop it into the fridge for later.

Snacks & Appetizers

Almond & Apricot Biscotti

Portions Provided: 24 servings
Time Required: 1 hour 5 minutes
Nutritional Statistics (Each Portion):
- Protein Counts: 2 grams
- Carbohydrates: 12 grams
- Fat Content: 2 grams
- Sugars: 6 grams
- Fiber Content: 1 gram
- Sodium: 17 mg
- Calories: 75

Essential Ingredients:
- Meal or flour - whole-wheat (.75 cup)
- A.P. flour (.75 cup)
- Brown sugar - tightly packed (.25 cup)
- Baking powder (1 tsp.)
- 1 % Milk - l.f. (2 tbsp.)
- Eggs (2)
- Dark honey (2 tbsp.)
- Canola oil (2 tbsp.)
- Almond extract (.5 tsp)
- Almonds (.25 cup)
- Dried apricots (.66 cup)

Preparation Method:
1. Set the oven temperature setting to 350° Fahrenheit/177° Celsius.
2. Sift or whisk each type of flour with baking powder and brown sugar.
3. Lightly whisk and mix in the eggs, milk, canola oil, honey, and almond extract. Mix till the dough is formed.
4. Chop and add the almonds and apricots - mixing till the dough is formed.
5. Scoop the dough onto a layer of plastic wrap. Knead it into a log (12x3-inches wide and about one inch high). Discard the plastic wrap to invert the dough onto a nonstick baking tray.
6. Bake till it's lightly browned (25-30 min.) and place it on another baking tray to cool for ten minutes.
7. Put the cooled 'log' onto a cutting board and slice the bread crosswise on the diagonal (one-half-inch wide). Arrange the (24) slices, cut-side down, onto the baking tray.
8. Bake till the cuts are crispy (15-20 min.).
9. Arrange the biscotti's pan onto a wire rack to thoroughly cool.

Asparagus & Horseradish Dip

Portions Provided: 16 servings
Time Required: 15 minutes
Nutritional Statistics (Each Portion):
2 spears + 1 tbsp. dip per serving:
- Protein Counts: 1 gram
- Carbohydrates: 3 grams (Net: 1 gram)
- Fat Content: 5 grams
- Sugars: 1 gram
- Dietary Fiber: -0- grams
- Sodium: 146 mg
- Calories: 63

Essential Ingredients:
- Fresh asparagus spears (32/910 g/about 2 lb.)
- Reduced-fat mayonnaise (1 cup)
- Parmesan cheese (.25 cup)
- Prepared horseradish (1 tbsp.)
- Worcestershire sauce (.5 tsp.)

Preparation Method:
1. Prepare a big saucepan with one inch of water and a steamer basket. Trim and add the asparagus.
2. Once boiling, place a top on the pot to steam till they're still crispy and fork-tender (2-4 min.).
3. Dump the cooked asparagus into a container of ice water to impede the cooking process. Pour them into a colander to drain - dab them dry using a few paper towels.
4. Combine the rest of the fixings. Serve with the chilled asparagus.

Baked Brie Envelopes

Portions Provided: 12 servings
Time Required: 30 minutes
Nutritional Statistics (Each Portion):
- Protein Counts: 4 grams
- Carbohydrates: 9 grams (Net: 5 grams)
- Fat Content: 7 grams
- Sugars: 4 grams
- Dietary Fiber: -0- grams
- Sodium: 133 mg
- Calories: 116

Essential Ingredients:
- Cranberries - frozen/fresh (.5 cup)
- Orange (half of 1 medium)
- Sugar (2 tbsp.)

- Cinnamon (1 stick)
- Puff pastry dough (1 sheet)
- Brie cheese (170 g/6 oz.)
- Water (2 tbsp.)
- Egg white (1)

Preparation Method:

1. Warm the oven to reach 425° Fahrenheit/218° Celsius.
2. Warm a small sauté pan using the med-high temperature setting - lightly coating it with a spritz of cooking spray. Adjust the temp to low.
3. Quarter the orange. Toss the orange pieces, cranberries, cinnamon stick, and sugar into the heated pan to simmer for about ten minutes, constantly stirring till the cranberries are softened (The mixture should be thick by now.).
4. Transfer the pan to the countertop for cooling. Discard the orange pieces and stick of cinnamon.
5. Cut the puff pastry into (12) ¼-ounce/7-gram squares. Roll out each square of pastry.
6. Cut the cheese into ½-ounce/14-gram cubes. Put a cube of cheese and cranberry mixture (1 tsp.) onto each square.
7. Whisk the egg white with the water in a mixing container. Dab egg wash over the pastry's inside using a pastry brush.
8. Pull one corner of the pastry at a time around the cheese and cranberry mixture to make an envelope.
9. Use a brush to baste the top of the pastry with the egg wash mixture. Continue the process till done.
10. Arrange the prepared and closed envelopes on a baking tray - bake until golden brown (10-12 min.).

Basil-Pesto Stuffed Mushrooms

Portions Provided: 20 servings
Time Required: 25 minutes
Nutritional Statistics (Each Portion):

- Fat Content: 3 grams
- Protein Counts: 2 grams
- Carbs: 4 grams
- Sodium: 80 mg
- Calories: 59

Essential Ingredients:

- Crimini mushrooms (20)

The Topping:

- Fresh parsley (3 tbsp.)
- Panko breadcrumbs (1.5 cups)
- Butter (.25 cup)

The Filling:

- Kosher salt (.5 tsp.)
- Basil - fresh leaves (2 cups)
- Parmesan cheese - freshly grated (.25 cup)
- Pumpkin seeds (2 tbsp.)
- Fresh garlic (1 tbsp.)
- Lemon juice (2 tsp.)
- Olive oil (1 tbsp.)

Preparation Method:

1. Heat the oven to 350° Fahrenheit/177° Celsius.
2. Rinse, remove the stems, and arrange the mushroom caps (upside down) on a baking tray.
3. Chop the basil and parsley. Mince the garlic. Melt the butter.
4. Combine the panko with parsley and butter - set it aside.
5. Make the filling by loading the food processor with the basil, pumpkin seeds, cheese, oil, garlic, salt, and lemon juice - pulsing till it's evenly mixed.
6. Generously stuff the mushroom caps with the freshly prepared filling.
7. Dust the mushroom caps with the panko topping (1 tsp. each.).
8. Gently pat down the topping.
9. Set a timer to bake till they're golden brown (10-15 min.)
10. Serve and enjoy!

Chickpea Polenta with Olives

Portions Provided: 8 servings @ 2 wedges each
Time Required: 2 hours - approximate & varies
Nutritional Statistics (Each Portion):

- Protein Counts: 8 grams
- Carbohydrates: 20 grams
- Fat Content: 5 grams
- Sugars: 4 grams
- Dietary Fiber: 3 grams
- Sodium: 160 mg
- Calories: 157

Essential Ingredients:

For the Polenta:

- Chickpea flour (1.75 cups)
- Olive oil (.5 tbsp.)
- Plain soy milk (2 cups)

- Broth or stock - chicken or vegetable (1 cup)
- Garlic (3 cloves)
- Fresh oregano/basil/thyme (1 tbsp.) *or* dried (1 tsp.)
- Black pepper (.25 tsp.)
- Dry mustard (1 tsp.)
- Egg whites (3)
  The Topping:
- Olive oil - EVOO (.5 tbsp.)
- Yellow onion (half of 1)
- Kalamata olives - pitted (.25 cup)
- Sun-dried tomatoes - dry-packed (.25 cup)
- Parmesan cheese - grated (2 tbsp.)
- Italian - fresh parsley - flat-leaf (2 tbsp.)
  Also Needed:
- Electric mixer
- Food processor or blender
- Baking pan (9x13-inch/9x33-cm)

Preparation Method:

1. Soak the tomatoes in water to rehydrate. Then, drain and chop.
2. Chop the onion, parsley, and garlic. Coarsely chop the olives.
3. Load the blender with soy milk, flour, stock, oil, thyme, garlic, pepper, and mustard. Blend till incorporated - pour the mixture into a big mixing container. Pop it in the fridge to chill for an hour or so.
4. Meanwhile, set the oven temperature setting to reach 425° Fahrenheit/218° Celsius. Spritz the baking pan using a tiny bit of cooking oil spray.
5. In another big mixing container, use an electric mixer on its high-speed setting, beat the egg whites until stiff peaks form. Gently mix the egg whites into the batter.
6. Dump the batter into the prepared baking pan. Bake till it's puffed and lightly browned around the edges (15 min.). Wait for it to cool (another 15 min.).
7. Warm the oven broiler - arranging the rack about four inches from the heat source.
8. Use a small skillet to heat the oil using a med-high heat setting.
9. Toss in the onion to sauté till it's lightly browned and softened (6 min.).
10. Mix in tomatoes and olives and tomatoes sautéing for another minute. Transfer the pan to a cool spot. Add the onion mixture over the baked polenta and dust it using the cheese. Broil till it's lightly browned (1

min.). Lightly garnish using parsley. Put the pan on a wire rack to cool (ten min.).
11. Slice it into eight squares, then slice them diagonally to make 16 wedges.
12. Serve promptly for the most flavorful results.

Roasted Root Vegetables with Goat Cheese Polenta

Portions Provided: 2 servings
Time Required: 35 minutes
Nutritional Statistics (Each Portion):

- Protein Counts: 9.1 grams
- Fat Content: 27.7 grams
- Sugars: 7.7 grams
- Carbohydrates: 41.4 grams
- Dietary Fiber: 7.7 grams
- Sodium: 589.4 mg
- Calories: 442

Essential Ingredients:

  Polenta:
- Vegetable or chicken broth - l.s. (2 cups)
- Polenta/corn grits/ - fine cornmeal (.5 cup)
- Goat cheese (.25 cup)
- Olive oil or butter (1 tbsp.)
- Black pepper and kosher salt (.25 tsp. each)
  Vegetables:
- Olive oil or butter (1 tbsp.)
- Garlic (1 clove)
- Roasted root vegetables - see the recipe (2 cups)
- Torn fresh sage (1 tbsp.)
- Prepared pesto (2 tsp.)
- For Garnish: Fresh parsley

Preparation Method:

1. Warm the broth in a saucepan. Adjust the temperature setting to low - slowly mix in the polenta, whisking vigorously. Place atop onto the pan to simmer (10 min.).
2. Mix in goat cheese, pepper, salt, and butter.
3. Warm butter to prepare the veggies using the medium-temperature setting in a skillet. Mash and toss the garlic into the pan to sauté till it's fragrant (1 min.).
4. Stir in the roasted vegetables and simmer until they're thoroughly heated (2-4 min.).
5. Mix in sage and continue to simmer till it's also fragrant (1 min.).
6. Serve the veggies over the polenta topped with pesto and parsley to your liking.

Fish & Seafood

Baked Cod

Portions Provided: 4 servings
Time Required: 20 minutes
Nutritional Statistics (Each Portion):
- Calories: 90
- Protein Counts: 20 grams
- Carbohydrates: trace grams
- Fat Content: 1 gram
- Sodium: 220 mg

Essential Ingredients:
- Cod fillets (4 @ 4 to 5 oz./140 g each)
- Lemon (1)
- Seasoning blend - ex. Old Bay (1 tsp.)

Preparation Method:
1. Set the oven temperature at 350° Fahrenheit or 177° Celsius. Cut the lemon into four wedges.
2. Lightly coat four squares of aluminum foil with cooking spray and add a piece of fish.
3. Sprinkle the fillets with a spritz of lemon and a dusting of the seasoning.
4. Wrap the fish in the foil pieces. Put them into the oven.
5. Bake until the fish is opaque (10 min.). Serve promptly for the best flavor results.

Baked Parchment-Packed Tuna Steaks & Veggies with Sauce

Portions Provided: 4 servings
Time Required: 30 minutes
Nutritional Statistics (Each Portion):
1 cup veggies + 4 oz. fish portion:
- Protein Counts: 36.4 grams
- Carbohydrates: 14 grams
- Fat Content: 11.3 grams
- Sugars: 2.4 grams
- Dietary Fiber: 1.7 grams
- Sodium: 511.6 mg
- Calories: 312

Essential Ingredients:
- Honey (1 tsp.)
- Mayonnaise (.25 cup)
- Dijon mustard (2 tsp.)
- Ground turmeric (.5 tsp.)
- Fresh parsley (1 tbsp.)
- Yukon Gold potatoes (2 cups)
- Salt (.5 tsp. divided)
- Ground pepper (.125 or ⅛ tsp. + .25 tsp. divided)
- Kale (4 cups)
- Tuna (1.25 lb./570 g)

Preparation Method:
1. Warm the oven to 450° Fahrenheit/232° Celsius.
2. Cut four large sheets of parchment baking paper (each about 16x12 in.).
3. Chop the parsley and thinly slice the potatoes (⅛-inch).
4. Chop the kale and slice the tuna into (4) one-inch-thick pieces.
5. Whisk the mayonnaise with mustard, parsley, turmeric, and honey in a mixing container.
6. Make the packets by laying the parchment sheets on the countertop (long sides closest to you). Fold each packet in half - leaving it open to fill.
7. Scoop the potatoes (½ cup) on one side of each parchment piece - dust each one using pepper (⅛ tsp.) and salt (¼ tsp.).
8. Add kale to each (1 cup), a piece of tuna, and the rest of the pepper and salt - brush them using the mayo mixture.
9. Close the packets - sealing the edges using tight folds. Arrange the packs on a big baking tray.
10. Bake till the fish is "just cooked" (10-15 min.).
11. Set each packet on a serving dish. Wait for about three minutes before opening. Use a pair of scissors to make an "x" in the package. Carefully open to serve.

Broiled Sea Bass

Portions Provided: 2 servings
Time Required: 15 minutes
Nutritional Statistics (Each Portion):
- Calories: 102
- Protein Counts: 21 grams
- Carbohydrates: <1 gram
- Fat Content: 2 grams
- Dietary Fiber: 10 grams
- Sodium: 77 mg

Essential Ingredients:
- White sea bass fillets (2 @ 110 g/4 oz. each)

- Lemon juice (1 tbsp.)
- Herb seasoning blend - salt-free (.25 tsp.)
- Freshly cracked black pepper (as desired)
- Garlic (1 tsp.)

Preparation Method:

1. Warm a grill/oven broiler. Place the roasting rack about four inches from the heating element/grill.
2. Lightly spritz a baking tray using a portion of cooking oil spray. Arrange the fillets in the pan.
3. Mince the garlic with a sprinkle of lemon juice, pepper, and herbed seasoning - scatter it over the fish.
4. Grill or broil the fillets until they're easily flaked when tested with a fork (8-10 min.). Serve as desired.

Charred Shrimp & Pesto Buddha Bowls - Diabetic-Friendly

Portions Provided: 4 servings @ 2 ½ cups each
Time Required: 25 minutes
Nutritional Statistics (Each Portion):

- Protein Counts: 30.9 grams
- Carbohydrates: 29.3 grams
- Fat Content: 22 grams
- Sugars: 5 grams
- Dietary Fiber: 7.2 grams
- Sodium: 571.4 mg
- Calories: 429

Essential Ingredients:

- Olive oil (1 tbsp.)
- Prepared pesto (.33 cup)
- Balsamic vinegar (2 tbsp.)
- Black pepper (.25 tsp.)
- Salt (.5 tsp.)
- Jumbo shrimp (1 lb./16-20 count)
- Cherry tomatoes (1)
- Arugula (4 cups)
- Cooked quinoa (2 cups)
- Avocado (1)

Preparation Method:

1. Whisk the pesto with the oil, vinegar, pepper, and salt in a big mixing container. Reserve four tablespoons of the mixture in a holding container - set both to the side for now.
2. Warm a big cast-iron skillet using a medium-high temperature setting.
3. Peel and devein the shrimp. Pat them dry and toss them into the skillet to sauté till

they're slightly charred (4-5 min.). Scoop them onto a platter.

4. Add quinoa and arugula in a big mixing container with vinaigrette - toss to coat.
5. Portion the mixture into four serving dishes.
6. Slice the tomatoes into halves and dice the avocado - adding it to the shrimp - add to the serving dishes.
7. Spritz each serving using a tablespoon of the reserved pesto mixture.

Chimichurri Meal-Prep Noodle Bowls - Diabetic-Friendly

Portions Provided: 4 servings @ 3 cups each
Time Required: 20 minutes
Nutritional Statistics (Each Portion):

- Protein Counts: 24.8 grams
- Carbohydrates: 28.1 grams
- Fat Content: 19.9 grams
- Sugars: 4.8 grams
- Dietary Fiber: 4.6 grams
- Sodium: 376.8 mg
- Calories: 377
  - *Diabetic Exchanges*:
- Vegetable: 1
- Starch: 1 ½
- Lean Protein: 2 ½
- Fat: 3

Essential Ingredients:

- *The Sauce*:
- Garlic (5 cloves)
- Flat-leaf parsley (2 cups)
- Fresh oregano (1 tbsp.) or dried (1 tsp.)
- Salt (.5 tsp.)
- Optional: Red pepper - crushed (.5 tsp.)
- Black pepper (.25 tsp.)
- Lemon juice (3 tbsp.)
- Olive oil (.5 cup)
  - *The Bowls*:
- Zucchini noodles (3 medium zucchini/8 cups)
- Whole-grain spaghetti (110 g/4 oz.)
- Peeled cooked shrimp (340 g/12 oz.)
- Crumbled feta cheese (.25 cup)

Preparation Method:

1. Prepare a big pot of boiling water for the pasta.
2. Load a food processor with garlic, parsley, lemon juice, oregano, black pepper, crushed red pepper, and salt to make the sauce. Puree the mixture until it's smooth. Drizzle the oil into the sauce with the motor

running - scraping the sides until it's thoroughly incorporated.

3. If prepping, portion two tablespoons of the sauce in four small, lidded containers and refrigerate.

4. Prepare the bowls. Cook spaghetti in the boiling water per its package instructions. Dump the pasta into a colander to rinse using cold tap water. Transfer it to a big mixing container. Toss in the zucchini noodles.

5. Gently toss the spaghetti and zoodles until mixed. Portion them into four individual containers with lids. Lastly, add three ounces of shrimp and feta (1 tbsp.).

6. Seal the containers for storage. When serving, toss with chimichurri sauce.

7. Meal Prep Tips: Refrigerate for up to four days. For frozen or pre-cooked shrimp, wait to defrost at serving time.

Coconut Shrimp

Portions Provided: 6 servings @ 2 shrimp each
Time Required: 20 minutes
Nutritional Statistics (Each Portion):
- Carbs: 4 grams
- Protein Counts: 5 grams
- Fat Content: 4 grams
- Sugars: 2 grams
- Dietary Fiber: -0- grams
- Sodium: 396 mg
- Calories: 75

Essential Ingredients:
- Sweetened coconut (.25 cup)
- Panko breadcrumbs (.25 cup)
- Kosher salt (.5 tsp.)
- Coconut milk (.5 cup)
- Jumbo shrimp (12)

Preparation Method:
1. Warm the oven to 375° Fahrenheit/191° Celsius.
2. Spray a baking tray using a spritz of cooking oil spray.
3. Peel and devein the shrimp.
4. Load a food processor with the panko, coconut, and salt - pulse till it's consistent.
5. Dump the panko mixture in a mixing container.
6. Pour the milk into a separate container.

7. Dip each shrimp in the milk and panko - place on the baking tray.
8. Lightly spritz the tops of the shrimp with a misting of cooking oil spray.
9. Bake till the shrimp are browned to your liking (10-15 min.) to serve.

Creamy Lemon Pasta with Shrimp

Portions Provided: 4 servings @ 1.5 cups
Time Required: 20 minutes
Nutritional Statistics (Each Portion):
- Protein Counts: 28.3 grams
- Carbohydrates: 45.5 grams
- Fat Content: 13.9 grams
- Sugars: 3 grams
- Dietary Fiber: 5.8 grams
- Sodium: 396.3 mg Calories: 403
  Diabetic Exchanges:
- Fat: 2 Starch: 2 ½
- Lean Protein: 2 ½

Essential Ingredients:
- Whole-wheat fettuccine (8 oz.)
- Olive oil (1 tbsp.)
- Sustainably sourced raw shrimp (12 oz. @ 26-30 per lb.)
- Unsalted butter (2 tbsp.)
- Crushed red pepper (.25 tsp.)
- Garlic (1 tbsp.)
- Arugula - packed loosely (4 cups)
- Whole-milk yogurt - plain (.25 cup)
- Lemon zest (1 tsp.)
- Lemon juice (2 tbsp.)
- Salt (.25 tsp.)
- Parmesan cheese - grated (.33 cup + more for garnish)
- Thinly sliced fresh basil (.25 cup)

Preparation Method:
1. Peel and devein the shrimp.
2. Bring seven cups of water to a boil. Add fettuccine, stirring to separate the noodles. Cook until just tender (6-9 min.). Reserve 1/2 cup of the cooking water and drain the remainder.
3. Warm oil in a big nonstick skillet using a med-high temperature setting. Toss in the shrimp and sauté them, occasionally stirring, till pink and curled (2-3 min.). Scoop the shrimp into another bowl.
4. Lower the temperature to medium and melt the butter.

5. Mince and add garlic and crushed red pepper - sauté till the garlic is fragrant (1 min.).

6. Fold in the arugula and cook, stirring, until wilted (1 min.). Adjust the temperature setting to low.

7. Add the fettuccine, lemon zest, reserved cooking water (1/4 cup at a time), and the yogurt, thoroughly mixing till the fettuccine is fully covered and creamy.

8. Fold in the shrimp, salt, and lemon juice -, tossing to coat the fettuccine. Place the pan on a cool burner and toss with parmesan.

9. Serve the fettuccine topped with basil and additional parmesan as desired.

Crispy Oven-Fried Fish Tacos

Portions Provided: 4 servings - 2 each
Time Required: 45 minutes
Nutritional Statistics (Each Portion):
- Protein Counts: 27.3 grams
- Carbohydrates: 65.4 grams
- Fat Content: 17.6 grams
- Sugars: 6.5 grams
- Dietary Fiber: 15.2 grams
- Sodium: 472.3mg
- Calories: 496
  Diabetic Exchanges:
- Vegetable: 1
- Lean Protein: 2
- Fat: 2 ½
- Starch: 3 ½

Essential Ingredients:
- Corn tortillas (8 warmed)
- Cod (1 lb.)
- Cooking spray (as needed)
- Avocado oil (2 tbsp.)
- Dry whole-wheat breadcrumbs (.75 cup)
- Whole-grain cereal flakes (1 cup)
- Garlic powder (.5 tsp.)
- Black pepper - divided (.75 tsp.)
- Paprika (.5 tsp.)
- Salt - divided (.5 tsp.)
- A.P. flour (.5 cup)
- Water (2 tbsp.)
- Egg whites (2 large)
- Rice vinegar - unseasoned (2 tbsp.)
- Avocado (1)
- Pico de Gallo (as desired)
- Coleslaw mix (3 cups)

Preparation Method:

1. Set the oven temperature to reach 450° Fahrenheit/232° Celsius.

2. Arrange a wire baking rack on a cookie tray and spritz with a little cooking oil spray.

3. Slice the cod in half horizontally - if it is thick - and into strips (½ x 3-inch). Load a food processor with the cereal flakes, pepper (.5 tsp.), breadcrumbs, garlic powder, salt (.25 tsp.), and paprika - mixing till the mixture is finely ground. Pour it into a shallow dish.

4. Put flour in a second shallow bowl.

5. Whisk/beat water with egg whites in one additional container.

6. Dip the fish pieces in the flour, egg mix - coating each side with the breadcrumb mixture. Arrange them on the baking rack.

7. Lightly spritz each fish's side with a little cooking oil spray.

8. Bake till the fish breading is crispy and nicely browned (10 min.).

9. In the meantime, whisk the oil with the vinegar and the remaining (0.25 tsp. each) pepper and salt in a mixing container. Fold in the coleslaw mix - thoroughly toss to cover.

10. Dice the avocado. Serve the fish with the coleslaw mix and avocado into the heated tortillas.

11. Add a portion of Pico de Gallo to your liking.

Garlic Shrimp & Spinach - Diabetic-Friendly

Portions Provided: 4 servings @ 1 cup each
Time Required: 25 minutes
Nutritional Statistics (Each Portion):
- Protein Count: 26.4 grams
- Carbohydrates: 6.1 grams
- Fat Content: 11.6 grams
- Fiber Count: 2.7 grams
- Sugars: 0.7 grams
- Sodium: 444 mg
- Calories: 226

Essential Ingredients:
- Olive oil (3 tbsp. - divided)
- Garlic - divided (6 medium cloves)
- Spinach (1 lb.)
- Salt (.25 tsp. + ⅛ tsp. - divided)
- Lemon: Juice (1 tbsp.) + zest (1.5 tsp.)

- Shrimp (1 lb./21-30 count)
- Crushed red pepper (.25 tsp.)
- Fresh parsley (1 tbsp.)

Preparation Method:
1. Warm oil (1 tbsp.) in a large pot using a medium temperature setting. Mince and add half the garlic and sauté it till it's beginning to brown (1-2 min.).
2. Add spinach and salt (¼ tsp.) and toss to coat. Fold it a couple of times till it's mostly wilted (3-5 min.). Move the pan to a cool burner - mix in the lemon juice. Scoop it into a holding container and keep it warm for now.
3. Raise the temperature setting to med-high. Pour in the rest of the oil (2 tbsp.) into the cooking pot.
4. Toss in the remaining garlic and simmer till it's starting to brown (1-2 min.).
5. Peel, devein - fold in the shrimp, crushed red pepper, and the rest of the salt (⅛ tsp.). Sauté till the shrimp are thoroughly heated (3-5 min.).
6. Finely chop the parsley. Serve the shrimp over the spinach, sprinkled with lemon zest and parsley.

Grilled Fish with Peperonata - Diabetic-Friendly

Portions Provided: 4 servings
Time Required: 45 minutes
Nutritional Statistics (Each Portion):
6 oz. fish + 1 cup of peperonata:
- Protein Counts: 31.2 grams
- Carbohydrates: 10.9 grams (Net: 2.1 grams)
- Fat Content: 24.6 grams
- Fiber: 3.7 grams
- Sugars: 5.1 grams
- Sodium: 461.5 mg
- Calories: 396

Essential Ingredients:
- Olive oil (4 tbsp. divided)
- Fennel seed (1 tbsp.)
- Garlic (3 cloves)
- Crushed red pepper (1 pinch)
- Medium red onion (1)
- Fresh thyme and oregano (1 tsp. each)
- Paprika (1 tsp.)
- Any color bell peppers (8 cups)
- Capers (.25 cup)
- Sherry vinegar (2 tbsp.)

- Skinned banded rudderfish/swordfish/mahi-mahi (1.5 lb.)
- Mixed tender fresh herbs as desired - parsley, basil, or mint (.25 cup)
- Kosher salt (.5 tsp.)
- Fennel (.25 cup)

Preparation Method:
1. Heat oil (2 tbsp.) in a big pot using a med-low temperature setting.
2. Thinly chop or mince and add the fennel seed, crushed red pepper, and garlic - sauté till it's fragrant and the garlic is browning (2-3 min.). Chop and mix in the onion - sautéing till it's softened (5 min.).
3. Chop and mix in paprika, thyme, and oregano.
4. Dice and mix in the bell peppers. Lower the temperature setting to low. Rinse, slice, and add the capers and vinegar. Simmer for two minutes more.
5. Meanwhile, warm the grill to med-high. Oil the grill rack.
6. Brush the fish with the remaining oil (2 tbsp.) and dust using a little salt.
7. Grill the fish, turning once halfway through the cycle until the flesh is opaque (6-10 min. - depending on thickness).
8. Transfer the fish to a chopping block and cut it into four servings.
9. Put the fish over the peperonata and garnish using the freshly prepared herbs and fennel.
10. Meal Prep Tip: Refrigerate the peperonata (step one) for up to one day.

Grits & Shrimp

Portions Provided: 8 servings
Time Required: 30 minutes
Nutritional Statistics (Each Portion):
- Carbohydrates: 17 grams
- Protein Counts: 17 grams
- Fat Content: 7 grams
- Dietary Fiber: 2 grams
- Sodium: 637 mg
- Calories: 199

Essential Ingredients:
The Grits:
- Unsalted chicken stock (3 cups)
- Butter (1 tbsp.)
- Grits (1 cup)

The Topping:

- Olive oil (1 tbsp.)
- Shrimp (1 lb. at about 16-20 per lb.)
- Black & stuffed green olives (5 slices of each)
- Crumbled goat cheese (2 tbsp.)
- Green onions** (1 bunch)
- Large garlic cloves (2)
- Sun-dried tomatoes (1 tbsp.) or (5 cherry tomatoes)
- Red/green bell pepper (.25 cup)
- Capers (1 tbsp.)
- Parsley - chopped (2 tbsp.)
- Black pepper (as desired)
- Optional: Lemon wedges

Preparation Method:
1. Prepare and measure the ingredients. Peel and devein the shrimp
2. Use a saucepan to heat the broth using a med-high temperature setting.
3. Slowly whisk in the grits to avoid clumping.
4. Lower the temperature setting and add a top. Simmer and stir intermittently until thickened (10-15 min.). Move the pan to a cool burner, and add the butter. Put a top back on the pan to keep it warm.
5. Heat oil using the medium-temperature setting in a big skillet.
6. Pat the oil from the tomatoes.
7. Mince the garlic, tomatoes, and green onions and toss them into the skillet. Sauté them until fragrant. (For cherry tomatoes, crush them once they're heated and mix them into the onion/garlic mixture.)
8. Dice and add the peppers. Toss in the shrimp.
9. Sauté the mixture until the shrimp are pink. Mix in sliced olives and capers to heat.
10. Pour about ¼ cup grits and add a portion of the shrimp mixture into the plates.
11. Garnish them using a few crumbs of cheese, a dusting of pepper, and a bit of parsley. Serve with a couple of lemon wedges.
12. *Note**For the onions - include the green top. Slice the onion into half-inch pieces.*

Peppered Sole

Portions Provided: 4 servings
Time Required: 25 minutes
Nutritional Statistics (Each Portion):
- Calories: 174
- Protein Counts:23 grams
- Carbohydrates: 4 grams (Net: 1 gram)
- Fat Content: 7 grams
- Sugars: 2 grams
- Fiber: 1 gram
- Sodium: 166 mg

Essential Ingredients:
- Sole fillets (4 @ 110 g/4 oz. each)
- Paprika (.25 tsp.)
- Lemon-pepper seasoning (.25 tsp.)
- Cayenne pepper (.125 or ⅛ tsp.)
- Medium tomato (1)
- Green onions (2)
- Butter (2 tbsp.)
- Fresh mushrooms (2 cups)
- Garlic (2 cloves)

Preparation Method:
1. Warm a skillet using the med-high temperature setting to melt the butter.
2. Slice and toss the mushrooms into the pan to sauté till they're tender.
3. Mince and toss in the garlic to sauté for one minute.
4. Place the fillets over the mushrooms—dust with the lemon pepper, paprika, and cayenne.
5. Cook with a lid on the skillet using the medium-temperature setting till the fish easily flakes when poked with a fork (5-10 min.).
6. Chop the tomatoes and thinly slice the onions. Garnish the fish to serve.

Peppery Barbecue-Glazed Shrimp with Vegetables & Orzo

Portions Provided: 4 servings @ 2 cups each
Time Required: 30 minutes
Nutritional Statistics (Each Portion):
- Protein Counts: 30.1 grams
- Carbohydrates: 40.6 grams
- Fat Content: 8.9 grams
- Sugars: 7.2 grams
- Fiber: 9.5 grams
- Sodium: 553.8 mg
- Calories: 360

Essential Ingredients:
- Jumbo shrimp (1 lb.)
- Cayenne pepper (.125 or ⅛ tsp.)
- Oregano - dry & crushed (.5 tsp.)
- Garlic powder (.5 tsp.)
- Paprika (1 tsp.)
- Black pepper (.25 tsp.)

- Whole-grain orzo (1 cup)
- Scallions (3)
- Olive oil (2 tbsp. divided)
- Zucchini (2 cups)
- Bell pepper (1 cup)
- Celery (.5 cup)
- Cherry tomatoes (1 cup)
- Salt (.5 tsp.)
- Barbecue sauce (2 tbsp.)
- Lemon wedges for serving

Preparation Method:

1. Thaw the shrimp if frozen.
2. Peel, devein the shrimp - toss them into a mixing container with paprika, garlic powder, oregano, pepper, and cayenne.
3. Toss them thoroughly to cover - set aside.
4. Prepare a big saucepan of boiling water. Prepare the orzo per its package instructions and drain. Cover the pot and keep the fixings warm.
5. Slice the scallions, separating white and green parts.
6. Coarsely chop the pepper and zucchini. Thinly slice the celery and slice the tomatoes in half.
7. Warm oil (1 tbsp.) in a skillet using a med-high temperature setting.
8. Toss in the zucchini, scallion whites, celery, and bell pepper - sauté them occasionally stirring - till the veggies are fork-tender (5 min.).
9. Add tomatoes and simmer until softened (2-3 min.).
10. Add the salt and veggies to the cooking pot with the orzo.
11. Use the same pan to warm the remaining oil (1 tbsp.) using a medium-temperature setting. Toss in the shrimp and simmer - turning once until it's opaque (4-6 min.).
12. Sprinkle them using the barbecue sauce and simmer until the shrimp are covered and heated (1 min.).
13. Serve the shrimp with the veggie mixture - garnish them using scallion greens and serve with lemon wedges as desired.
14. Meal Prep Tip: Frozen shrimp will thaw if placed in a big bowl filled with ice water (20 min.).

Provençal Baked Fish with Roasted Potatoes & Mushrooms

Portions Provided: 4 servings
Time Required: 60 minutes
Nutritional Statistics (Each Portion):

- Protein Counts: 24.4 grams
- Carbs: 25.3 grams
- Fat Content: 8.8 grams
- Fiber: 2.8 grams
- Sugars: 2.6 grams
- Sodium: 218.9 mg
- Calories: 276

Essential Ingredients:

- Yukon Gold or red potatoes (450 g/1 lb.)
- Mushrooms - shiitake/cremini/oyster/other fresh mushrooms (1 lb.)
- Virgin olive oil (2 tbsp. divided)
- Ground pepper & salt (.25 tsp. each)
- Garlic (2 cloves)
- Halibut/grouper or cod fillet (14 oz./400 g - cut into four servings)
- Lemon juice (4 tbsp.)
- Herbs de Provence (1 tsp.)
- To Garnish: Fresh thyme
- Also Suggested: 9x13-inch/23-33-cm baking dish

Preparation Method:

1. Warm the oven ahead of baking time to reach 425° Fahrenheit/218° Celsius.
2. Cube the potatoes and mince the garlic. Trim and slice the mushrooms - tossing both into a big mixing container with oil (1 tbsp.), pepper, and salt. Scoop the mixture into a baking dish.
3. Roast till the veggies are tender (30-40 min.).
4. Mix in the garlic and add the fish on top with a spritz of lemon juice and the rest of the oil (1 tbsp.). Dust them using the herbs de Provence.
5. Bake till the fish flakes easily (10-15 min.).
6. Mince and garnish with thyme as desired.

Seared Scallops & White Bean Ragu with Charred Lemon

Portions Provided: 4 servings
Time Required: 25 minutes
Nutritional Statistics (Each Portion):

- Protein Counts: 21.4 grams
- Carbohydrates: 21 grams
- Fat Content: 8.3 grams

- Sugars: 1.4 grams
- Dietary Fiber: 5.3 grams
- Sodium: 589.6 mg
- Calories: 255

Essential Ingredients:

- Olive oil (3 tsp. divided)
- Mature spinach or white chard (450 g/1 lb.)
- Garlic (2 cloves)
- Capers (1 tbsp.)
- Black pepper (.5 tsp. divided)
- Chicken broth - l.s. (1 cup)
- Cannellini beans - no salt (540 g/15 oz. can)
- Butter (1 tbsp.)
- Dry sea scallops (430 g/1 lb.)
- Dry white wine (.33 cup)
- Lemon (1 halved)
- Fresh parsley (2 tbsp.)

Preparation Method:

1. Toss the beans into a colander to rinse and drain.
2. Remove the tough side muscle from the scallops.
3. Warm two teaspoons of oil in a big frying pan using a med-high temperature setting.
4. Trim and thinly slice the spinach/chard. Rinse and chop the capers.
5. Toss in the greens and cook, often stirring until wilted (4 min.).
6. Mince and stir in the garlic with the capers and pepper (¼ tsp.) - simmer and stir it intermittently till it is fragrant (30 sec.).
7. Add broth, beans, and wine - wait for it to simmer. Adjust the temperature setting to maintain a low simmer. Put a top on the pot and cook it for five minutes.
8. Transfer the pan to a cool burner and mix in the butter.
9. Put a top on the pot so it will remain warm.
10. Meanwhile, sprinkle the scallops with the rest of the pepper (¼ tsp.).
11. Warm the remaining one teaspoon oil in a big skillet using a med-high temperature setting.
12. Fold in the scallops and simmer till they're browned to your liking on each side (4 min. total). Scoop them into a platter and set them aside.
13. Arrange lemon halves into the pan (cut-side down) and cook till they're charred (1 min.). Now, slice them into wedges.
14. Sprinkle the scallops and the bean ragu with chopped parsley - serve with the lemon wedges.

Shrimp Orzo & Feta

Portions Provided: 4 servings
Time Required: 25 minutes
Nutritional Statistics (Each Portion):

- Protein Counts: 33 grams
- Carbohydrates: 40 grams
- Fat Content: 12 grams
- Sugars: 2 grams
- Dietary Fiber: 9 grams
- Sodium: 307 mg
- Calories: 406

Essential Ingredients:

- Uncooked shrimp (1.25 lb./26-30-count per lb.)
- Minced fresh cilantro (2 tbsp.)
- Pepper (.25 tsp.)
- Uncooked whole-wheat orzo pasta (1.25 cups)
- Olive oil (2 tbsp.)
- Medium tomatoes (2)
- Garlic cloves (2)
- Lemon juice (2 tbsp.)
- Crumbled feta cheese (.5 cup)

Preparation Method:

1. Peel and devein the uncooked shrimp.
2. Cook the orzo (7-10 min.). In the meantime, prep a big pan to warm the oil using a medium-temperature setting.
3. Mince and add the garlic. Sauté for one minute.
4. Chop and mix in the tomatoes and lemon juice.
5. Once boiling, mix in the shrimp. Adjust the temperature setting to simmer with the lid off until the shrimp turn pink (4-5 min.).
6. Drain the orzo and toss it with pepper and cilantro. Toss it into the shrimp mixture. Heat and sprinkle with feta cheese.

Shrimp Scampi Zoodles

Portions Provided: 4 servings
Time Required: 30 minutes
Nutritional Statistics (Each Portion):

- Protein Counts: 27.4 grams
- Carbohydrates: 8.1 grams
- Fat Content: 15.4 grams
- Sugars: 4.7 grams
- Dietary Fiber: 2 grams

- Sodium: 530.4 mg
- Calories: 286

Essential Ingredients:
- Medium zucchini (4-6 trimmed/2.25-2.5 lb.)
- Butter (2 tbsp.)
- Salt (.5 tsp. divided)
- Olive oil (2 tbsp. - divided)
- Wine - dry white suggested (.33 cup)
- Garlic (1 tbsp.)
- Raw shrimp (1 lb.)
- Lemon juice (1 tbsp.)
- Fresh parsley (.25 cup)
- Parmesan cheese - grated (.25 cup)
- Black pepper (.25 tsp.)
- To Serve: Lemon wedges

Preparation Method:
1. Using a vegetable peeler, prepare the zucchini - slicing it lengthwise into long - thin strips.
2. Toss the "zoodles" into a colander and generously toss with salt (¼ tsp.). Set them aside to drain for 15 minutes to ½ hour - and gently squeezing to remove any excess liquid.
3. Prepare a big skillet using a med-high temperature setting to warm the butter and oil (1 tbsp.). Mince and toss in garlic - sauté (½ min.).
4. Carefully stir in the wine - wait for it to boil.
5. Use 16 to 20 count shrimp for each pound, leaving tails left on if desired. Devein and peel the shrimp - toss them into the pan - stirring till the shrimp are pink (3-4 min.). Transfer the skillet to a cool burner.
6. Mix in the pepper, parsley, lemon juice, and rest of the salt (¼ tsp.). Scoop them into a big container and place them on the side for now.
7. Warm oil (1 tbsp.) in the skillet using a med-high temperature setting. Toss in the zucchini - stirring till it's heated (3 min.).
8. Gently combine the shrimp mixture with the zucchini.
9. Chop the parsley and dust the shrimp adding a lemon squeeze.

Spicy Jerk Shrimp

Portions Provided: 4 servings
Time Required: 55 minutes

Nutritional Statistics (Each Portion):
5 oz. shrimp + 1 cup pineapple mix:
- Protein Counts: 33.5 grams
- Carbohydrates: 37.2 grams
- Fat Content: 8.5 grams
- Sugars: 12.1 grams
- Dietary Fiber: 5.1 grams
- Sodium: 411.3 mg
- Calories: 351
  Diabetic Exchanges:
- Fruit: ½
- Starch: 1 Vegetable: 2
- Lean Protein: 4

Essential Ingredients:
- Jamaican jerk seasoning (1 tbsp.)
- Fresh/frozen large shrimp (680 g/1.5 lb.)
- Red sweet pepper (2 cups)
- Fresh jalapeño chili pepper (1)
- Peeled and cored - fresh pineapple - halved - 4 - (6-mm or ¼-inch thick slices)
- Red onions (2 cups)
- Olive oil (2 tbsp.)
  portion of brown rice:
- Fresh cilantro (.5 cup)
- Brown rice - cooked (1.33 cups)
- Lime wedges
- Also Needed: Two 15x10-inch baking pans

Preparation Method:
1. Thaw the shrimp if it's frozen.
2. Set the oven temperature to reach 425° Fahrenheit/218° Celsius.
3. Prepare the baking trays with a piece of tin foil.
4. Prep the peppers and onions into bite-sized strips. Slice (lengthwise) and remove the seeds from the jalapeno.
5. Peel and remove the veins from each of the shrimp - leave the tails intact if desired. Use cool water to rinse the shrimp and dab them dry using several paper towels.
6. Use a big mixing container to toss the shrimp with the next six ingredients (through jerk seasoning up to the line ****), tossing them gently to coat.
7. Scoop the mixture into the prepared baking pans. Roast until shrimp are opaque (15 min.).
8. Enjoy the shrimp with a portion of brown rice and dusting of cilantro with a side of freshly sliced lime wedges.

Spinach-Stuffed Sole

Portions Provided: 2 servings
Time Required: 25-30 minutes
Nutritional Statistics (Each Portion):
- Calories: 157
- Protein Counts: 27 grams
- Carbohydrates: 1 gram
- Sodium: 140 mg

Essential Ingredients:
- Spinach leaves (2 cups)
- Garlic (2 tsp.)
- Butter (.5 tsp.)
- Olive oil (1 tsp.)
- Sole/flounder fillets (2 @ 140 g or 5-oz. each) - Black pepper (as desired)

Preparation Method:
1. Lightly spray a coat of a nonstick cooking spray to a baking pan/dish.
2. Set the oven temperature to reach 400° Fahrenheit/204° Celsius.
3. Use the stovetop and warm a skillet to heat the oil using the medium-temperature setting. Mince the garlic and tear the spinach as desired.
4. Once heated, toss in the pepper, spinach, and garlic. Sauté about two or three minutes or until the spinach starts to wilt.
5. Put the fillets on the prepared baking container. Arrange about ½ of the spinach mix into the middle of each fillet and roll them up. Put them into the pan with the seam side down - brushing with the butter. Bake till the fish is opaque (8-10 min.).

Steamed Trout with Mint & Dill Dressing

Portions Provided: 2 servings
Time Required: 35 minutes
Nutritional Statistics (Each Portion):
- Protein Counts: 43 grams
- Carbohydrates: 25 grams
- Fat Content: 10 grams
- Sugars: 12 grams
- Dietary Fiber: 7 grams
- Sodium: 0.5 mg
- Calories: 378

Essential Ingredients:
- New potatoes (120 g/4.2 oz.)
- Asparagus spears (170 g/6 oz. pack)
- Vegetable bouillon powder made up to 8 oz./225 ml with water (1.5 tsp.)
- Green beans (80 g/2.8 oz.)
- Frozen peas (80 g)
- Skinless trout fillets (2)
- Lemon (2 slices)
  The Dressing:
- Bio yogurt (4 tbsp.)
- Cider vinegar (1 tsp.)
- Dry/English mustard powder (.25 tsp.)
- Mint (1 tsp.)
- Dill (2 tsp.)

Preparation Method:
1. Slice the potatoes into halves and put them on to simmer in a pan of boiling water until tender.
2. Trim the green beans. Cut the asparagus in half to shorten the spears and slice the ends without the tips. Finely chop the mint and dill.
3. Tip the bouillon into a wide non-stick pan.
4. Arrange the asparagus in the pan with the beans. Place a top on the pan to simmer them (5 min.).
5. Stir the peas into the mixture and top with the trout and lemon slices. Cover again and continue to cook until the fish flakes easily but is still juicy (5-6 min.).
6. Whisk the yogurt with mustard powder, vinegar, mint, and dill.
7. Whisk in fish cooking juices (2-3 tbsp.).
8. Serve the veggies and any remaining pan juices into serving bowls, top with the fish and herb dressing, and serve with the potatoes.

Sweet Chili & Pistachio Mahi Mahi

Portions Provided: 4 servings
Time Required: 45 minutes
Nutritional Statistics (Each Portion):
½ cup quinoa + 1 fish fillet:
- Protein Counts: 27.5 grams
- Carbohydrates: 28.3 grams
- Fat Content: 11.5 grams
- Sugars: 10.4 grams
- Dietary Fiber: 4.3 grams
- Sodium: 328.3 mg
- Calories: 322
  Diabetic Exchanges:
- Other Carbohydrate: ½
- Fat: 1

- Starch: 1 ½
- Lean Protein: 3

Essential Ingredients:

- Fresh or frozen mahi-mahi fillets (4 @ 4-5 oz. each)
- Lime (1)
- Warmed honey (5 tsp. divided)
- Olive oil (2 tsp.)
- Black pepper and salt (.25 tsp. each)
- Whole almonds/dry roasted salted pistachio nuts (.5 cup)
- Onion powder (.25 tsp.)
- Chili powder (.75 tsp.)
- Paprika (.25 tsp.)
- Quinoa - cooked (1.33 cups)
- Red onion (.25 cup)
- Red bell pepper (.5 cup)
- Fresh cilantro sprigs (.25 cup + more to garnish)

Preparation Method:

1. Thaw the fish if it's frozen. Chop the peppers, onions, and cilantro.
2. Set the oven to reach 325° Fahrenheit/163° Celsius.
3. Cover a baking tray using a layer of parchment baking paper.
4. Prepare the lime dressing by finely shredding the lime peel and squeezing its juice - combine with oil, honey (2 tsp.), pepper, and salt in a mixing container - set it aside.
5. Combine the nuts with the onion powder, chili powder, paprika, and honey (1 tsp.) in a mixing container and spread them over the baking tray.
6. Bake until toasted (12 min.) and cool. Toss the nut mixture in a food processor and mix till they're finely crushed.
7. Raise the oven temperature to 425° Fahrenheit/218° Celsius. Cover the baking tray with another layer of parchment baking paper and set it to the side for now.
8. Rinse the fish with tap water and dab it dry using a few paper towels.
9. Brush the fish tops with the remainder of the honey (2 tsp.). Sprinkle with the crushed nut mixture, pushing gently to adhere, and arrange the fish on the baking tray.
10. Bake till the fish flakes easily using a fork (10-15 min.).
11. Meanwhile, toss the quinoa with bell pepper, onions, and chopped cilantro in a mixing container. Stir in the reserved lime dressing.
12. When ready, serve the fish with the quinoa mixture and a sprinkle of cilantro sprigs.

Swordfish with Roasted Lemons

Portions Provided: 4 servings
Time Required: 1 hour 15 minutes
Nutritional Statistics (Each Portion):

- Protein Counts: 34 grams
- Fat Content: 12 grams
- Carbohydrates: 9 grams (Net: 5 grams)
- Sugars: 4 grams
- Dietary Fiber: trace grams
- Sodium: 287 mg
- Calories: 280

Essential Ingredients:

- Lemons (2)
- Sea salt (.25 tsp.)
- Sugar (1 tbsp.)
- Swordfish (4 fillets @ 170 g/6 oz. each)
- Canola oil (.5 tsp.)
- Chopped garlic (.5 tsp.)
- Chopped parsley (.25 cup)

Preparation Method:

1. Set the oven temperature at 375° Fahrenheit/191° Celsius.
2. Quarter, remove the seeds, and toss the lemon wedges, salt, and sugar in a mixing container.
3. Put the lemons in a shallow baking container. Place a foil layer over the dish and roast until soft and slightly browned (1 hr.).
4. Warm the grill or oven broiler (four inches from the heating element). Lightly spritz a baking tray using a cooking oil spray.
5. Arrange the fish in the pan and lightly brush with a portion of the oil and garnish it using garlic. Grill/broil it till the fish is opaque (5 min. per side).
6. Serve the fish with a squeeze of lemon wedge over the fillets and dusting of parsley.
7. Add a roasted wedge of lemon to the side if desired.

Tilapia on the Grill with Salsa

Portions Provided: 8 servings
Time Required: 20 minutes

Nutritional Statistics (Each Portion):
- Calories: 131
- Protein Counts: 21 grams
- Carbohydrates: 6 grams (Net: 1 gram)
- Fat Content: 3 grams
- Sugars: 4 grams
- Dietary Fiber: 1 gram
- Sodium: 152 mg

Essential Ingredients:
- Fresh pineapple (2 cups)
- Green onions (2)
- Green pepper (.25 cup)
- Fresh cilantro (.25 cup)
- Lime juice - divided (4 tsp. + 2 tbsp.)
- Cayenne pepper (1 dash)
- Salt - divided (.125 tsp. + .25 tsp. - divided)
- Canola oil (1 tbsp.)
- Tilapia fillets (8 @ 110 g/4 oz. of each)
- Pepper (.125 or 1/8 tsp.)

Preparation Method:
1. Cube and add the pineapple with the finely chopped green onions, green pepper, cilantro, lime juice (4 tsp.), cayenne, and salt (1/8 tsp.). Refrigerate until serving.
2. Mix oil and the rest of the lime juice (2 tbsp.) to drizzle over fillets. Dust them with the rest of the pepper and salt as desired.
3. Use an oily paper towel to grease the grill rack.
4. Grill the fish with the lid on using the medium-temperature setting or broil in the oven (4 inches from the heating source) till the fish "just begins" to easily flake (2-3 min.).
5. Enjoy the fish with a bit of salsa.

Turkish Seared Tuna with Bulgur & Chickpea Salad

Portions Provided: 4 servings
Time Required: 45 minutes
Nutritional Statistics (Each Portion):
One steak + 3/4 cup salad:
- Protein Counts: 35.9 grams
- Carbohydrates: 43.2 grams
- Fat Content: 16.2 grams
- Fiber: 8.2 grams
- Sugars: 2.1 grams
- Sodium: 556.6 mg
- Calories: 459

Essential Ingredients:
- Bulgur (.5 cup)
- Olive oil (.75 cup - divided)
- Lemon zest (4 tsp. divided)
- Lemon juice (.5 cup divided
- Salt - divided (.5 tsp.)
- Ground pepper (.25 tsp.)
- Chickpeas - no salt (430 g/15 oz. can)
- Fresh mint (.25 cup)
- Fresh Italian parsley (.25 cup)
- Tuna (1 lb. or 4 steaks)
- Medium yellow onion (1)
- Fresh dill (.25 cup)

Preparation Method:
1. Rinse and drain the chickpeas in a colander. Chop the mint, parsley, and dill. Zest and juice a lemon. Thinly slice the onion.
2. Prepare a pot of boiling water. Put the bulgur in a big container (heat-proof). Add boiling water to cover it by two inches. Wait for about 1/2 hour and drain any excess water.
3. Mix the bulgur with oil (2 tbsp.), lemon juice (1/4 cup), lemon zest (2 tsp.), and salt and pepper (1/4 tsp. each).
4. Mix in the parsley, chickpeas, and mint - stirring to combine. Set to the side for now.
5. Warm the rest of the oil (2 tbsp.) in a big skillet using a med-high temperature setting. Place the steaks in the pan and sear till they're lightly browned on one side (2-3 min.). Flip them over and continue cooking till they're as desired on the second side. Plate the steaks.
6. Adjust the temperature to medium. Toss in the onion to the pan and sauté it till it's translucent (5 min.). Lower the temperature setting to medium-low.
7. Place the steaks in the pan with a top - turning them once till the tuna is easily flaked when tested with a fork (3-4 min. per side).
8. Toss the dill with the rest of the lemon juice (1/4 cup) and salt (1/4 tsp.) in a mixing container
9. Move the tuna onto a serving platter. Scoop the onions over the tuna with a drizzle of the lemon juice-dill mixture. Garnish using the rest of the lemon zest (2 tsp.) to serve with the bulgur salad.

Meal Prep Suggestions: Prepare the bulgur (step one) and refrigerate for up to two days.

The Ultimate Fish Tacos - Diabetic-Friendly

Portions Provided: 6 servings @ 2 tacos per portion
Time Required: 30 minutes
Nutritional Statistics (Each Portion):
- Protein Counts: 35 grams
- Carbohydrates: 26 grams
- Fat Content: 5 grams Sugars: 2 grams
- Dietary Fiber: 4 grams
- Sodium: 278 mg Calories: 284

Essential Ingredients:
- Olive oil (.25 cup)
- Cardamom - ground (1 tsp.)
- Paprika (1 tsp.)
- Black pepper and salt (1 tsp. each)
- Mahi-mahi fillets (6 @ 170 g/6 oz. each)
- Corn tortillas (12 @ 6-inches each)
- Red cabbage (2 cups)
- Fresh cilantro (1 cup)
- Optional: Salsa verde
- Limes - cut into wedges (2 medium)
- Hot pepper sauce (Tapatio preferred)
- Suggested: 13x9-inch/33x23-cm baking dish

Preparation Method:
1. Chop the cabbage and cilantro.
2. Whisk and add the first five fixings into a baking dish (oil, cardamom, salt, & pepper). Add the fillets - turn to coat. Refrigerate - covered for ½ hour.
3. Drain the fish and discard the marinade. On an oiled grill rack, grill the mahi-mahi, *covered*, using the med-high temperature setting (or broil about four inches from the heat) till it flakes easily with a fork (4-5 min. per side). Remove fish.
4. Put the tortillas on the grill rack - heat 30-45 seconds. Keep warm.
5. Portion the fish into each tortilla - layer with cilantro, red cabbage, and, if desired, salsa verde. Squeeze a little lime juice and hot pepper sauce over the fish mixture - fold sides of the tortilla over the mixture.
6. Serve with lime wedges and additional pepper sauce.

Chili-Lime Salmon with Peppers & Potatoes in a Sheet-Pan

Portions Provided: 4 servings
Time Required: 25 minutes
Nutritional Statistics (Each Portion):
One piece of fish + 1 ¼ cups veggies:
- Protein Counts: 35.4 grams
- Carbohydrates: 25.9 grams
- Fat Content: 17.4 grams
- Sugars: 3.5 grams
- Dietary Fiber: 3 grams
- Sodium: 516.6 mg
- Calories: 405

Essential Ingredients:
- Olive oil (2 tbsp. divided)
- Potatoes - Yukon Gold (450 g/1 lb.)
- Ground cumin (1 tsp.)
- Chili powder (2 tsp.)
- Black pepper (.25 tsp.)
- Salt (.75 tsp. - divided)
- Garlic powder (.5 tsp.)
- Lime (1 zested & quartered)
- Any color bell peppers (2 medium)
- Center-cut salmon fillet (570 g/1.25 lb.)
- Suggested: Large rimmed baking sheet

Preparation Method:
1. Warm the oven to reach 425° Fahrenheit/218° Celsius.
2. Coat the baking tray using a spritz of cooking oil spray.
3. Slice the potatoes into ¾-inch pieces - toss them with oil (1 tbsp.) and pepper and salt (¼ tsp. each) in a mixing container.
4. Gently toss them into the pan and roast for 15 minutes.
5. Whisk the chili powder with the garlic powder, cumin, lime zest, and the remainder of the salt (½ tsp.) in a mixing container.
6. Slice the bell peppers in a mixing container - tossing with the rest of the oil (1 tbsp.) and ½ tablespoon of the spice mixture. Thoroughly toss to cover the fixings.
7. Skin the salmon and portion it into four servings. Cover it using the remainder of the spice mixture. Set a timer to bake it for 15 minutes.
8. At that point, toss in the peppers to roast for another five minutes.
9. Scoot the veggies aside and place the salmon in the pan.

10. Roast till the salmon is ready (6-8 min.). Serve as desired with lime wedges.

Dijon Salmon with Green Bean Pilaf

Portions Provided: 4 servings
Time Required: 30 minutes
Nutritional Statistics (Each Portion):
- Protein Counts: 32.2 grams
- Carbohydrates: 21.6 grams
- Fat Content: 24.8 grams
- Sugars: 1.7 grams
- Dietary Fiber: 3.8 grams
- Sodium: 605.2 mg
- Calories: 442

Essential Ingredients:
- Wild salmon (570 g/1.25 lb.)
- Olive oil - divided (3 tbsp.)
- Garlic (1 tbsp.)
- Salt (.75 tsp.)
- Whole-grain mustard (2 tsp.)
- Mayonnaise (2 tbsp.)
- Black pepper - divided (.5 tsp.)
- Thin-cut green beans (340 g/12 oz.)
- Pine nuts (2 tbsp.)
- Lemon (1 small - zested + 4 wedges)
- Precooked brown rice (230 g/8 oz. pkg.)
- Water (2 tbsp.)
- To Garnish: Freshly chopped fresh parsley
- Suggested: Rimmed baking sheet

Preparation Method:
1. Set the oven to 425° Fahrenheit/218° Celsius.
2. Cover the baking tray using a sheet of foil or parchment paper.
3. Remove the skin and slice the salmon into four portions.
4. Lightly brush salmon with oil (1 tbsp.) and place on the prepared baking tray.
5. Mash the garlic and salt into a paste with the side of a chef's knife or a fork. Combine a scant one teaspoon of the garlic paste in a small bowl with the mustard, mayonnaise, and pepper (¼ tsp.).
6. Spread the mixture over the fish.
7. Roast the salmon until it flakes easily with a fork in the thickest part (6-8 min. per inch of thickness).
8. Warm the rest of the oil (2 tbsp.) in a big skillet using a med-high temperature setting.
9. Slice the green beans into thirds and toss with the lemon zest, pine nuts, the rest of the garlic paste, and pepper (¼ tsp.) - cook and stir till the beans are tender (2-4 min.)
10. Adjust the temperature setting to medium. Pour in the rice and water - cooking while stirring till it's heated (2-3 min.).
11. Sprinkle the salmon with parsley. Serve with the green bean pilaf and lemon wedges.

Easy Low-Sodium Salmon with Lime & Herbs

Portions Provided: 4 servings
Time Required: 20 minutes
Nutritional Statistics (Each Portion):
- Protein Counts: 24 grams
- Carbohydrates: 7 grams
- Fat Content: 15 grams
- Dietary Fiber: 2 grams
- Sodium: 70 mg
- Calories: 260

Essential Ingredients:
- Fresh salmon fillets (4)
- Limes (2)
- Fresh thyme (12 sprigs)
- Dillweed (fresh @ 2 tsp. or dried @ 1 tsp.)

Preparation Method:
1. Place two fillets on a layer of foil.
2. Squeeze the juice of one lime over the fish and gently rub it with dill weed.
3. Thinly slice the second lime and arrange the slices over the fish.
4. Put thyme sprigs over the top and gently fold aluminum foil over to create pouches.
5. Place the pouches on a grill to cook using the medium-temperature setting (12-15 min.), rotating once after seven minutes.
6. The fish will easily flake when it's done.

Honey Mustard Salmon with Mango Quinoa

Portions Provided: 2 servings
Time Required: 30 minutes
Nutritional Statistics (Each Portion):
3.5 oz. salmon + 2/3 cup quinoa mix:
- Protein Counts: 26.4 grams
- Carbohydrates: 26.6 grams
- Fat Content: 12.2 grams
- Sugars: 12.3 grams
- Dietary Fiber: 3 grams
- Sodium: 281.2 mg
- Calories: 326

Diabetic Exchanges:
- Fruit: ½
- Starch: 1
- Fat 1 ½
- Lean Protein: 3

Essential Ingredients:
- Fresh/frozen salmon fillet - skinless (8 oz./230 g)
- Garlic (1 large clove)
- Olive oil (1 tsp.)
- Mustard - spicy brown (2 tsp.)
- Honey (2 tsp.)
- Unchilled cooked quinoa (.66 or 2/3 cup)
- Frozen - thawed/fresh mango (.5 cup)
- Seeded & finely chopped fresh jalapeño chili pepper (1-2 tbsp)
- Sliced almonds - toasted (1 tbsp.)
- Black pepper and salt (.125 or 1/8 tsp. each)
- Freshly chopped cilantro (2 tbsp.)

Preparation Method:
1. Cook the quinoa beforehand. Chop the mango and jalapenos. Mince the garlic.
2. Thaw the salmon if it is frozen. Rinse the fish and dab it dry using a few paper towels.
3. Whisk the honey, mustard, and garlic in a mixing container. Brush each side of the salmon with the honey mixture.
4. Arrange the salmon on the grill rack (gas or charcoal) and cook using a medium-temperature setting. Cover and grill **till the salmon starts flaking when tested with a fork - flip it one time during grilling time.
5. Meanwhile, combine quinoa with mango, almonds, jalapeño pepper, olive oil, black pepper, and salt. Garnish it using a bit of fresh cilantro. Serve the salmon with a portion of warm quinoa.
6. ** For the fish, cook for four to six minutes per 'each' ½-inch thickness.

Lemon-Herb Salmon with Caponata & Spelt - Diabetic-Approved

Portions Provided: 4 servings
Time Required: 50 minutes
Nutritional Statistics (Each Portion):
4 oz. salmon + ½ cup spelt + 1 cup veggies:
- Protein Counts: 34.8 grams
- Carbohydrates: 41.2 grams
- Fat Content: 17.3 grams
- Sugars: 12.5 grams
- Dietary Fiber: 8.2 grams

- Sodium: 562.1 mg
- Calories: 450
Diabetic Exchanges:
- Lean Protein: 4
- Fat: 2
- Veg: 3
- Starch: 1 1/2

Essential Ingredients:
- Water (2 cups)
- Spelt (.66 or 2/3 cup)
- Eggplant (1 medium)
- Bell pepper (1 red)
- Summer squash (1)
- Onion (1 small)
- Cherry tomatoes (1.5 cups)
- Capers (2 tbsp.)
- Olive oil (3 tbsp.)
- Salt (.75 tsp. divided)
- Black pepper (.5 tsp. divided)
- Honey (2 tsp.)
- Wild salmon (570 g/1.25 lb.)
- Lemon zest (1 tsp.)
- Italian seasoning (.5 tsp.)
- Red-wine vinegar (1 tbsp.)
- Lemon wedges for serving

Preparation Method:
1. Set the oven temperature at 450° Fahrenheit/232° Celsius.
2. Cut the peppers, eggplant, onions, and squash into one-inch cubes.
3. Position racks in the lower and upper 1/3 of the oven.
4. Cover two rimmed baking sheets with foil and a spritz of cooking oil spray.
5. Fill a pot of water. Toss in the spelt and wait for it to boil. Adjust the temperature setting to low - put a top on the cooking pot - simmer till it's tender (½ hour). Drain as needed.
6. Toss eggplant with the squash, bell pepper, tomatoes, and onion with salt (½ tsp.), oil, and pepper (¼ tsp.) in a big mixing container. Divide between the baking trays.
7. Roast, stirring once halfway through the cycle till the veggies are fork-tender and beginning to brown (25 min.). Return them to the bowl.
8. Rinse, chop, and mix in capers, vinegar, and honey.
9. Slice the salmon into four portions and season it using Italian seasoning, lemon zest,

and the rest of the pepper and salt (¼ tsp. each). Arrange them on one of the baking trays.

10. Roast on the lower rack until just cooked through (6-12 min.) depending on thickness.
11. Serve the salmon with the vegetable caponata, farro, and a side of lemon wedges.

Roasted Salmon

Portions Provided: 4 servings
Time Required: 30 minutes
Nutritional Statistics (Each Portion):
- Calories: 251
- Protein Counts: 34 grams
- Carbohydrates: 10 grams (Net: 1 gram)
- Fat Content: 10 grams
- Sugars: 9 grams
- Dietary Fiber: trace grams
- Sodium: 150 mg

Essential Ingredients:
- Wild salmon fillets (4 @ 6 oz./170 g each)
- Black pepper (as desired)
- Garlic cloves (4 cloves)
- Fresh dill (.25 cup)
- Lemon (1)

Preparation Method:
1. Use a nonstick cooking spray to coat a glass baking dish.
2. Warm the oven temperature to reach 400° Fahrenheit/204° Celsius.
3. Cut the lemon into wedges.
4. Add the salmon to the dish and squeeze the lemon over them.
5. Mince the garlic and dill to drizzle over the fish with a sprinkle of black pepper.
6. Bake till the center of the salmon is opaque (20-25 min.).

Roasted Salmon with Olives - Garlic & Tomatoes

Portions Provided: 4 servings
Time Required: 35 minutes
Nutritional Statistics (Each Portion):
- Protein Counts: 29.1 grams
- Carbohydrates: 4.9 grams
- Fat Content: 15.1 grams
- Sugars: 2 grams
- Dietary Fiber: 1.1 grams
- Sodium: 545 mg
- Calories: 276

Essential Ingredients:
- Cherry tomatoes (1 pint)
- Kalamata olives (.25 cup)
- Olive oil (2 tbsp. divided)
- Garlic (4 tsp.)
- Fresh thyme (1 tbsp.)
- Ground pepper & salt - divided (.5 tsp. each)
- Salmon fillet (1.25 lb.)

Preparation Method:
1. Set the oven temperature setting in advance at 400° Fahrenheit/204° Celsius.
2. Slice the tomatoes into halves, mince the garlic, and quarter the olives.
3. Cut the salmon into four servings and chop the thyme.
4. Stir tomatoes, one tablespoon of oil, olives, garlic, thyme, ¼ teaspoon of each - pepper and salt - in a mixing container. Spread the mixture on half of a large rimmed sheet pan.
5. Brush the rest of the oil (1 tbsp.) over the salmon pieces.
6. Mix in the remainder of the salt and pepper (¼ tsp. each) - putting them on one side of the sheet pan.
7. Bake till the tomatoes have broken down, and the salmon is flaky (12-15 min.).
8. Serve the tomato mixture atop the salmon.

Roasted Salmon with Maple Glaze

Portions Provided: 6 servings
Time Required: 45 minutes
Nutritional Statistics (Each Portion):
- Protein Counts: 30 grams
- Carbohydrates: 10 grams
- Fat Content: 10 grams
- Added Sugars: 9 grams
- Dietary Fiber: trace grams
- Sodium: 150 mg
- Calories: 250

Essential Ingredients:
- Maple syrup (.25 cup)
- Garlic clove (1)
- Balsamic vinegar (.25 cup)
- Salmon fillets (2 lb./910 g @ 6 servings)
- Black pepper (.125 tsp.)
- Kosher salt (.25 tsp.)
- For a Garnish: Fresh parsley/mint

Preparation Method:
1. Warm the oven to reach 450° Fahrenheit/232° Celsius.

2. Lightly spritz a baking pan with a tiny bit of cooking oil spray.
3. Mince the garlic and mint/parsley.
4. Use a small saucepan (low-temperature setting) to whisk the maple syrup, garlic, and balsamic vinegar.
5. Warm the mixture till it's heated and remove the pan off of the burner.
6. Pour about ½ of the mixture into a mixing container to use for basting - reserve the rest for later.
7. Use a few paper towels to dab dry the salmon - arrange it skin-side down on the baking tray - brush it using the maple syrup mixture.
8. Bake about ten minutes, baste it again with the syrup - continue baking for five minutes.
9. Continue the process till the fish easily flakes (20-25 min. total).
10. Plate the salmon and dust with a bit of pepper and salt - garnish it with the rest of the syrup mixture. Sprinkle it with fresh mint/parsley to serve.

Roasted Salmon with Smoky Chickpeas & Greens

Portions Provided: 4 servings
Time Required: 40 minutes
Nutritional Statistics (Each Portion):
- Protein Counts: 37 grams
- Carbohydrates: 23.4 grams
- Fat Content: 21.8 grams
- Sugars: 2.2 grams
- Dietary Fiber: 6.4 grams
- Sodium: 556.7 mg
- Calories: 447

Essential Ingredients:
- E.V. olive oil (2 tbsp. - divided)
- Smoked paprika (1 tbsp.)
- Salt - divided (.5 tsp. + a pinch)
- Chickpeas - no-salt (430 g/15 oz. can)
- Buttermilk (.33 cup)
- Mayonnaise (.25 cup)
- Fresh chives or dill - chopped (.25 cup + more for garnishing)
- Garlic powder (.25 tsp.)
- Black pepper - divided (.5 tsp.)
- Water (.25 cup)
- Kale (10 cups - chopped)
- Wild salmon (570 g/1.25 lb.)

Preparation Method:
1. Position racks in the upper third and middle of the oven.
2. Warm the oven to reach 425° Fahrenheit/218° Celsius.
3. Slice the salmon into four portions.
4. Combine oil (1 tbsp.) with paprika and salt (¼ tsp.) in a mixing container.
5. Rinse the chickpeas in a colander and dab dry using a few paper towels. Toss them with the paprika mixture. Scatter the mixture over a rimmed baking tray.
6. Bake the chickpeas on the upper rack - stirring twice (½ hour).
7. Puree buttermilk with mayonnaise, pepper (¼ tsp.), herbs, and garlic powder in a blender till it's creamy smooth.
8. Warm the rest of the oil (1 tbsp.) in a big skillet using a medium-temperature setting. Add kale and cook, occasionally stirring (2 min.).
9. Add water and cook till the kale is tender (5 min./as needed). Remove from the burner and stir in a pinch of salt.
10. Transfer the chickpeas from the oven and scoot them aside in the pan.
11. Arrange the salmon on the other side and season with the rest of the pepper and salt (¼ tsp. each).
12. Bake till the salmon is flaky (5-8 min.).
13. Drizzle the dressing over the salmon, and garnish with additional herbs - serve with the chickpeas and kale as desired.

Salmon & Asparagus with Lemon-Garlic Butter Sauce

Portions Provided: 4 servings
Time Required: 25 minutes
Nutritional Statistics (Each Portion):
One salmon piece + 5 asparagus spears:
- Protein Counts: 25.4 grams
- Carbohydrates: 5.6 grams
- Fat Content: 16.5 grams
- Sugars: 2.2 grams
- Dietary Fiber: 2.5 grams
- Sodium: 350.5 mg

Essential Ingredients:
- Center-cut salmon fillet - preferably wild (1 lb.)
- Trimmed fresh asparagus (1 lb.)
- Salt and black pepper (.5 tsp. each)

- Butter (3 tbsp.)
- Olive oil (1 tbsp.)
- Grated garlic (.5 tbsp.)
- Lemon: juice (1 tbsp.) + grated zest (1 tsp.)
- Also Needed: Large rimmed baking sheet

Preparation Method:
1. Set the oven temperature to reach 375° Fahrenheit/191° Celsius.
2. Prepare the baking tray using a spritz of cooking oil spray.
3. Fillet the fish into four portions.
4. Arrange the asparagus on one side and salmon on the opposite side of the prepared baking tray. Sprinkle them using pepper and salt.
5. Warm the oil with the butter, lemon zest, garlic, and lemon juice in a skillet using a medium-temperature setting till the butter is melted.
6. Drizzle the butter mixture over the asparagus and salmon.
7. Bake till the salmon is thoroughly cooked, and the asparagus is just-tender (12-15 min.). Serve as desired.

Salmon with Cilantro-Pineapple Salsa

Portions Provided: 4 servings
Time Required: 30 minutes
Nutritional Statistics (Each Portion):
- Protein Counts: 23.4 grams
- Carbohydrates: 13.2 grams
- Fat Content: 12.4 grams
- Sugars: 8.6 grams
- Dietary Fiber: 1.9 grams
- Sodium: 218.6 mg
- Calories: 257

Essential Ingredients:
- Skinless salmon fillet - fresh/frozen (1 lb. @ 1-inch thickness)
- Red onion (.25 cup)
- Fresh pineapple (2 cups)
- Green/red bell pepper (.5 cup)
- Lime peel (.5 tsp.)
- Lime juice (3 tbsp. - divided)
- Fresh jalapeño chili pepper (1 small)
- Parsley or cilantro (2 tbsp. - divided)
- Salt (.25 tsp.)
- Chili powder (.5 tsp.)
- Cayenne pepper (1 pinch)
- Lime (4 wedges)
- Torn lettuce (4 leaves)

Preparation Method:
1. If the fish is frozen, it's important to thaw it first. Rinse it and dab it dry using a few paper towels.
2. Chop the pineapple, onion, and bell pepper. Discard the seeds and finely dice the jalapeno. Finely chop the parsley or cilantro. Shred the lime for zest and juice the rest of the lime. Cut another lime into four wedges.
3. Make the salsa by combining the pineapple with red onion, bell pepper, lime juice (2 tbsp.), cilantro/parsley (1 tbsp.), and chili pepper in a mixing container - set it aside.
4. Toss the lime peel with the rest of the lime juice (1 tbsp.), the rest of the cilantro/parsley (1 tbsp.), salt, chili powder, and cayenne pepper in a mixing container. Cover each side of the fish with the mix using a pastry brush.
5. Thoroughly grease a wire grill basket. Arrange the fish in the basket, tucking under any thin edges for an even thickness. Put the basket on the rack (without the dome) to grill over medium coals.
6. Grill till the fish easily flakes, carefully turning once halfway through its grilling cycle (8-12 min.).
7. Slice the fish into four serving-size pieces and serve with a garnish of salsa on a bed of lettuce and a side of lime wedges.

Salmon & Edamame Cakes

Portions Provided: 4 servings
Time Required: 55-60 minutes
Nutritional Statistics (Each Portion):
- Calories: 267
- Protein Counts: 21 grams
- Carbohydrates: 5 grams
- Fat Content: 1 gram
- Dietary Fiber: 1 gram
- Sodium: 166 mg

Essential Ingredients:
- Cooked flaky salmon (2 cups/approx. 13 oz.)
- Egg whites (2 large)
- Panko (Japanese-style breadcrumbs (.25 cup)
- Scallion (1 green & white parts)
- Fresh ginger (1 tbsp.)
- Fresh cilantro (1 tbsp.)
- Thawed frozen edamame (.5 cup)
- Garlic (1 clove)

- Canola oil spray (as needed)
- To Serve: Lime wedges

Preparation Method:

1. Finely chop the scallion and cilantro. Peel and mince the ginger and run the garlic through a press to crush.
2. Prepare a platter with some waxed paper.
3. Combine the panko with the salmon, ginger, egg whites, garlic, cilantro, and scallion in a medium mixing container. Mix in the edamame.
4. Form the mixture into four cakes at 3.5-inches wide. Add to the platter and place them in the refrigerator (15 min. to ½ hr.).
5. Use the cooking spray in a pan, and set the stovetop using the medium-temperature setting. Place the cakes in the pan, cooking for three to four minutes. Flip them over and continue cooking for about three to four additional minutes.
6. Serve piping hot with a lime wedge or two as desired.

Spicy Salmon

Portions Provided: 8 servings
Time Required: 20 minutes
Nutritional Statistics (Each Portion):

- Protein Counts: 20 grams
- Carbohydrates: 5 grams
- Fat Content: 17 grams
- Sugars: 5 grams
- Sodium: 330 mg
- Calories: 256

Essential Ingredients:

- Soy sauce (1 tbsp.)
- Butter (1 tbsp.)
- Olive oil (1 tbsp.)
- Dill weed (.25 tsp.)
- Brown sugar - tightly packed (2 tbsp.)
- Dried tarragon - cayenne - salt (1 dash each)
  Spices to Add at 0.5 tsp each:
- Garlic powder
- Ground mustard
- Paprika
- Pepper
- Salmon fillet (2 lb.)

Preparation Method:

1. Melt the butter. Measure each of the fixings.
2. Combine everything except for the salmon and brush over the salmon.
3. Put the salmon on an oiled grill rack or a

4. lightly oiled baking tray (skin side down).
5. Grill with the lid on using the medium temperature setting. *Option 2*: Broil the fish four inches from the heat source till the salmon just begins to flake easily (10-15 min.). Serve as desired.

Poultry

Balsamic Roasted Chicken

Portions Provided: 8 servings
Time Required: 30-35 minutes
Nutritional Statistics (Each Portion):
- Calories: 364
- Protein Counts: 51 grams
- Carbohydrates: 3 grams
- Fat Content: 13 grams
- Sugars: 3 grams
- Dietary Fiber: trace grams
- Sodium: 257 mg

Essential Ingredients:
- Garlic (1 clove)
- Fresh rosemary (1 tbsp.) or Dried (1 tsp.)
- Olive oil (1 tbsp.)
- Whole chicken (4 lb.)
- Freshly cracked black pepper (.125 or ⅛ tsp.)
- Brown sugar (1 tsp.)
- Fresh rosemary (8 sprigs)
- Balsamic vinegar (.5 cup)

Preparation Method:
1. Mince the garlic and rosemary in a mixing container.
2. Set the oven temperature to 350° Fahrenheit/177° Celsius.
3. Loosen the chicken flesh and rub it with the herbal mixture and oil.
4. Flavor the chicken with pepper and put two sprigs of rosemary into the chicken's cavity.
5. Tie the chicken.
6. Bake the bird for twenty to twenty-five minutes for each pound; approximately an hour and 20 minutes. The temperature of the chicken should be 175°F internally.
7. Saturate the bird with the leftover juices from the pan.
8. Place the chicken onto a platter when browned.
9. Blend the brown sugar and vinegar in a saucepan. Don't boil but heat until warmed.
10. Remove the skin and carve the chicken, topping it with the vinegar mixture. Use the remainder of rosemary sprigs as a garnish.

BBQ Basil Turkey Burgers

Portions Provided: 4 servings
Time Required: 30 minutes

Nutritional Statistics (Each Portion):
- Calories: 315
- Protein Counts: 27 grams
- Carbohydrates: 29 grams
- Fat Content: 11 grams
- Sugars: 8 grams
- Dietary Fiber: 4 grams
- Sodium: 482 mg

Essential Ingredients:
- Lean ground turkey (1 lb.)
- Garlic clove (1)
- Fresh basil (.25 cup)
- BBQ sauce - mesquite smoke-flavor (3 tbsp.)
- Oat bran/quick-cooking oats (2 tbsp.)
- Black pepper (.125 or 1/8 tsp.)
- Garlic salt (.25 tsp.)
- Multigrain/Whole-wheat burger buns - split (4)
  Optional Garnishes:
- Red onion slices- Sliced tomato
- Sliced provolone cheese
- Additional barbecue sauce
- Fresh basil leaves

Preparation Method:
1. Mince the garlic. Combine freshly chopped basil with the barbecue sauce, garlic, oats, pepper, and garlic salt.
2. Mix in the turkey, shaping it into four patties (½-inch-thick). Lightly grease a grill rack.
3. Grill the burgers with the top *on* using the medium-temperature setting until a thermometer reads 165° Fahrenheit/74° Celsius (5-7 min. per side).
4. Slice the buns and grill them using the medium-temperature setting with the cut side down until toasted (30 sec. to 1 min.)
5. Serve the burgers using the toppings of your choice.

Cabbage Lo Mein - Heart Healthy

Portions Provided: 4 servings @ 2 cups each
Time Required: 50 minutes
Nutritional Statistics (Each Portion):
- Protein Counts: 26.1 grams
- Carbohydrates: 26.6 grams (Net: 4.1 grams)
- Fat Content: 23.4 grams
- Sugars: 17.5 grams
- Dietary Fiber: 5 grams
- Sodium: 551.7 mg
- Calories: 414

Essential Ingredients:
- Sesame oil (2 tbsp. + 2 tsp. - divided)
- Soy sauce - reduced-sodium (3 tbsp.)
- Crushed red pepper (.25 tsp.)
- Chicken breast (340 g/12 oz.)
- Lo mein noodles (230 g/8 oz. pkg.)
- Vegetable oil - divided (3 tbsp.)
- Chile-garlic sauce (1 tsp.)
- Mushrooms (140 g/5 oz.)
- Garlic (4 cloves)
- Ginger (2 tbsp.)
- Scallions (1 bunch)
- Snow peas (1 cup)
- Small broccoli florets (2 cups/about 1 big crown)
- Red bell pepper (1)
- Napa cabbage (4.5 cups/half of 1 head)
- Unsalted chicken broth (.75 cup)
- Cornstarch (1 tsp.)

Preparation Method:
1. Thinly slice the mushrooms, peppers, cabbage, and scallions. Mince the garlic and ginger. Break the broccoli into florets. Cut the snow peas into halves.
2. Trim the chicken - removing fat and bones, and cut it into ¼-inch slices.
3. Combine soy sauce with sesame oil (2 tbsp.) and crushed red pepper in a big mixing container. Add chicken, tossing thoroughly to coat, and set it to the side for now.
4. Prepare a big pot of boiling water. Prepare the noodles per their package directions (8-10 min.). Drain, toss them in a big mixing container with the remaining two teaspoons of sesame oil and chili-garlic sauce. Set to the side for now.
5. Warm oil (1 tbsp.) in a big wok/skillet using a med-high temperature setting till it's shimmering.
6. Toss in and sauté the mushrooms till they're tender (4-5 min.).
7. Mix in the ginger, garlic, and scallions - cook until fragrant (1 min.). Scoop it into a mixing container.
8. Add oil (1 tbsp.) to the pan and warm it using the medium-high temperature setting till it's shimmering.
9. Add bell pepper, broccoli, and snow peas. Sauté till they're tender and crispy (2-3 min.).

10. Fold in cabbage and sauté it till it has wilted (2 min.). Scoop it into the bowl with the mushroom mixture.
11. Warm the last one tablespoon of oil in the pan using the med-high temperature setting. Toss in the reserved chicken, leaving the sauce in the bowl. Sauté the chicken till it's done (2-3 min.).
12. Meanwhile, toss the broth and cornstarch with the reserved sauce and mix thoroughly. Pour the sauce into the pan with the chicken to simmer till it's thickened (1-2 min.).
13. Toss the vegetable mixture into the pan to mix.
14. Combine the chicken and veggies in the bowl with the noodles and toss it gently before serving.

Chicken Cutlets & Sun-Dried Tomato Cream Sauce

Portions Provided: 4 servings
Time Required: 20 minutes
Nutritional Statistics (Each Portion):
3 oz chicken + ¼ cup of sauce:
- Protein Counts: 25 grams
- Carbohydrates: 8.4 grams (Net: 5.6 grams)
- Fat Content: 18.9 grams
- Sugars: 1.8 grams
- Dietary Fiber: 1 gram
- Sodium: 249.5 mg
- Calories: 324

Essential Ingredients:
- Chicken cutlets (1 lb.)
- Salt & black pepper (.25 tsp. each - divided)
- Dry white wine (.5 cup)
- Heavy cream (.5 cup)
- Sun-dried tomatoes - oil-packed & slivered (.5 cup + 1 tbsp. oil from the jar)
- Shallots (.5 cup)
- Fresh parsley (2 tbsp.)

Preparation Method:
1. Sprinkle chicken with pepper and salt (⅛ tsp. each).
2. Warm the oil (from the sun-dried tomato) in a big skillet using a medium-temperature setting on the stovetop.
3. Toss the chicken into the pan and simmer - flipping it once till it's nicely browned and it reaches an internal temp of 165°

Fahrenheit/74° Celsius (6 min. total). Plate the chicken.

4. Finely chop and add the shallots and tomatoes to the skillet. Simmer it for one minute. Adjust the temperature setting to reach high - stir in the wine. Simmer while scraping the browned bits till the liquid has mostly evaporated (2 min.).

5. Lower the temperature setting to medium and mix in any accumulated juices from the chicken, the cream, and the rest of the pepper and salt (⅛ tsp. each). Simmer the mixture for about two minutes.

6. Scoop the chicken into the skillet with the sauce to cover - garnishing it using a portion of freshly chopped parsley to serve.

Chicken Fajitas - Party Pack

Portions Provided: 12 servings
Time Required: 35 minutes
Nutritional Statistics (Each Portion):
- Protein Counts: 30 grams
- Carbohydrates: 16 grams (Net: 6 grams)
- Fat Content: 4 grams
- Dietary Fiber: 10 grams
- Sodium: 380 mg
- Calories: 220

Essential Ingredients:
- Lime juice (.25 cup)
- Garlic (1-2 cloves)
- Ground cumin (.5 tsp.)
- Chili powder (1 tsp.)
- Chicken breasts (3 lb./1.4 kg.)
- Large onion (1)
- Red & green sweet bell pepper (half of 1 each)
- Low-fat - whole-wheat (12 tortillas @ 8-inch/20-cm each)
- Salsa (.5 cup)
- Cheddar cheese - low-fat - shredded (.5 cup)
- Sour cream - fat-free (.5 cup)

Preparation Method:
1. Mince the garlic. Combine the first four ingredients (garlic, lime juice, cumin, and chili powder) in a large mixing container.

2. Prepare the chicken removing all skin and bones, cutting it into ¼-inch strips. Fold in the sliced chicken - stirring till it's thoroughly covered. Marinate for 15 minutes.

3. Prepare the chicken on a grill or a skillet on the stovetop till it's done - not pink (3 min.).

4. Mince and stir in peppers and onions - sauté till they're as desired. Scatter the mixture over the tortillas.

5. Garnish them using salsa (2 tsp.), a portion of sour cream, and shredded cheese (3-5 min.).

6. Roll them up and serve.

Chicken Souvlaki Kebabs & Mediterranean Couscous

Portions Provided: 4 servings
Time Required: 2 hours 20 minutes
Nutritional Statistics (Each Portion):
Two kabobs + 3/4 cup of couscous:
- Protein Counts: 32.1 grams
- Carbohydrates: 27.7 grams
- Fat Content: 9.4 grams
- Sugars: 6.4 grams
- Dietary Fiber: 2.3 grams
- Sodium: 360: mg
- Calories: 332
  Diabetic Exchanges:
- Fat: ½
- Lean Protein: 3 ½
- Starch: 1
- Vegetable: 2

Essential Ingredients:
  The Kabobs:
- Chicken breast halves (1 lb.)
- Fennel (1 cup)
- Dry white wine (.33 cup)
- Lemon juice (.25 cup)
- Canola oil (3 tbsp.)
- Garlic (4 cloves)
- Dried oregano (2 tsp. - crushed)
- Salt (.5 tsp.)
- Black pepper (.25 tsp.)
- Lemon wedges
  The Couscous:
- Olive oil (1 tsp.)
- Israeli (large pearl) couscous (.5 cup)
- Water (1 cup)
- Snipped dried tomatoes (not oil-packed (.5 cup)
- Red sweet pepper (.75 cup)
- Cucumber (.5 cup)
- Red onion (.5 cup)
- Plain fat-free Greek yogurt (.33 cup)
- Fresh basil leaves (.25 cup)
- Fresh parsley (.25 cup)
- Lemon juice (1 tbsp.)
- Black pepper & salt (.25 tsp. each)
- Also Needed: Eight 10-12-inch skewers

Preparation Method:

1. Trim the chicken removing all bones and fat. Slice them into ½-inch strips.
2. Chop the sweet pepper, red onion, and cucumber. Trim the parsley and chop it with the basil.
3. Slice the fennel, saving the leaves if desired. Mince the garlic and crush the oregano.
4. Toss the prepared chicken and fennel in a zipper-type plastic bag set in a shallow dish.
5. Prepare the marinade in a mixing container by mixing the lemon juice with the wine, oil, oregano, garlic, pepper, and salt.
6. Scoop out ¼ cup of the marinade and reserve it for later.
7. Dump the rest of the marinade over the chicken and close the bag to cover it with its marinade.
8. Marinate in the fridge for 1.5 hours, turning the bag once.
9. Meanwhile, if using wooden skewers, soak the skewers in water for ½ hour.
10. Drain the chicken - trash the fennel and marinade.
11. Thread chicken onto skewers. Grill the chicken with the lid on/covered using the med-high temperature setting till the chicken is done (not pink), turning once (6-8 min.).
12. Remove the skewered chicken from the grill and brush with the reserved marinade (¼ cup).
13. Prepare couscous in a small saucepan. Warm olive oil (1 tsp.) using the medium-temperature setting.
14. Add the couscous (½ cup) and simmer till it's lightly browned (4 min.). Add one cup of water, wait for it to boil, and lower the temperature setting.
15. Simmer it with a top on for about ten minutes or till the couscous is tender and liquid is absorbed.
16. Mix in the dried tomatoes (½ cup) during the last five minutes - cool.
17. Scoop the couscous into a big mixing container with the red sweet pepper (¾ cup), ½ cup each of the cucumber and c red onion), Greek yogurt (1/3 cup), 1/4 cup each of the basil leaves and parsley, lemon

juice (1 tbsp.), and 1/4 teaspoon each of the black pepper and salt.
18. Serve and enjoy the kebabs with a portion of the couscous, lemon wedges, and fennel leaves.

Chicken-Spaghetti Squash Bake

Portions Provided: 8 servings
Time Required: 1 hour 40 minutes
Nutritional Statistics (Each Portion):

- Protein Counts: 25.4 grams
- Carbohydrates: 18.5 grams
- Fat Content: 11.5 grams
- Sugars: 6.1 grams
- Dietary Fiber: 4.6 grams
- Sodium: 493.5 mg
- Calories: 273

Essential Ingredients:

- Broccoli florets (4 cups)
- Spaghetti squash (1 medium/3 lb./1.4 kg.)
- Canola oil (1 tbsp.)
- Mushrooms (10 oz./280 g pkg.)
- Onion - finely chopped (1 medium)
- Garlic (2 cloves)
- Dried thyme (.5 tsp.)
- Ground pepper (.5 tsp.)
- Condensed cream of mushroom soup - ex. Campbell's 25% Less-Sodium (2 - 10 oz./280 g cans)
- Chicken breasts (680 g/1.5 lb.)
- Cheddar shredded cheese - extra-sharp (.5 cup)
- Also Needed: Baking dishes or foil pans (2 @ 8-inch/20-cm square each)

Preparation Method:

1. Set the oven temperature to reach 375° Fahrenheit/191° Celsius.
2. Spray the baking dishes with a tiny bit of cooking oil spray.
3. Slice the squash in half and remove its seeds. Place it (sliced side facing downward - uncovered) into a microwave-safe dish with water (2 tbsp.).
4. Set it on high and microwave till the flesh is easily scraped away using a fork (10-12 min.). Scrape the strands into a holding container and place them to the side for now.
5. Put the broccoli florets in the same microwaveable dish with water (1 tbsp.) and cover with a paper towel or layer of plastic. Microwave them using the high setting till

they're tender (2-3 min.). Empty the broccoli into a colander, setting them to the side to cool.

6. Warm oil in a big skillet using a med-high temperature setting. Slice and toss in the mushrooms to sauté till they've released their juices (8 min.).

7. Chop and add the onion. Sauté till the mushrooms are lightly browned, and the onions are tender (8 min.).

8. Chop or mince and mix in the garlic, thyme, and pepper - sauté them for about ½ minute and toss for another ½ minute or so. Stir in soup (*don't dilute* with water) and wait till it's thoroughly heated.

9. Trim the chicken - discarding its fat and bones. Chop it into one-inch chunks.

10. Mix in the prepared chicken and the reserved broccoli and squash, tossing to thoroughly mix.

11. Portion the mixture into the baking dishes with ¼ cup of cheddar. Cover one using a layer of foil and label if you're prepping them. Freeze one casserole for up to one month.

12. Bake the remaining casserole until bubbling (25 min.). Remove the cover to continue baking till it's lightly browned along the edges (10-15 min.) Wait for about ten minutes before serving.

13. Meal Prep Tips: This double-batch recipe makes one casserole for tonight and one to freeze for up to one month (see step six).

14. At mealtime, put the package in the refrigerator compartment - overnight. Spoon off any liquid that has accumulated in the pan. Bake as directed in step seven.

Chicken & Spinach Skillet Pasta with Lemon & Parmesan

Portions Provided: 4 servings @ 2 cups each
Time Required: 25 minutes
Nutritional Statistics (Each Portion):
- Protein Counts: 28.7 grams
- Carbohydrates: 24.9 grams
- Fat Content: 12.3 grams
- Sugars: 1.1 grams
- Dietary Fiber: 2 grams
- Sodium: 499.2 mg
- Calories: 335

Essential Ingredients:
- Olive oil (2 tbsp.)
- G. F. penne pasta/whole-wheat penne pasta (8 oz./230 g)
- Chicken breast or thighs (1 lb./450 g)
- Salt (.5 tsp.)
- Black pepper (.25 tsp.)
- Garlic (4 cloves)
- Dry white wine (.5 cup)
- Juice and zest (1 lemon)
- Freshly chopped spinach (10 cups)
- Parmesan cheese - grated (4 tbsp. divided)
- Suggested: Large - high-sided skillet

Preparation Method:
1. Prepare the pasta per its package instructions. Drain it into a colander and set them to the side.
2. Warm oil in the skillet using a med-high temperature setting.
3. Trim the skin and bones from the chicken, cutting it into bite-sized chunks. Toss it into the pan with pepper and salt. Cook till it is just cooked through (5-7 min.).
4. Mince and toss in the garlic - sauté it till it's fragrant (1 min.).
5. Stir in lemon juice, wine, and the zested lemon - wait for it to boil.
6. Transfer the pan from the hot burner.
7. Stir in the cooked pasta and spinach.
8. Put a lid on the pot and wait till the spinach is wilted.
9. Portion it into four plates with a garnish of parmesan to serve.

Chicken - Spring Pea & Farro Risotto with Lemon

Portions Provided: 2 servings
Time Required: 45 minutes
Nutritional Statistics (Each Portion):
4 oz. chicken + ¾ cup risotto:
- Protein Counts: 36.4 grams
- Carbohydrates: 34.6 grams
- Fat Content: 8.4 grams
- Sugars: 4.2 grams
- Dietary Fiber: 4.6 grams
- Sodium: 574.8 mg
- Calories: 371

Diabetic Exchanges:
- Vegetable: 1
- Starch: 2

- Lean Protein: 4

Essential Ingredients:
- Chicken broth - l.s. (1 cup)
- Water (.5 cup)
- Light butter with canola oil (4 tsp.)
- Shallots (.25 cup)
- Fresh mushrooms (1.25 cups)
- Semi-pearled farro (6 tbsp.)
- Garlic (2 cloves minced)
- Fresh/frozen-thawed peas (.25 cup)
- Lemon-pepper seasoning- salt-free (.5 tsp.)
- Chicken breast (8 oz.)
- Cooking oil spray (as needed)
- Fresh parmesan cheese (2 tbsp. - grated)
- Finely shredded lemon peel (.5 tsp. + 1 twist)
- Freshly snipped thyme (1 tsp.)

Preparation Method:
1. Trim the chicken, removing all bones and skin fat. Slice it in half - horizontally.
2. Combine broth and the water in a saucepan and warm it using the high-temperature setting - not to boiling. Reduce the temperature to low and keep warm.
3. Prepare a saucepan using the medium-temperature setting to melt three teaspoons of butter.
4. Quarter and add mushrooms and finely chop the shallots; toss them into the pan to cook till they're tender (3-5 min.).
5. Mince and toss in the garlic and farro to sauté for five minutes - frequently stirring. Adjust the setting to medium-low.
6. Carefully add the warm broth mixture (½ cup), stirring to loosen brown bits from the saucepan's bottom. Once it's boiling, adjust the temperature to low.
7. Simmer, uncovered until the farro has absorbed the liquid (6-7 min.).
8. Add another ½ cup portion of the broth mixture. Simmer for another six to seven minutes until the farro has absorbed the liquid.
9. Continue adding broth mixture, a half cup at a time, and simmering till all of the liquid has been absorbed before adding more, often stirring (25-30 min. total.) Stir the peas in with the final addition of the broth mixture. In the meantime, sprinkle lemon-pepper seasoning over the chicken and rub it in thoroughly.
10. Spray a big skillet with a spritz of cooking oil spray - warming using the medium temperature setting.
11. Add the chicken and cook until it's done - not pink in the center (6 min.) and it has reached an internal temp of 165° Fahrenheit/74° Celsius), flipping it one time about halfway through cooking time. Cut the chicken into ½-inch-thick slices.
12. Once the farro is thoroughly cooked and slightly firm, transfer the pan from the burner and mix in the rest of the butter (1 tsp.), thyme, the parmesan, and the lemon peel (½ tsp.).
13. Portion the farro mixture into two serving dishes, garnish using the slices of chicken, and more lemon peel as desired.

Chicken Stir-Fry with Basil - Eggplant & Ginger

Portions Provided: 4 servings @ 2 cups each
Time Required: 25 minutes
Nutritional Statistics (Each Portion):
- Protein Counts: 29 grams
- Carbohydrates: 14 grams (Net: 3 grams)
- Fat Content: 10 grams
- Sugars: 7 grams
- Dietary Fiber: 4 grams
- Sodium: 395 mg
- Calories: 262

Essential Ingredients:
- Freshly chopped mint (3 tbsp.)
- Coarsely chopped fresh basil (.25 cup)
- Chicken stock or broth - low-sodium (.75 cup - divided)
- Spring onions - green tops too (3 total - 2 coarsely chopped & 1 thinly sliced)
- Fresh ginger (1 tbsp.)
- Garlic cloves (2)
- Eggplant (1 small/about 4 cups)
- Yellow onion (1 @ about 0.5 cup)
- Yellow & red bell pepper (1 of each)
- Chicken breasts (1 lb.)
- Olive oil (2 tbsp. - divided)
- Soy sauce - l.s. (2 tbsp.)

Preparation Method:
1. Remove the peeling from the eggplant and dice it.
2. Slice and discard the seeds from the peppers and julienne them.

3. Load a food processor to mix the basil with the mint, stock (¼ cup), roughly chopped garlic, ginger, and green onions. Combine till the mixture is minced - not pureed. Put it to the side for now.

4. Use a big skillet to warm the olive oil (1 tbsp.) using a med-high temperature setting.

5. Peel, dice, and mix in the eggplant, bell peppers, and onion.

6. Sauté them till the veggies are tender (8 min.). Transfer them into a storage container and cover them with a foil tent or towel to keep the mixture warm.

7. Add the remainder of the oil (1 tbsp.) into the pan and warm it using the med-high temperature setting.

8. Mix in the basil mixture - sauté it one minute.

9. Trim the bones and fat from the chicken. Cut it into strips ½-inch wide & 2 inches long. Toss the chicken strips with soy sauce.

10. Sauté the mixture till the chicken is almost done and opaque (2 min.).

11. Add the remaining stock (½ cup). Wait for it to boil.

12. Return the eggplant mixture to the pan - stirring till it's thoroughly heated (3 min.).

13. Transfer it to a plate and garnish using the sliced green onion. Serve and enjoy it promptly for the most flavorful results.

Chicken & Vegetable Penne with Parsley-Walnut Pesto

Portions Provided: 4 servings @ 2 cups each
Time Required: 30 minutes
Nutritional Statistics (Each Portion):
- Protein Counts: 31.4 grams
- Carbohydrates: 43.4 grams
- Fat Content: 26.6 grams
- Sugars: 4.8 grams
- Dietary Fiber: 8.6 grams
- Sodium: 556.6 mg
- Calories: 514

Essential Ingredients:
- Walnuts (.75 cup)
- Parsley leaves - lightly packed (1 cup)
- Garlic (2 cloves)
- Black pepper and salt (1/8 tsp. up to .5 tsp. - to taste)
- Olive oil (2 tbsp.)
- Parmesan cheese (⅓ cup grated)
- Cooked chicken breast - sliced or shredded (230 g/8 oz.)
- Whole-wheat penne/fusilli pasta (170 g/6 oz./1.75 cups)
- Green beans (8 oz./2 cups)
- Cauliflower florets (8 oz.)

Preparation Method:
1. Prepare a big pot of boiling water.
2. Chop and toss the walnuts into a container and microwave using the high setting till it's fragrant and lightly toasted (2-2.5 min.). OR - toast the walnuts in a dry skillet using a med-low temperature setting, continuously stir till it's fragrant (2-3 min.).
3. Transfer the nuts onto a plate and let cool - set aside ¼ of a cup of them for topping.
4. Peel and crush the garlic. Trim and halve the green beans.
5. Combine the remaining ½ of a cup of walnuts with garlic, pepper, salt, and parsley in a food processor. Work the mixture till the nuts are ground.
6. Slowly add in the oil through the "feed tube" with the motor running. Add the parmesan pulsing to mix. Scrape the pesto into a big mixing container and add the chicken.
7. Prepare the pasta in boiling water (4 min.). Toss in the cauliflower and green beans. Place a top on the cooking pot. Simmer till the pasta is al dente, and the veggies are fork tender (5-7 min.).
8. Before draining, remove ¾ of a cup of the cooking water to use later.
9. Stir the reserved water into the pesto-chicken mixture to warm it slightly.
10. Dump the pasta and veggies into a colander to drain. Thoroughly toss them into the pesto-chicken mixture.
11. Divide into four pasta bowls and top each portion using one tablespoon of the reserved walnuts and serve.

Cinnamon Carrots & Chicken Sheet Pan Favorite - Meal Prep

Portions Provided: 4 servings

Time Required: 1 hour 5 minutes
Nutritional Statistics (Each Portion):
- Protein Counts: 26 grams
- Carbohydrates: 24 grams
- Fat Content: 3 grams
- Sugars: 6 grams
- Dietary Fiber: 5 grams
- Sodium: 237 mg
- Calories: 234

Essential Ingredients:
- Frozen, sliced carrots (10 oz./283.5 pkg.)
- Cut - frozen sweet potatoes (10 oz./283.5 pkg.)
- Frozen chicken breasts (2 breasts or 1 lb.)
- Ground cinnamon (1 tsp.)
- Ground cloves (.25 tsp.)
- Dried parsley (1 tbsp.)
- Ground ginger (.25 tsp.)
- Oil (about 1/3 cup for cooking)
- Also Needed: 1-gallon freezer bag - zipper-top

Preparation Method:
1. Combine each of the fixings in the freezer bag (except the oil) - tossing to combine.
2. Store in the freezer for about four months. When ready to prepare, warm the oven to 350° Fahrenheit/177° Celsius.
3. Open the bag and pour in the oil. Close it and toss it thoroughly to coat.
4. Pour the contents of the bag out onto a sheet pan with edges.
5. Bake for one hour or until the chicken reaches at least 165° Fahrenheit/74° Celsius on a meat thermometer.
6. Cool slightly to serve.

Creamy Chicken & Mushrooms

Portions Provided: 4 servings
Time Required: 30 minutes
Nutritional Statistics (Each Portion):
- Protein Counts: 29.1 grams
- Carbohydrates: 4.2 grams
- Fat Content: 19.6 grams
- Sugars: 2.5 grams
- Dietary Fiber: 0.8 grams
- Sodium: 329.2 mg
- Calories: 325

Essential Ingredients:
- Chicken cutlets (4 @ 5 oz./140 g each)
- Mixed mushrooms (4 cups - sliced if needed)
- Dry white wine (.5 cup)
- Heavy cream (.5 cup)
- Fresh parsley (2 tbsp.)

Preparation Method:
1. Season the chicken using pepper and kosher salt (¼ tsp. each).
2. Add a tablespoon of oil to a big skillet to warm using a medium-temperature setting. Add and fry the chicken till it's browned and just cooked through (7-10 min.). Transfer it onto a plate.
3. Add oil (1 tbsp.) and mushrooms to the skillet to sauté till the liquid has evaporated (4 min.).
4. Adjust the temperature setting to high, pour in the wine, and simmer till it has mostly evaporated (4 min.).
5. Lower the temperature setting to medium - stir any accumulated juice from the chicken, the cream, pepper, and salt (¼ tsp. each).
6. Scoop the chicken back into the pan and mix it thoroughly with the sauce.
7. Serve the saucy chicken. Chop and sprinkle with parsley.

Easy Low-Sodium Chicken Breast

Portions Provided: 2 servings
Time Required: 17 minutes
Nutritional Statistics (Each Portion):
- Protein Counts: 13 grams
- Carbohydrates: <1 gram
- Fat Content: 3 grams
- Dietary Fiber: -0- grams
- Sodium: 70 mg
- Calories: 80

Essential Ingredients:
- Olive oil (1 tsp.)
- Chicken breasts (2)
- Vinegar - white wine suggested (2 tbsp.)
- Onion powder (.5 tsp.)
- Parsley flakes (1 tsp.)
- Garlic powder (.25 tsp.)
- Black pepper (.5 tsp.)

Preparation Method:
1. Trim the chicken of all fat and bones, then pound it to reach a ½-inch to ¾-inch thickness.
2. Load a zipper-type plastic bag with the rest of the fixings and shake the bag. Add the chicken to the marinade and pop it into the refrigerator to marinate for at least one hour.

3. Spray a grill pan using a spritz of cooking oil spray - set the temperature setting to high and let it heat.

4. Set the oven temperature to 375° Fahrenheit/191° Celsius.

5. When the grill pan is heated, add the chicken using a pair of tongs. Don't move or touch it for "exactly 1½ minutes"; and flip it over to grill the other side for "exactly 1½ minutes".

6. Bake it all in the oven (8-10 min.) till its internal temp is 165° Fahrenheit/74° Celsius.

7. Plate it and wait for about five minutes before serving.

Greek Chicken with Roasted Spring Vegetables & Lemon Vinaigrette

Portions Provided: 4 servings
Time Required: 50 minutes
Nutritional Statistics (Each Portion):
- Protein Counts: 29.5 grams
- Carbohydrates: 12.1 grams
- Fat Content: 15.1 grams
- Sugars: 3.6 grams
- Dietary Fiber: 1.6 grams
- Sodium: 431.5 mg
- Calories: 306

Essential Ingredients:
   The Vinaigrette:
- Olive oil (1 tbsp.)
- Lemon (1)
- Feta cheese - crumbled (1 tbsp.)
- Honey (.5 tsp.)
   The Greek Chicken & Veggies:
- Chicken breast halves - cut in half lengthwise (2 @ 230 g/8 oz. each)
- Light mayonnaise (.25 cup)
- Garlic (6 minced cloves)
- Panko breadcrumbs (.5 cup)
- Parmesan cheese - grated (3 tbsp.)
- Kosher salt & black pepper (.5 tsp. each)
- Nonstick olive oil cooking spray (as needed)
- Asparagus (2 cups @ 1-inch/3-cm pieces)
- Fresh cremini mushrooms - sliced (1.5 cups)
- Grape tomatoes (1.5 cups)
- Olive oil (1 tbsp.)
- Fresh dill
- Also Needed: 15x10-inch/38x25-cm baking pan

Preparation Method:
1. Prepare the lemon for juice (1 tbsp.) and zest (.5 tsp.). Whisk the lemon zest and juice with the remainder of the fixings in a mixing container - set aside.

2. Prepare chicken and vegetables: Put the baking pan in the oven and set the oven temperature setting to reach 475° Fahrenheit/246° Celsius.

3. Trim the chicken and remove all bones and fat.

4. Use a meat mallet to flatten the chicken between two plastic wrap pieces until it reaches a ½-inch thickness.

5. Toss the chicken in a mixing container with the mayo and garlic cloves (2) - stirring to cover thoroughly.

6. In a shallow dish, toss the breadcrumbs with the cheese and ¼ of a teaspoon of salt and pepper.

7. Dredge the chicken through crumb mixture, turning to cover. Lightly coat the tops of the chicken with a spritz of cooking oil spray.

8. Slice the tomatoes into halves. Use a big container to combine the asparagus, tomatoes, mushrooms, oil, the rest of the garlic cloves (4) with pepper and salt (¼ of a tsp. each).

9. Arrange the chicken in one end of the heated pan and put the asparagus mixture in the opposite end of the pan.

10. Roast until chicken is done for 18-20 minutes (165° Fahrenheit/74° Celsius) and veggies are fork-tender.

11. Drizzle the chicken and vegetables with vinaigrette and dusting of dill.

Greek Meatball Mezze Bowls - Meal Prep

Portions Provided: 4 servings @ 2.5 cups each
Time Required: 35 minutes
Nutritional Statistics (Each Portion):
- Protein Counts: 32.4 grams
- Carbohydrates: 29.3 grams
- Fat Content: 17.2 grams
- Sugars: 5.3 grams
- Dietary Fiber: 5.6 grams
- Sodium: 542.5 mg
- Calories: 392

Essential Ingredients:

- Frozen spinach (1 cup)
- Ground turkey - 93%-lean (1 lb.)
- Feta cheese - crumbled (.5 cup)
- Dried oregano (.5 tsp.)
- Garlic powder (.5 tsp.)
- Black pepper and salt (⅜ tsp. divided)
- Cooked quinoa - cooled (2 cups)
- Lemon juice (2 tbsp.)
- Olive oil (1 tbsp.
- Mint (3 tbsp.)
- Fresh parsley (.5 cup)
- Sliced cucumber (2 cups)
- Cherry tomatoes (1 pint)
- Tzatziki (.25 cup)

Preparation Method:

1. Before you begin, chop the parsley and mint.
2. Thaw and squeeze excess moisture from spinach - chop it.
3. Toss the spinach with feta, turkey, oregano, garlic powder, pepper & salt (⅛ tsp. each) in a mixing container till thoroughly combined.
4. Shape it into twelve meatballs. Warm a big skillet using a medium-temperature setting. Lightly cover using a spritz of cooking spray.
5. If needed, work in batches - place the meatballs in the skillet to cook till they're nicely browned with an internal temperature @ 165° Fahrenheit/74° Celsius (10-12 min.).
6. Put the meatballs aside to cool.
7. Combine quinoa with oil, parsley, lemon juice, mint, and the rest of the pepper and salt in a medium mixing container.
8. Portion it into four individual-serving containers with lids.
9. Top each with three meatballs, cucumbers, and cherry tomatoes (½ cup each).
10. Pour the tzatziki into four separate containers. Close the containers and pop them into the fridge to chill. Enjoy them for up to four days. Before serving, place the meatballs into a microwave-safe container. Warm them till they're steaming. Serve as desired.

Greek Turkey Burgers with Spinach - Feta & Tzatziki

Portions Provided: 4 servings
Time Required: 30 minutes
Nutritional Statistics (Each Portion):

- Protein Counts: 30 grams
- Carbohydrates: 28.5 grams
- Fat Content: 17 grams
- Sugars: 5.4 grams
- Dietary Fiber: 4.9 grams
- Sodium: 677.5 mg
- Calories: 376

Essential Ingredients:

- Frozen chopped spinach (1 cup)
- Ground turkey - 93% lean (1 lb.)
- Feta cheese - crumbled (.5 cup)
- Garlic powder (.5 tsp.)
- Oregano - dried (.5 tsp.)
- Salt and black pepper (.25 tsp. each)
- Small burger buns - whole-wheat (4 split)
- Tzatziki (4 tbsp.)
- Cucumber (12 slices)
- Red onions (8 thick rings @ about .25-inches)

Preparation Method:

1. Preheat the grill using a med-high temperature setting. Oil the grill rack.
2. Thaw and squeeze excess moisture from spinach.
3. Toss the spinach with feta, turkey, garlic powder, oregano, pepper, and salt in a mixing container till thoroughly combined.
4. Shape the mixture into four (four-inch) patties.
5. Grill the patties until done - the pink center is gone (5-6 min. each side reaching an internal temp of 165° Fahrenheit/74° Celsius.).
6. Place the burgers on the buns with tzatziki (1 tbsp.), three cucumber slices, and two onion rings.

Harissa Chicken & Vegetables Sheet-Pan

Portions Provided: 4 servings
Time Required: 45 minutes
Nutritional Statistics (Each Portion):
1.25 cups veggies + 3 oz. chicken & 2 tbsp. of sauce:

- Protein Counts: 31.8 grams
- Carbohydrates: 15.6 grams
- Fat Content: 13.9 grams

- Sugars: 9 grams
- Dietary Fiber: 4.7 grams
- Sodium: 460.7 mg
- Calories: 314

Essential Ingredients:

- Cauliflower florets (4 cups)
- Orange/red/yellow bell peppers or a mix (4 cups)
- Olive oil (3 tbsp. divided)
- Kosher salt (.25 tsp. + .5 tsp. divided)
- Harissa paste (2 tsp + 0.5 tsp. divided)
- Brown sugar (1 tsp.)
- Garlic (1 minced clove)
- Chicken breasts (2 @ 8-ounce each)
- Plain Greek yogurt (.5 cup)
- Lemon (1): Zest (1 tsp.) & juice (2 tbsp.)
- Ground pepper (.125 or ⅛ tsp.)

Preparation Method:

1. Set the oven temperature setting at 400° Fahrenheit/204° Celsius.
2. Toss sliced peppers and cauliflower with oil (2 tbsp.) and salt (¼ tsp.) in a big mixing container. Scoop them into a big rimmed baking tray to roast (15 min.).
3. Trim the chicken to remove all fat and bones.
4. Meanwhile, combine two teaspoons of harissa paste with the garlic, brown sugar, the remaining oil (1 tbsp.), and salt (½ tsp.) in a mixing container. Rub the chicken thoroughly using the harissa mixture.
5. Stir the veggies and toss the chicken into the pan.
6. Roast till it reaches an internal temp of 165° Fahrenheit/74° Celsius (20 min.).
7. Mix the lemon zest and juice with the yogurt rest of the harissa paste (½ tsp.), parsley, and pepper in a mixing container - drizzle it over the chicken and veggies, or serve on the side for dipping.

Lemon-Thyme Roasted Chicken with Fingerlings

Portions Provided: 4 servings
Time Required: 30 minutes
Nutritional Statistics (Each Portion):
¾ cup of potatoes + 1 breast half:

- Protein Counts: 28.6 grams
- Carbohydrates: 20.7 grams
- Fat Content: 6 grams
- Sugars: 1 gram

- Fiber: 2.6 grams
- Sodium: 307.2 mg
- Calories: 255
  Diabetic Exchanges:
- Lean Meat: 3 ½
- Starch 1 ½

Essential Ingredients:

- Olive or canola oil (4 tsp. divided)
- Black pepper (.25 tsp.)
- Kosher salt (.5 tsp.) or regular salt (.25 tsp.)
- Crushed dried thyme (1 tsp. divided)
- Fingerling potatoes or tiny new red or white potatoes (1 lb.)
- Chicken breast halves (4 small @ 1-1.25 lb. total)
- Garlic (2 cloves)
- Lemon (1 thinly sliced)

Preparation Method:

1. Slice the potatoes into halves - lengthwise.
2. Use a big skillet to warm two teaspoons of oil using the medium-temperature setting. Sprinkle in thyme (½ tsp.), pepper, and salt into the oil. Add potatoes - tossing till they're thoroughly covered.
3. Place a top on the pan, stir, and sauté them for 12 minutes.
4. Stir the potatoes - pushing them to one side of the skillet. Pour in the rest of the oil (2 tsp.). Trim the chicken to remove all fat and bones.
5. Place the breast halves on the other side of the skillet.
6. Cook with the top off for five minutes. Flip the chicken.
7. Mince and spread garlic over the halves and sprinkle with the rest of the thyme (½ tsp.).
8. Arrange lemon slices over the chicken. Cover and cook till it's done - not pink - (7-10 min.) or reaches an internal temp of 170° Fahrenheit/77° Celsius. The potatoes should also be tender.

Mediterranean Chicken Quinoa Bowls

½ cup quinoa + 3 oz. chicken + 1/4 cup of sauce:
Portions Provided: servings
Time Required: 30 minutes
Nutritional Statistics (Each Portion):

- Protein Counts: 34.1 grams
- Carbohydrates: 31.2 grams
- Fat Content: 26.9 grams
- Fiber: 4.2 grams

- Sugars: 2.5 grams
- Sodium: 683.5 mg
- Calories: 519

Essential Ingredients:
- Chicken breasts (1 lb./450 g)
- Ground pepper & salt (.25 tsp. each)
- Roasted red peppers (7 oz./200 g jar)
- Slivered almonds (.25 cup)
- Olive oil - divided (4 tbsp.)
- Garlic clove (1 small) crushed
- Ground cumin (.5 tsp.)
- Paprika (1 tsp.)
- Red pepper - crushed (.25 tsp. - optional)
- Cooked quinoa (2 cups)
- Kalamata olives - pitted & chopped (.25 cup)
- Red onion - finely chopped (.25 cup)
- Cucumber - diced (1 cup)
- Feta cheese - crumbled (.25 cup)
- Fresh parsley (2 tbsp.)

Preparation Method:
1. Position a rack in the upper third of the oven.
2. Warm the broiler unit using the high-temperature setting.
3. Cover a rimmed baking tray using a foil layer.
4. Trim the chicken and remove the bones and skin. Dust it using a bit of pepper and salt. Arrange it on the baking tray. Broil, turning once till its internal temp reaches 165° Fahrenheit/74° Celsius (14-18 min.).
5. Place the chicken on a chopping block and shred or slice it.
6. Finely chop the parsley. Rinse and add the peppers, almonds, oil (2 tbsp.), garlic, cumin, crushed red pepper, and paprika into a food processor and puree.
7. Chop and combine the olives with the quinoa, red onion, and the rest of the oil (2 tbsp.) into a medium mixing container.
8. To serve, portion the quinoa mixture into four serving bowls and top with chicken, cucumber, and pepper sauce. Dust them using a bit of feta and parsley.

Mushroom-Swiss Turkey Burgers

Portions Provided: 4 servings **Time Required:** 30 minutes

Nutritional Statistics (Each Portion):
- Protein Counts: 33.5 grams
- Total Carbs: 10.3 grams (Net: 1.4 grams)
- Fat Content: 18.4 grams
- Dietary Fiber: 2.9 grams
- Sugars: 6 grams
- Sodium: 503.5 mg
- Calories: 332

Essential Ingredients:
- Olive oil (2 tbsp.)
- Garlic (1 clove)
- Ground pepper (.75 tsp. divided)
- Salt (.5 tsp. divided)
- Portobello mushroom caps (8)
- Lean ground turkey (1 lb.)
- Dijon mustard (1 tsp.)
- Worcestershire sauce - G.F. (2 tsp.)
- Swiss cheese (4 slices)
- Tomato (1 small)
- Baby arugula (3 cups)

Preparation Method:
1. Warm a grill using a med-high temperature setting (400° Fahrenheit/204° Celsius to 450° Fahrenheit/232° Celsius).
2. Discard the gills and stems from the mushrooms.
3. Mince and stir the garlic with the oil, pepper, and salt (¼ tsp. each) in a small mixing container. Brush the mushroom caps with the oil mixture - set aside to marinate for ten minutes (the countertop if fine).
4. Meanwhile, combine the turkey with the mustard, Worcestershire, and rest of the pepper (½ tsp.) and salt (¼ tsp.) in a mixing container. (Don't overmix it.) Shape the mixture into four patties (¾-inch-thick) and set aside.
5. Oil the grill rack and arrange the mushrooms with the cap-side downwards on the oiled grill rack. Grill them with the lid 'on' until tender (4 min. each side).
6. Plate the mushrooms and cover them with a layer of foil to keep warm.
7. Oil the rack again and add the patties.
8. Grill with a lid on the rack till the patties are lightly charred with an internal temp of 165° Fahrenheit/74° Celsius (4-5 min. each side).
9. Put a cheese slice on each burger during the last minute of cooking.
10. Transfer the patties to a plate and wait for five minutes before preparing it to serve.
11. Note: If your grill is large enough, grill the portobello caps and the patties simultaneously.
12. Thinly slice the tomato.

13. Place each patty on the stem side of a portobello cap - adding arugula and the fresh tomato slices. Cover with the rest of the portobello caps, stem-side down, and serve promptly.

1-Pan Chicken & Asparagus Bake - Heart & Diabetic Friendly

Portions Provided: 4 servings
Time Required: 35 minutes
Nutritional Statistics (Each Portion):
1 chicken piece + 6 spears + ¾ dup potato/carrot mix:
- Protein Counts: 27.6 grams
- Carbohydrates: 30.7 grams
- Fat Content: 13.8 grams
- Sugars: 8 grams
- Dietary Fiber: 5.7 grams
- Sodium: 599.4 mg
- Calories: 352

Essential Ingredients:
- Chicken breasts - cut in half crosswise (2 @ 230 g/8 oz. each)
- Baby Yukon Gold potatoes (340 g/12 oz.)
- Carrots (8 oz.)
- Olive oil (3 tbsp. divided)
- Ground coriander (2 tsp. divided)
- Salt (.75 tsp. divided)
- Ground pepper (.5 tsp. divided)
- Lemon juice (2 tbsp.)
- Shallot - chopped (2 tbsp.)
- Honey (2 tsp.)
- Dijon mustard - whole-grain (1 tbsp.)
- Fresh asparagus (1 lb. trimmed)
- Fresh dill (1 tbsp.)
- Fresh parsley - flat-leaf (2 tbsp.)
- Lemon wedges

Preparation Method:
1. Warm the oven to reach 375° Fahrenheit/191° Celsius.
2. Diagonally slice the carrots into one-inch pieces.
3. Trim the chicken and remove the bones and fat and place it on a chopping block. Cover it using a layer of plastic wrap - pound it using a meat mallet to reach a ½-inch thickness. Put it on half of a large rimmed baking tray.
4. Slice the potatoes - lengthwise and chop the carrots. Arrange them single-layered on the rest of the pan. Sprinkle the mixture with oil (1 tbsp.) and sprinkle with coriander (1 tsp.), salt (½ tsp.), and pepper (¼ tsp.).

5. Bake for 15 minutes.
6. Whisk the lemon juice with the honey, shallot, mustard, the rest of the oil (2 tbsp.), coriander (1 tsp.), and ¼ of a teaspoon each - pepper and salt - in a mixing container.
7. Transfer the pan to the countertop. Adjust the oven setting to broil.
8. Fold in the potato-carrot mixture and put the asparagus in the middle of the baking tray. Scoop the lemon juice-shallot mixture over the veggies and chicken.
9. Broil till they're lightly browned, asparagus is tender, and an internal temp of 165° Fahrenheit/74° Celsius (10 min.).
10. Finely chop the dill and parsley to sprinkle over the baked chicken. Serve with a couple of lemon wedges.

Orange Rosemary Roasted Chicken

Portions Provided: 6 servings
Time Required: 1 hour 5 minutes
Nutritional Statistics (Each Portion):
- Calories: 204
- Protein Counts: 31 grams
- Carbohydrates: 2 grams
- Fat Content: 8 grams
- Dietary Fiber: trace
- Sodium: 95 mg

Essential Ingredients:
- Fresh rosemary (3 tsp.) or Dried rosemary (1 tsp.)
- Garlic cloves (2)
- Olive oil (1.5 tsp.)
- Chicken breast halves (3 @ 8 oz. each) ***
- Chicken legs & thighs (3 @ 8 oz. each) ***
- Black pepper (.125 or ⅛ tsp.)
- Orange juice (.33 cup)
- *** Skinless & bone-in

Preparation Method:
1. Heat the oven to 450° Fahrenheit/232° Celsius.
2. Lightly spritz a baking tray using a portion of cooking oil spray. Mince the garlic and rosemary (as needed).
3. Rub the chicken with garlic and oil. Sprinkle it with pepper and rosemary. Arrange the pieces of chicken into the baking tray, adding the juice over its top.
4. Place a layer of foil over the pan to bake for ½ hour. Flip the chicken and continue

baking until it's nicely browned (approx. 10-15 min.).

5. Use the pan juices to baste the chicken as needed for extra moisture.

6. Plate the chicken and serve with the orange sauce.

Paella with Chicken Leeks & Tarragon

Portions Provided: 4 servings
Time Required: 1.5 hours
Nutritional Statistics (Each Portion):
- Calories: 378
- Protein Counts: 35 grams
- Carbohydrates: 46 grams
- Fat Content: 6 grams
- Dietary Fiber: 7 grams
- Sodium: 182 mg

Essential Ingredients:
- Olive oil (1 tsp.)
- Onion (1 small)
- Large tomatoes (2)
- Leeks - whites parts only (2)
- Garlic (3 cloves)
- Chicken breast (1 lb.)
- Red pepper (1)
- Long-grain brown rice (2/3 cup)
- Unsalted chicken broth - fat-free (2 cups)
- Frozen peas (1 cup)
- Tarragon (1 tsp./to your liking)
- Freshly chopped parsley (.25 cup)
- Lemon (1 cut into 4 wedges)

Preparation Method:
1. Warm the oil in a big skillet using the medium temperature setting.
2. Chop the tomatoes. Thinly slice the leeks, peppers, onions, peppers, and leeks, and mince the garlic.
3. Trim the fat and bones from the chicken - slice it into strips (2 x ½-inches).
4. Toss the chicken, garlic, leeks, and onions into the skillet. Sauté the mixture until the veggies are done, and the chicken is slightly browned (5 min.).
5. Toss in the pepper slices and tomatoes. Sauté them for another five minutes.
6. Mix in the broth, tarragon, and rice. Wait for it to boil.
7. Lower the temperature setting and place a top on the pan to simmer (10 min.). Mix in the peas and continue cooking uncovered

till the broth is entirely absorbed and the rice is tender (45 min. to one hr.).

8. When you are ready to eat, portion the meal into plates with a lemon wedge and parsley.

Pineapple Chicken Stir-Fry

Portions Provided: 4 servings
Time Required: 20-25 minutes
Nutritional Statistics (Each Portion):
½ cup rice + 1 cup stir-fry:
- Protein Counts: 17 grams
- Carbohydrates: 44 grams
- Fat Content: 5 grams
- Sugars: -0- grams
- Dietary Fiber: 4 grams
- Sodium: 325 mg
- Calories: 289

Essential Ingredients:
For the Marinade:
- Rice vinegar (1 tsp.)
- Soy sauce - l.s. (1 tsp.)
- Fresh ginger (.5 tsp.)
- Chicken breast (.5 lb.)
For the Rice:
- Water (1.33 cups water)
- Brown rice (.66 or 2/3 cup)
For the Sauce:
- Unsweetened pineapple juice (3 tbsp.)
- Rice vinegar (1 tsp.)
- Garlic (2 cloves)
- Fresh ginger (1 tsp.)
- Soy sauce - l.s. (1.5 tbsp.)
- Cornstarch (1.5 tbsp.)
For the Stir-fry:
- Peanut oil (1 tbsp. - divided)
- Red bell pepper (1 cup)
- Carrot (1 small)
- Snow peas (1 cup)
- Bok choy (1 cup)
- Green onion (.5 cup)
- Canned unsweetened pineapple chunks (1 cup)

Preparation Method:
1. Mince/grate the garlic and ginger. Trim the fat from the chicken and chop it into one-inch chunks. Slice the carrot into diagonal strips. Chop the bok choy.
2. Cut the pepper into ½-inch strips. Slice the green onion.
3. Whisk the vinegar with the soy sauce and ginger in a mixing container. Empty it into a zipper-type plastic bag with the chicken pieces. Securely close the bag and place it in the refrigerator till ready for it.

4. Meanwhile, pour water into a saucepan and wait for it to heat over a burner using the med-high temperature setting. Put a lid on the pan and wait for it to boil.
5. Measure and pour in the rice. Adjust the temperature setting to low.
6. Simmer till the water is absorbed - setting it to the side for now. Keep it warm.
7. Prepare the sauce in a separate container - toss all of its fixings and set aside.
8. Measure the rest of the fixings for the stir-fry.
9. Use a big wok to warm the peanut oil (.5 tbsp.) using the med-high temperature setting.
10. Add red pepper and carrots to stir-fry (2-3 min.).
11. Toss in the pineapple and bok choy - stir-fry for one minute.
12. Mix in the peas and onions - stir-fry for one minute. Remove the vegetables from the wok into a big mixing container and put it to the side for now.
13. Place the wok on the hot burner and pour in peanut oil (.5 tbsp.) and the marinated chicken. Stir-fry till the chicken is thoroughly cooked (3 min.) to reach internal temperature should be 165° Fahrenheit/74° Celsius). Add the cooked veggies - stir them for another minute.
14. Whisk the sauce mixture till the cornstarch is thoroughly dissolved. Pour the sauce into the wok - wait for it to boil. Simmer till the sauce has thickened and appears shiny (1 min.).
15. To serve, add rice (.5 cup each) into four dinner plates. Portion the stir-fry mix into each one and enjoy right away.

Roasted Red Pepper Chicken Wrap

Portions Provided: 2 servings
Time Required: 20-25 minutes
Nutritional Statistics (Each Portion):
- Protein Counts: 21 grams
- Carbohydrates: 50 grams
- Fat Content: 8 grams
- Dietary Fiber: 5 grams
- Sodium: 415 mg
- Calories: 356

Essential Ingredients:
- Chicken breast (4 oz./25-cm)
- Flour tortillas - pesto-flavored/your preference (2 @ 10-inch each)
- Hummus (2 tbsp.)
- Chopped tomatoes (.5 cup)
- Roasted red bell pepper (1)
- Lettuce (1 cup)

Preparation Method:
1. Spray a skillet using a spritz of cooking oil spray.
2. Peel and slice the peppers, and shred the lettuce as desired.
3. Trim the chicken and remove all fat and skin. Slice it into strips (0.5x2-inches).
4. Place the chicken in the skillet and sauté it using a med-high temperature setting until it's opaque and lightly browned. Set it to the side for now.
5. Warm a big, dry frying pan using a medium-temperature setting.
6. Place one of the tortillas onto the hot skillet and warm it till it's softened (20 seconds on each side). Repeat with the other tortilla.
7. Prepare the warmed tortilla with one tablespoon of hummus. Add ½ of the lettuce, chicken, cooked peppers, and tomatoes to prepare each wrap.
8. Tuck in the sides and tuck the bottom of the tortilla as you roll it over the filling. Roll them and securely close. Slice each wrap in half crosswise and serve promptly.

Roasted Turkey

Portions Provided: 12 servings
Time Required: varied - 1 hour 20 minutes
Nutritional Statistics (Each Portion):
- Protein Counts: 56 grams
- Fat Content: 9 grams
- Total Carbs: 8 grams (Net: 4 grams)
- Dietary Fiber: 1 gram
- Sugars: 3 grams
- Sodium: 161 mg
- Calories: 337

Essential Ingredients:
- Carrots (2)
- Celery (2 stalks)
- Yellow onions (2)
- Shallot (about 2 tbsp./1 medium)
- Garlic (4 cloves)
- Coarse ground black pepper (as desired)

- Turkey (12 lb. - whole & thawed)
- Roma tomatoes (8)

Preparation Method

1. Warm the oven temperature setting in advance to reach 400° Fahrenheit/204° Celsius.
2. Peel, finely chop, and add the shallots with minced garlic and black pepper in a mixing container. Thoroughly combine and set to the side for now.
3. Chop and arrange the carrots, onion, and celery in the roasting pan.
4. Open the giblet/turkey package and discard giblets and fatty tissues. Keep the neck for preparing the stock.
5. Slice the tomatoes into halves through the stem.
6. Thoroughly rinse the turkey and pay it to dry using a few paper towels.
7. Arrange it on the roasting pan over the veggies (breast-side up). Push the wing tips behind the turkey.
8. Rub the turkey with the shallot mixture and place tomatoes around the border of the turkey. (Don't cover it.)
9. Place the pan into the centermost oven rack.
10. Set a timer to bake it for 20 minutes.
11. Adjust the oven temperature to 325° Fahrenheit/163° Celsius. Roast it for 3-3.5 hours.
12. Test for doneness. Pierce it using a skewer. If the juices run clear or the internal temp reaches (180° Fahrenheit/82° Celsius to 185 Fahrenheit, or 82 C to 85 Celsius); it is done.
13. Transfer the turkey to a platter.
14. Place the vegetables around the turkey. Tent the turkey and veggies tightly with aluminum foil. Wait for it to steam for 20 minutes before carving.
15. Carve the turkey, serve, and enjoy it with your favorite side dishes.

Sesame Ginger Chicken Stir-Fry with Cauliflower Rice

Portions Provided: 6 servings
Time Required: 40 minutes
Nutritional Statistics (Each Portion):
- Protein Counts: 25 grams
- Carbohydrates: 11 grams
- Fat Content: 9 grams
- Dietary Fiber: 4 grams
- Sodium: 415 mg
- Calories: 225

Essential Ingredients:
- Cauliflower (2 lb./910 g/1 small head)
- Coconut oil (1 tbsp.)
- Chicken bone broth (2 tbsp.)
- Sea salt (.25 tsp.)
  The Stir-Fry:
- Bone broth - chicken (1.5 cups)
- Tapioca starch (2 tbsp.)
- Organic crushed red pepper (.25 tsp.)
- Coconut oil (1 tbsp.)
- Chicken breasts (450 g/1 lb.)
- Medium red bell pepper (1)
- Asparagus (1 lb.)
- Shiitake mushrooms (110 g/4 oz.)
- Garlic (3 cloves)
- Grated fresh ginger (1 tbsp.)
- Sea salt (.5 tsp.)
- Organic toasted sesame seeds (2 tbsp.)

Preparation Method:

1. Trim the chicken to remove all fat and bones to slice it into thin strips.
2. Slice the mushrooms. Trim the pepper and asparagus into one-inch strips.
3. Cut florets from the cauliflower and pulse them in batches in a food processor until the cauliflower resembles rice's texture.
4. Warm oil in a big skillet using a med-high temperature setting.
5. Toss in and sauté the cauliflower (2 min.).
6. Mix in the bone broth and sea salt, simmer five more minutes till the cauliflower is tender. Set aside - keeping it warm.
7. *For the Stir-Fry* - mix bone broth with the tapioca and crushed red pepper in a small mixing container till it's smooth. Set aside.
8. Warm coconut oil in a big skillet using a med-high temperature setting. Add chicken and stir-fry till browned (5 min.). Remove from the skillet.
9. Mince the garlic. Add vegetables, garlic, ginger, and sea salt - stir fry for three minutes or until tender-crisp.
10. Stir bone broth mixture. Add to a skillet and constantly stir, waiting for it to boil using the medium-temperature setting (2 min. till thickened).
11. Add chicken and stir fry until heated as desired. Sprinkle with sesame seeds.

12. Serve with cauliflower rice as desired.

Skillet Lemon Chicken & Potatoes with Kale

Portions Provided: 4 servings
Time Required: 50 minutes
Nutritional Statistics (Each Portion):
One thigh + 1 cup of veggies:
- Protein Counts: 24.7 grams
- Carbohydrates: 25.6 grams
- Fat Content: 19.3 grams
- Sugars: 1.8 grams
- Dietary Fiber: 2.9 grams
- Sodium: 377.9 mg
- Calories: 374
  Diabetic Exchanges:
- Vegetable: ½
- Starch: 1 ½
- Fat: 2
- Lean-Protein: 3

Essential Ingredients:
- Olive oil (3 tbsp. divided)
- Chicken thighs (1 lb.)
- Black pepper and salt (.5 tsp. each - divided)
- Baby Yukon Gold potatoes (1 lb.)
- Chicken broth - l.s. (.5 cup)
- Lemon - sliced & seeds removed (1 large)
- Garlic (4 cloves)
- Fresh tarragon (1 tbsp.)
- Baby kale (6 cups)

Preparation Method:
1. Warm the oven to reach 400° Fahrenheit/204° Celsius.
2. Slice the potatoes into halves - lengthwise.
3. Trim the chicken, removing all the bones and fat.
4. Heat oil (1 tbsp.) in a big cast-iron skillet using a med-high temperature setting. Season the chicken using ¼ of a teaspoon of each - pepper and salt.
5. Cook until browned on both sides - flipping it once (5 min.). Plate it for now.
6. Add the rest of the oil (2 tbsp.), potatoes, and the rest of the pepper and salt (¼ tsp. each) to the skillet.
7. Cook the potatoes, cut-side down, till browned (3 min.).
8. Mince the garlic and tarragon. Stir in broth, garlic, lemon, tarragon, and chicken into the pan.

9. Roast till the potatoes are tender, and chicken is thoroughly cooked (15 min.).
10. Fold the kale into the pan and roast until it has wilted (3-4 min.) and serve.

Thai Chicken & Pasta Skillet

Portions Provided: 6 servings @ 1 - 1/3 cup portions
Time Required: 30 minutes
Nutritional Statistics (Each Portion):
- Calories: 403
- Protein Counts: 25 grams
- Carbohydrates: 43 grams
- Fat Content: 15 grams
- Sugars: 15 grams
- Dietary Fiber: 6 grams
- Sodium: 432 mg

Essential Ingredients:
- Whole-wheat spaghetti - uncooked (170 g/6 oz. pkg.)
- Carrots (2 cups/about 8 oz./230 g)
- Chicken - shredded & cooked (2 cups)
- Fresh sugar-snap peas (280 g/10 oz. pkg.)
- Thai peanut sauce (1 cup)
- Cucumber (1 medium)
- Canola oil (2 tsp.)
- Optional: Fresh cilantro

Preparation Method:
1. Cook the spaghetti (8-10 min.) and dump it into a colander to drain.
2. In the meantime, prepare a big skillet to warm the oil (med-high).
3. Halve the cucumber, discard the seeds, and slice it diagonally—Julienne the carrots. Trim the peas and cut them into thin diagonal pieces.
4. Mix the peas and carrots to the skillet - stir-fry till they're crispy and tender (6-8 min.). Fold in the chicken, peanut sauce, and spaghetti, tossing to heat, and combine.
5. Scoop it onto a plate and top using a portion of cucumber. Chop and add the cilantro as desired.

Zucchini Noodles & Quick Turkey Bolognese - Meal Prep

Portions Provided: 4 servings
Time Required: 35 minutes
Nutritional Statistics (Each Portion):

- Protein Counts: 18.7 grams
- Carbohydrates: 15.6 grams (Net: 2.6 grams)
- Fat Content: 10.1 grams
- Sugars: 9.3 grams
- Dietary Fiber: 3.7 grams
- Sodium: 555.3 mg
- Calories: 216
  Diabetic Exchanges:
- High-Fat Protein: ½
- Fat: ½
- Lean Protein 1 ½
- Vegetables: 3

Essential Ingredients:
- Zucchini noodles (3 medium-sized/8 cups)
- *"Quick Turkey Meat Sauce"* (3 cups)[2]
- Parmesan cheese - grated (.5 cup)

Preparation Method:
1. Prepare the meat sauce.
2. While the sauce is simmering, portion the zucchini noodles among four single-serving containers with tops (approx. two cups in each container).
3. Add ¾ cup of the sauce and parmesan (2 tbsp.) to each container. Securely close each of the containers and pop them in the fridge for up to four days.
4. When you are ready to use them, set the lid ajar, and microwave using the high setting till the noodles are tender, and the sauce is steamy (2.5-3 min.).

The Quick & Delicious Turkey Meat Sauce

Portions Provided: 12 servings @ ½ cup each
Time Required: 35 minutes
Nutritional Statistics (Each Portion):
- Protein Counts: 8.8 grams
- Carbohydrates: 7.1 grams (Net: 1.6 grams)
- Fat Content: 4.6 grams
- Sugars: 3.9 grams
- Dietary Fiber: 1.6 grams
- Sodium: 249.3 mg
- Calories: 100
  Diabetic Exchanges:
- Medium-Fat Protein: 1
- Vegetable: 1 ½

Essential Ingredients:
- Garlic (4 cloves)
- Large onion (1)

- Olive oil (1 tbsp.)
- Lean ground turkey (450 g or 1 lb.)
- Mushrooms (230 g or 8 oz.)
- Salt (.5 tsp.)
- Crushed tomatoes (790 g or 28 oz. can)
- Italian seasoning (1 tbsp.)
- Parsley or basil (.5 cup)

Preparation Method:
1. Warm oil in a big skillet using a medium-temperature setting. Chop and add onion to sauté - stirring till it's softened (5 min.).
2. Mince and stir in garlic and Italian seasoning -sauté another minute till it's fragrant.
3. Chop the mushrooms and parsley/basil.
4. Add the mushrooms, turkey, and salt. Cook the mixture, crumbling the meat as it cooks till it's done (not pink) and the mushrooms are cooked (10 min.).
5. Raise the temperature setting to med-high. Stir in tomatoes and simmer till thickened (5 min.). Stir in parsley (or basil) to serve.

---

[2] - see next recipe

Meats

Beef & Bean Sloppy Joes - Diabetic & Heart-Friendly

Portions Provided: 4 servings
Time Required: 20 minutes
Nutritional Statistics (Each Portion):
- Protein Counts: 25.8 grams
- Carbohydrates: 43.8 grams
- Fat Content: 15 grams
- Sugars: 12.2 grams
- Dietary Fiber: 8.4 grams
- Sodium: 537.5 mg
- Calories: 411
  Diabetic Exchanges:
- Fat: 1
- Vegetable: 1 ½
- Starch: 2
- Lean-Protein: 3

Essential Ingredients:
- Olive oil (1 tbsp.)
- 90% lean ground beef (340 g/12 oz.)
- Black beans - no salt (1 cup)
- Onion (1 cup)
- Cayenne pepper (1 pinch)
- New Mexico chili powder/your favorite (2 tsp.)
- Garlic & onion powder (.5 tsp. each)
- Light brown sugar (1 tsp.)
- Ketchup (3 tbsp.)
- Spicy brown mustard (2 tsp.)
- Tomato sauce - no salt (1 cup)
- Worcestershire sauce - l.s. (1 tbsp.)
- Hamburger buns - whole wheat (4)

Preparation Method:
1. Warm oil in a big skillet using the med-high temperature setting. Put the beef in the pan and fry it while breaking it apart - till it's lightly browned - but not thoroughly cooked (3-4 min.).
2. Scoop the beef into a mixing container, reserving the drippings in the pan.
3. Rinse the beans in a colander. Toss them in the pan with chopped onions - cook, often stirring until the onion is softened (5 min.).
4. Add chili powder, onion powder, garlic powder, and cayenne - continually stirring for approximately ½ minute.
5. Mix in Worcestershire, ketchup, mustard, tomato sauce, and brown sugar. Toss the beef into the pan. Simmer till the sauce is thickened and beef is cooked as desired (5 min.).
6. Split the buns in half to toast. Serve the sloppy joes.

Beef & Blue Cheese Penne with Pesto

Portions Provided: 4 servings
Time Required: 30 minutes
Nutritional Statistics (Each Portion):
- Protein Counts: 35 grams
- Carbohydrates: 49 grams
- Fat Content: 22 grams
- Sugars: 3 grams
- Dietary Fiber: 9 grams
- Sodium: 434 mg
- Calories: 532

Essential Ingredients:
- Penne pasta - whole-wheat (2 cups - uncooked)
- Beef tenderloin steaks (2 @ 170 g/6 oz. each)
- Black pepper & salt (.25 tsp. each)
- Baby spinach (140 g/5 oz./about 6 cups)
- Grape tomatoes (2 cups)
- Prepared pesto (.33 cup)
- Walnuts (.25 cup)
- Crumbled Gorgonzola cheese (.25 cup)

Preparation Method:
1. Prepare the pasta per its package directions.
2. Sprinkle each of the steaks with a bit of pepper and salt.
3. Grill the steaks with the lid on using the medium-temperature setting.
4. Alternately, you can broil them four inches from the burner till the meat is as desired (5-7 min. per side) or (medium-rare is at 135° F or 57° C; medium will be at 140° F or 60° C; & medium-well will reach 145° F or 63° C).
5. Drain pasta and toss it into a big mixing container. Chop the walnuts into a bowl
6. Coarsely chop and add the spinach. Slice the tomatoes into halves and toss them in with the walnuts and pesto - tossing to cover.
7. Thinly slice the steak.
8. Serve the pasta with beef and a dusting of cheese.

Beef Stroganoff

Portions Provided: 4 servings
Time Required: 40 minutes
Nutritional Statistics (Each Portion):
- Calories: 273
- Protein Counts: 20 grams
- Carbohydrates: 37 grams
- Fat Content: 5 grams
- Dietary Fiber: 2 grams
- Sodium: 193 mg

Essential Ingredients:
- Boneless beef round steak (.5 lb. or 230 g)
- Onion (.5 cup)
- Yolkless egg noodles (4 cups - uncooked)
- Paprika (.5 tsp.)
- All-purpose flour (1 tbsp.)
- Water (.5 cup)
- Undiluted cream of mushroom soup - fat-free (half of 1 small can)
- Fat-free sour cream (.5 cup)

Preparation Method:
1. Trim the fat from the steak and slice it into ¾-inch thick slices.
2. Chop the onions and measure the rest of the fixings.
3. On the stovetop, using the medium-temperature setting, place a skillet with a spritz of cooking oil spray, adding the onions to sauté (5 min.).
4. Fold in the beef - sautéing till the beef is done (5 min.). Drain and set it to the side.
5. Prepare a big pot of water (¾ full of water).
6. After it's boiling, toss in the noodles and let them cook (10-12 min.). At that point, toss the pasta into a colander to drain.
7. Use another saucepan, mix the water with the soup and flour using the medium-temperature setting. Add the paprika and soup mixture to the beef in the frying pan.
8. Stir till they are thoroughly warmed. Take the pan from the burner and mix in the sour cream and serve as desired.

Chinese Ginger Beef Stir-Fry with Baby Bok Choy

Portions Provided: 4 servings @ 1¼ cups
Time Required: 25 minutes
Nutritional Statistics (Each Portion):
- Protein Counts: 25.5 grams
- Carbohydrates: 6.3 grams (Net: 2.1 grams)
- Sugars: 3.1 grams
- Fat Content: 12.8 grams
- Dietary Fiber: 1.1 grams
- Sodium: 568.5 mg
- Calories: 247

Essential Ingredients:
- Beef flank steak (12 oz.)
- Soy sauce - l.s. (1.5 tsp.)
- Dry sherry (1 tsp. + 1 tbsp. divided)
- Cornstarch (1 tsp.)
- Oyster-flavored sauce - ex. Lee Kum Kee Premium (2 tbsp.)
- Toasted sesame oil (1 tsp.)
- Vegetable oil (1 tbsp.)
- Fresh ginger (1 tbsp.)
- Baby bok choy (1 lb./about 8 cups)
- Unsalted chicken broth (3 tbsp.)
- Suggested: Stainless-steel skillet(12-inch) or flat-bottomed carbon-steel wok (14-inch)

Preparation Method:
1. Trim and slice the beef (*with the grain*) into two-inch-wide strips. Slice them (*across the grain*) into ¼-inch-thick slices.
2. Mince the ginger and trim the bok choy into two-inch pieces.
3. Combine the beef, one teaspoon of sherry, ginger, soy sauce, and cornstarch in a mixing container - stirring till the cornstarch is dissolved.
4. Pour in the sesame oil - stirring till the beef is lightly coated.
5. Whisk the oyster sauce and the rest of the sherry (1 tbsp.) in another mixing container and set it to the side for now.
6. Warm the wok/skillet using the high-temperature setting till it's sizzling hot. Pour in the vegetable oil.
7. Arrange the beef in the heated pan - simmer undisturbed till it begins to brown (1 min.). Stir-fry the mix until lightly browned - 30 seconds to one minute more. Plate it for now.
8. Add the broth and bok choy to the pan. Place a lid on the pan and simmer till the bok choy is bright green and most of the liquid is absorbed (1-2 min.).
9. Scoop the beef back into the skillet with the reserved sauce.
10. Stir-fry till the bok choy is tender, and the beef is cooked (30 sec. to 1 min.).

Low-Sodium Dash Meatloaf

Portions Provided: 10 servings
Time Required: 1 hour 10 minutes
Nutritional Statistics (Each Portion):
- Protein Counts: 13 grams
- Total Carbs: 5 grams
- Sugars: 3 grams
- Fat Content: 11 grams
- Sodium: 55 mg
- Calories: 170

Essential Ingredients:
- Lean ground beef (680 g/1.5 lb.)
- Panko breadcrumbs (.75 cup)
- No-salt-added ketchup - divided (.5 cup)
- Onion powder (1 tbsp.)
- Parsley flakes (1.5 tbsp.)
- Fresh oregano (2 tbsp.)
- Black pepper (1 tsp.)
- Garlic powder (.75 tsp.)
- Egg (1 large)
- Suggested Pan Size: Loaf pan 13x9-inch/13x23-cm

Preparation Method:
1. Set the oven temperature to reach 350° Fahrenheit/177° Celsius.
2. Combine all of the fixings in a mixing container (omit ¼ cup of the ketchup).
3. Shape the meat mixture and scoop it into a greased loaf pan.
4. Set a timer to bake it for 45 minutes. Brush the rest of the ketchup over meatloaf and bake another 15 minutes for a total of one hour. Its internal temp when done should be 165° Fahrenheit/74° Celsius.
5. Serve with your favorite DASH sides.

Philly Cheesesteak Stuffed Peppers

Portions Provided: 4 servings
Time Required: 40 minutes
Nutritional Statistics (Each Portion):
- Protein Counts: 29 grams
- Carbohydrates: 11.9 grams (Net: 3.2 grams)
- Fat Content: 7.5 grams
- Sugars: 5.8 grams
- Dietary Fiber: 2.9 grams
- Sodium: 464.7 mg
- Calories: 308

Essential Ingredients:
- Bell peppers (2 large)
- Olive oil (1 tbsp.)
- Onion (1 large)

- Mushrooms (8 oz. or 230 g pkg.)
- Top round steak (12 oz. or 340 g)
- Italian seasoning (1 tbsp.)
- Salt (.25 tsp.)
- Black pepper (.5 tsp.)
- Worcestershire sauce (1 tbsp.)
- Provolone cheese (4 slices)
- Suggested: Rimmed baking sheet

Preparation Method:
1. Preheat the oven temperature to 375° Fahrenheit/191° Celsius.
2. Slice the peppers into halves - lengthwise and discard its seeds.
3. Arrange the halves on the baking tray - baking till they're tender - yet holding their shape (½ hour).
4. Meanwhile, warm oil in a big skillet using the medium-temperature setting.
5. Cut the onion in half and slice it - toss it in the pan. Sauté it till it starts browning (4-5 min.).
6. Slice the mushrooms into halves, toss in the pan, and sauté them till they're softened (5 min.).
7. Thinly slice and add the steak, pepper, Italian seasoning, and salt. Simmer till the steak is just cooked through (3-4 min.).
8. Transfer the pan onto a cool burner and stir in Worcestershire.
9. Warm the oven broiler to high.
10. Portion the filling into the pepper halves and add a cheese slice.
11. Pop it in the oven and broil it about five inches from the heat till the cheese is lightly browned (2-3 min.).

Sesame - Garlic Beef & Broccoli with Whole-Wheat Noodles

Portions Provided: 4 servings @ 2 ½ cups each
Time Required: 60 minutes
Nutritional Statistics (Each Portion):
- Protein Counts: 31.1 grams
- Carbohydrates: 39.2 grams
- Fat Content: 9.7 grams
- Sugars: 3.3 grams
- Dietary Fiber: 6.2 grams
- Sodium: 335.6 mg
- Calories: 357
  Diabetic Exchanges:
- Vegetable: 1

- Fat: 1
- Starch: 2
- Lean Protein: 3

Essential Ingredients:
- Beef sirloin steak (450 g/1 lb.)
- Garlic (3 cloves)
- Lemon juice (2 tbsp.)
- Soy sauce - reduced-sodium (2 tbsp.)
- Toasted sesame oil (1 tbsp. + 2 tsp. divided)
- Ground ginger (1 tsp.)
- Crushed red pepper (.25 tsp.)
- Linguine - whole-wheat preferred (170 g/6 oz.)
- Onion (.5 cup)
- Broccoli florets (4 cups)
- Water (.5 cup)
- Ground pepper (.125 or ⅛ tsp.)
- Toasted sesame seeds (1 tsp.)
- To Serve: Lemon wedges

Preparation Method:
1. Trim the steak making sure to remove all of its bone. Thinly slice beef across the grain into short strips as desired. Toss it into a zipper-type plastic bag.
2. Thoroughly whisk the soy sauce with sesame oil (1 tbsp.), garlic, lemon juice, ginger, and red pepper in a mixing container - empty it over the beef. Securely close the bag - rotating it to cover the fixings. Pop it into the fridge for ½ hour - rotating the bag once during that time.
3. Prepare a big saucepan of boiling water to prepare the linguine (1 min. under the suggested pkg. time). Reserve ½ cup of the water and drain the remainder into a colander to thoroughly drain.
4. In the meantime, toss the broccoli and water in a wok/skillet till it boils using a med-high temperature setting. Cook until the water is evaporated (3-4 min.).
5. Mince and add onion, pepper, and the rest of the sesame oil (2 tsp.). Cook, occasionally stirring till the broccoli is tender (2-4 min.). Scoop the broccoli mixture into a mixing container and cover with a foil tent to keep it warm.
6. Set the marinade aside after you drain the beef. Mix ½ of the beef into the heated skillet and simmer - mixing till it's slightly pink in the middle (3-5 min.). Put it onto a platter and tent it with foil to keep it warm.
7. Continue the process with the rest of the beef and transfer it to the plate.

8. Mix the reserved cooking water and marinade in the skillet, and lastly, toss in the noodles.
9. Simmer them using the medium-temperature setting - stirring just until the sauce is thickened slightly and noodles are fork-tender to your liking (3-4 min.).
10. Portion the noodle mixture into four shallow bowls. Add the broccoli and beef mixture. Garnish with a few sesame seeds and a side of lemon wedges to your liking.

Skillet Steak with Mushroom Sauce - Diabetic-Friendly

Portions Provided: 4 servings
Time Required: 25 minutes
Nutritional Statistics (Each Portion):
2 ½ oz. meat + 1/3 cup sauce:
- Protein Counts: 26.5 grams
- Total Carbs: 16.4 grams (Net: 6.6 grams)
- Fat Content: 6.4 grams
- Dietary Fiber: 5.1 grams
- Sugars: 5.7 grams
- Sodium: 355.7 mg
- Calories: 226
  Diabetic Exchanges:
- Sauce: ½
- Fat: ½
- Lean Protein: 3
- Vegetable: 1

Essential Ingredients:
- Canola oil (2 tsp.)
- Beef top sirloin steak (340 g/12 oz. - 1-inch thick)
- Salt-free steak grilling seasoning (2 tsp.)
- Broccoli rabe (170 g/6 oz.)
- Sliced fresh mushrooms (3 cups)
- Frozen peas (2 cups)
- Unsalted beef broth (1 cup)
- Whole-grain mustard (1 tbsp.)
- Salt (.25 tsp.)
- Cornstarch (2 tsp.)
- Suggested: 12-inch/30-cm cast-iron skillet

Preparation Method:
1. Warm the oven temperature setting in advance to reach 350° Fahrenheit/177° Celsius.
2. Trim all bones from the steak.
3. Sprinkle the meat with steak seasoning.
4. In a skillet, warm the oil using a medium-high temperature setting.

5. When heated, add the meat and trimmed broccoli rabe. Let it cook for four minutes, turning the broccoli once (*don't turn the meat*).

6. Sprinkle the peas around the meat and pop the skillet into the oven.

7. Set a timer to bake for eight minutes or until meat is medium-rare at 145° Fahrenheit/63° Celsius.

8. Transfer the veggies and meat from the pan. Tent them using a sheet of aluminum foil to keep them warm. Make the sauce by adding the mushrooms to the pan's drippings. Sauté them using the med-high setting for three minutes, stirring intermittently.

9. Whisk the beef broth with cornstarch, salt, and mustard - mix into the mushrooms.

10. Simmer till it's thickened and piping hot (1 min.). Serve the veggies and meat with sauce.

Slow-Cooked Braised Beef with Carrots & Turnips

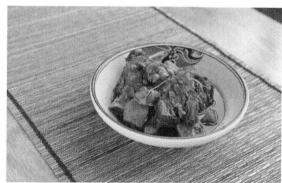

Portions Provided: 8 servings
Time Required: 4 hours
Nutritional Statistics (Each Portion):
3 oz. Beef + 1 Cup Vegetables:
- Protein Counts: 34.7 grams
- Carbohydrates: 12.8 grams
- Fat Content: 10.7 grams
- Sugars: 6.2 grams
- Dietary Fiber: 3.1 grams
- Sodium: 538.4 mg
- Calories: 318

Essential Ingredients:
- Kosher salt (1 tbsp.)
- Ground allspice (.5 tsp.)
- Cinnamon (2 tsp.)
- Black pepper (.5 tsp.)
- Ground cloves (.25 tsp.)

- Beef chuck roast - trimmed (3-3.5 lb./1.4-1.6 kg.)
- Olive oil (2 tbsp.)
- Medium onion (1)
- Red wine (1 cup)
- Whole tomatoes (28 oz./790 g can)
- Carrots (5 medium)
- Garlic cloves (3)
- Turnips (2 medium)
- For the Garnish: Chopped fresh basil
- Suggested: Five to Six-quart slow cooker

Preparation Method:

1. Combine salt with the allspice, cinnamon, pepper, and cloves in a mixing container. Rub the mixture over the beef.

2. Warm oil in a big skillet using a medium-temperature setting. Add the beef and cook until browned (4-5 min. per side). Scoop it into the slow cooker.

3. Cut the carrots into one-inch chunks. Peel and slice the turnips into ½-inch pieces - set aside.

4. Chop or mince and toss the garlic and onion into the pan.

5. Simmer for two minutes. Mix in the wine and tomatoes (with juices) - wait for it to boil, scraping up any browned bits and breaking up the tomatoes.

6. Pour the mixture into the slow cooker with carrots and turnips.

7. Cover and set the timer to cook (low for 8 hrs.) or (high for 4 hrs.).

8. Scoop the beef from the cooker and slice.

9. Serve the beef with the sauce and veggies, garnished with basil as desired.

Spaghetti & Quick Meat Sauce - Diabetic-Friendly

Portions Provided: 8 servings
Time Required: 30 minutes
Nutritional Statistics (Each Portion):
¾ cup of sauce + 1 cup of pasta:
- Protein Counts: 27.2 grams
- Carbohydrates: 53.8 grams
- Fat Content: 9 grams
- Fiber: 9.4 grams
- Sugars: 7.8 grams
- Sodium: 483.6mg
- Calories: 389

Essential Ingredients:
- Whole-wheat spaghetti (450 g or 1 lb.)
- Olive oil (2 tsp.)
- Onion (1 large)
- Celery (1 stalk)
- Carrot (1 large)
- Garlic (4 cloves)
- Italian seasoning (1 tbsp.)
- Lean ground beef (450 g/1 lb.)
- Crushed tomatoes (790 g/28 oz. can)
- Chopped flat-leaf parsley (.25 cup)
- Salt (.5 tsp.)
- Parmesan cheese - grated (.5 cup)

Preparation Method:
1. Prepare a big pot of boiling water. Toss in the pasta and simmer it per its package instructions (8-10 min.). Drain it into a colander.
2. Meantime, warm oil in a big skillet using a medium-temperature setting till it's hot.
3. Chop or mince the celery, carrots, and onion - sautéing them as you are mixing - till the onion has started browning (5-8 min.).
4. Mince and add Italian seasoning and garlic - simmer until it's fragrant (30 sec.).
5. Mix in the beef and continue to cook as you break it apart using a spoon till the pink is gone (3-5 min.). Raise the temperature setting to high.
6. Pour in tomatoes, parsley, and salt - simmer till it's thickened (4-6 min.).
7. Serve the sauce over the pasta with a serving of cheese.
8. Meal Prep Tips: Tightly cover the container and pop it into the fridge for up to three days.
9. You can also freeze the sauce for up to three months.

Spicy Orange Beef & Broccoli Stir-Fry

Portions Provided: 6 servings
Time Required: 30 minutes
Nutritional Statistics (Each Portion):
- Protein Counts: 21.1 grams
- Carbohydrates: 26.8 grams
- Fat Content: 6.1 grams
- Sugars: 12 grams
- Dietary Fiber: 5.8 grams
- Sodium: 343.1 mg
- Calories: 238

Essential Ingredients:
- Oranges (3)
- Cornstarch (1 tbsp.)
- Sugar (.5 tsp.)
- Soy sauce - l.s. (3 tbsp.)
- Chinese rice wine (1 tbsp.)
- Canola/peanut oil (3 tsp. divided)
- Beef sirloin (1 lb.)
- Minced garlic & ginger (2 tbsp. each)
- Dried red chiles (6-8 small)
- Broccoli florets (2 lb./6 cups)
- Water (.33 or 1/3 cup)
- Red bell pepper (1 seeded & sliced)
- Scallion greens - sliced (.5 cup)

Preparation Method:
1. Trim the beef and slice it against the grain to make ⅛-inch thick slices.
2. Carefully zest one of the oranges into one-inch strips.
3. Squeeze juice from all the oranges into another dish (¾ of a cup).
4. Whisk the soy sauce with the cornstarch, sugar, and wine - set aside.
5. Warm oil (1 tsp.) in a big skillet/wok using a high-temperature setting till it's almost smoking.
6. Add beef and stir-fry till the pink is gone (1 min.).
7. Scoop it into a paper-lined plate - setting it to the side for now.
8. Empty the remainder of the oil (2 tsp.) into the pan and warm till it's piping hot. Add garlic, chiles, the remainder of the orange zest, and ginger - stir-fry till it's fragrant (½ min.).
9. Mix in the broccoli and water. Put a lid on the pot and steam, stirring intermittently till the water is evaporated (3 min.). Toss in the peppers to stir-fry for one more minute.
10. Mix the reserved orange sauce into the wok. Wait for it to boil as you stir it till the sauce is slightly thickened (1-2 min.).
11. Mix in the scallion greens and the reserved beef - tossing to coat with sauce until it's thoroughly heated.

Veggie-Filled Meat Sauce with Zucchini Noodles

Portions Provided: 6 servings
Time Required: 55 minutes

Nutritional Statistics (Each Portion):

2/3 cup noodles + ¾ cup sauce:
- Protein Counts: 12.5 grams
- Carbohydrates: 17.8 grams
- Fat Content: 4.6 grams
- Sugars: 11.6 grams
- Dietary Fiber: 8.5 grams
- Sodium: 334.4 mg
- Calories: 158
  Diabetic Exchanges:
- Fat: ½
- Lean Protein: 1
- Vegetable: 3 ½

Essential Ingredients:

- 90%-lean ground beef (8 oz./230 g)
- Carrot (.5 cup)
- Garlic (2 cloves)
- Onion (.5 cup)
- Celery (.5 cup)
- Tomato sauce - no-salt (2 cans @ 8 oz. each)
- Diced tomatoes with garlic - oregano & basil - no-salt - drained (14.5 oz. can)
- Water (.25 cup)
- Dried Italian seasoning (1 tsp. crushed)
- Black pepper (.25 tsp.)
- Salt (.5 tsp.)
- Crushed red pepper (.125 tsp. to .25 tsp.)
- Medium zucchini (2 @ 10 oz./280 g each)
- Fresh mushrooms (8 oz. pkg.)
- Parmesan cheese (3 tbsp.)

Preparation Method:

1. Chop the celery, carrot, and onion. Mince the garlic and finely grate the parmesan.
2. Prepare the sauce by frying the beef with garlic, celery, carrots, and onions in a big skillet using a medium-temperature setting till the meat is browned (breaking it apart while cooking). The veggies should be tender.
3. Thoroughly drain the fat. Stir in tomato sauce, water, diced tomatoes, Italian seasoning, ground pepper, salt, and crushed red pepper. Wait for it to boil and lower the heat setting.
4. Simmer with the lid removed to reach the desired consistency, occasionally stirring (10-15 min.).
5. Meanwhile, use a julienne cutter, vegetable spiralizer, or mandoline to cut the zucchini into long - thin noodles.
6. Spritz an oversized skillet with a little cooking oil spray and warm it using a medium-high temperature setting.
7. Trim and slice the mushrooms to sauté till its liquid has evaporated (5 min.).
8. Fold in the zucchini and sauté them until just crisp-tender (2-3 min.). Drain the vegetable mixture in a colander.
9. Serve the meat sauce over the zucchini-mushroom mixture with a sprinkle of parmesan.

Pork Specialties

Brown Sugar Pork Tenderloin Stir-Fry

Portions Provided: 4 servings
Time Required: 2.5 hours - varies
Nutritional Statistics (Each Portion):
- Protein Counts: 26 grams
- Carbohydrates: 30 grams
- Fat Content: 9.1 grams
- Sugars: 12 grams
- Dietary Fiber: 3 grams
- Sodium: 502 mg
- Calories: 307

Essential Ingredients:
- Baby bok choy (6 cups)
- Sliced carrots (.5 cup)
- Garlic (1 tsp.)
- Green onions (2 tbsp.)
- Fresh ginger (1 tbsp.)
- Brown sugar (.25 cup)
- Cornstarch (2 tsp.)
- Salt (.25 tsp.)
- Pork tenderloin (1 lb.)
- Brown & white sushi rice (1.33 cups)
- Peanut oil (4 tsp.)

Preparation Method:
1. Use a sharp knife to remove any thick ends on the bok choy stems.
2. Mince the garlic, onions, and ginger.
3. Trim the pork and slice it into strips.
4. Whisk the brown sugar with green onions, ginger, garlic, salt, and cornstarch to make a marinade.
5. Toss the pork in the bowl and pop it into the fridge to marinate for two hours.
6. Meanwhile, cook the rice per its package instructions - set it aside.
7. Transfer the pork from the fridge to the countertop and wait for it to heat till it is at room temperature.
8. Use a wok (med-high temperature), and add peanut oil (2 tsp.).
9. After the oil is hot, toss in the pork. Stir-fry till the pork has reached 155° Fahrenheit/68° Celsius (7 min.).
10. Meanwhile, warm another big sauté pan using the med-high temperature setting.
11. Pour the remainder of the oil in the pan (2 tsp.) to warm.
12. Sauté the bok choy and carrots till tender (4 min.).
13. Serve with rice.

Irish Pork Roast with Roasted Root Vegetables

Portions Provided: 8 servings
Time Required: 1 hour 40 minutes
Nutritional Statistics (Each Portion):
3 oz. pork + 2/3 cup veggies:
- Protein Counts: 23.5 grams
- Carbohydrates: 22.9 grams
- Fat Content: 8.6 grams
- Sugars: 9.5 grams
- Dietary Fiber: 5.8 grams
- Sodium: 326.5 mg
- Calories: 272

Essential Ingredients:
- Carrots (1.5 lb./680 g)
- Parsnips (1.5 lb.)
- Olive oil (3 tbsp. divided)
- Fresh thyme (2 tsp. leaves - divided)
- Black pepper & salt (.75 tsp. each - divided)
- Boneless pork loin roast (2 lb./910 g)
- Dry hard cider (1 cup)
- Honey (1 tsp.)
- To Serve: Ploughman's chutney/Bramley applesauce

Preparation Method:
1. Warm the oven to 400° Fahrenheit/204° Celsius. Peel and slice the parsnips and carrots, cutting them into one-inch chunks - tossing them into a big mixing container with oil (2 tbsp.), thyme (1 tsp.), and ¼ teaspoon each of pepper and salt.
2. Spread the veggies in a roasting pan. Rub the pork using the rest of the oil (1 tbsp.) and sprinkle with the remainder of the thyme (1 tsp.) and ½ teaspoon each of the pepper and salt.
3. Arrange the pork (fat-side up) over the veggies.
4. Roast - occasionally stir the veggies until the internal temp reaches 145° Fahrenheit/63° Celsius (50-65 min.).
5. Scoop the pork onto a cutting block and layer it using a tent of foil. Wait for it to rest

for about 15 minutes. Scoop the veggies into a big mixing container and mix in honey.

6. Put the roasting pan over two burners using a high-temperature setting. Add cider and simmer while you scrape up any browned bits until the mix is reduced by half (3-5 min.).

7. Slice and serve the pork with sauce, vegetables, and chutney to your liking.

Pork Carnitas - Slow-Cooked

Portions Provided: 6 servings
Time Required: 4 hours 10 minutes
Nutritional Statistics (Each Portion):
Two tortillas + 1- 1/3 cups of meat:
- Protein Counts: 32 grams
- Carbohydrates: 24 grams
- Fat Content: 10 grams
- Sugars: 1 gram
- Dietary Fiber: 4 grams
- Sodium: 377 mg
- Calories: 318

Essential Ingredients:
- Pork shoulder roast - boneless (2 lb./910 g)
- Black pepper & salt (.25 tsp. each)
- Black peppercorns - whole (1 tbsp.)
- Cumin seeds (2 tsp.)
- Garlic (4 minced cloves)
- Dried oregano (1 tsp. crushed)
- Bay leaves (3)
- Chicken broth - l.s. (2 cans @14 oz./400 g each)
- Lime zest - grated (2 tsp.)
- Lime juice (2 tbsp.)
- Crispy corn tortillas (12 @ 41-cm/16-inch)
- Scallions (2 thinly sliced)
  Optional: (.33 cup each)
- Light dairy sour cream
- Purchased salsa
- Suggested: 3.5 to 4-quart slow cooker

Preparation Method:
1. Slice the pork into two-inch chunks.
2. Dust the prepared pork with pepper and salt - put it into the cooker.
3. To make a bouquet, cut a six-inch square from a double thickness of cheesecloth. Place garlic, peppercorns, oregano, cumin seeds, and bay leaves in the cheesecloth square center. Raise the corners of the cheesecloth to tie using kitchen string. Toss it into the slow cooker with the broth.

4. Securely close the lid and simmer using the low setting (10-12 hrs.) or high (4.5 to 5 hrs.).

5. Transfer the meat to a cutting block. Trash the bouquet and the cooking liquid.

6. Coarsely shred the meat while removing all of its excess fat.

7. Drizzle the meat with lime peel and juice - tossing to mix.

8. Serve it over tortillas garnished with sour cream, scallions, or salsa to your liking.

Pork & Cherry Tomatoes

Portions Provided: 4 servings
Time Required: 35 minutes
Nutritional Statistics (Each Portion):
- Protein Counts: 29.9 grams
- Carbohydrates: 16.5 grams
- Fat Content: 11.2 grams
- Sugars: 10 grams
- Dietary Fiber: 4.2 grams
- Sodium: 517.7 mg
- Calories: 288
  Diabetic Exchanges:
- Fat: 1 ½
- Lean Protein: 4
- Vegetable: 3

Essential Ingredients:
- Rutabaga (1 lb.)
- Olive oil (2 tbsp. divided)
- Black pepper and salt (.75 tsp. each - divided)
- Cherry tomatoes (4 cups - halved)
- Pork tenderloin (1.25 lb.)
- Ground coriander (.5 tsp.)
- Dried sage (.5 tsp.)
- Balsamic vinegar (3 tbsp.)

Preparation Method:
1. Warm the oven temperature setting to reach 425° Fahrenheit/218° Celsius.
2. Peel and slice the rutabaga into ½-inch wedges. Slice the pork into one-inch-thick medallions.
3. Toss rutabaga with oil (1 tbsp.) and ¼ teaspoon each of pepper and salt in a big mixing container. Scatter the mixture evenly over a rimmed baking tray.
4. Set a timer and roast for 15 minutes.
5. Combine the tomatoes with the remaining oil (1 tbsp.) and ¼ teaspoon each of the pepper and salt in a mixing container. Mix it with the rutabaga on the baking tray.

6. Season the pork with sage, coriander, and the remainder of the pepper and salt (¼ tsp. each). Scatter it over the vegetables.
7. Roast till the pork is cooked, and the veggies are deliciously tender (10-15 min.).
8. Scoop a portion of the pork to a serving plate. Spritz the vinegar over the vegetables and serve with the pork.

Pork Chops with Tomato Curry - Diabetic-Friendly

Portions Provided: 6 servings
Time Required: 40 minutes
Nutritional Statistics (Each Portion):
One pork chop + ¾ cup tomato mixture + 2/3 cup rice - no almonds:
- Protein Counts: 38 grams
- Carbohydrates: 50 grams
- Fat Content: 14 grams
- Sugars: 15 grams
- Dietary Fiber: 7 grams
- Sodium: 475 mg
- Calories: 478
  Diabetic Exchanges:
- Fat: ½
- Starch: 2
- Lean meat: 5
- Vegetable: 2
- Fruit: ½

Essential Ingredients
- Butter (4 tsp. - divided)
- Boneless pork loin chops (6 @ 6 oz./170 g each)
- Onion (1 small)
- Apples (3 medium/about 5 cups)
- Whole tomatoes - undrained (28 oz./790 g can)
- Salt (.5 tsp.)
- Curry powder (2 tsp.)
- Sugar (4 tsp.)
- Chili powder (.5 tsp.)
- Hot - cooked brown rice (4 cups)
- Optional: Toasted slivered almonds (2 tbsp.)
- Suggested: 6-qt./5.7-L. stockpot

Preparation Method:
1. Warm butter (2 tsp.) in the stockpot (med-high).
2. Brown the chops in batches. Remove them from the pan.
3. Warm the remainder of the butter using the medium temperature setting.

4. Finely chop and add the onion. Sauté them till tender (2-3 min.).
5. Thinly slice and fold in apples, tomatoes, sugar, curry powder, salt, and chili powder. Wait for it to boil - stir to break up tomatoes.
6. Return the chops to the pan. Lower the temperature setting and simmer with the lid *off* the pan (5 min.).
7. Flip the chops and simmer till a thermometer inserted in the pork's center reads 145° Fahrenheit/63° Celsius (3-5 min.).
8. Let it rest - standing for about five minutes.
9. Serve the delicious treat with a serving of rice and a sprinkle of almonds.

Pork Tenderloin with Apple-Thyme Sweet Potatoes

Portions Provided: 4 servings
Time Required: 60 minutes
Nutritional Statistics (Each Portion):
3.5 oz. meat + 1.25 cups potatoes:
- Protein Counts: 26.9 grams
- Carbohydrates: 44.2 grams
- Fat Content: 5.8 grams
- Sugars: 17.8 grams
- Dietary Fiber: 7.2 grams
- Sodium: 257.1 mg
- Calories: 342
  Diabetic Exchanges:
- Fruit: ½
- Vegetable: 1 ½
- Starch: 1 ½
- Lean Protein: 3

Essential Ingredients:
- Pork tenderloin - trimmed of fat (1 lb.)
- Black pepper (.25 tsp.)
- Kosher salt (.5 tsp.)
- Canola oil (1 tbsp.)
- Sweet potatoes (1 lb.)
- Sweet onions - ex. Vidalia (1 cup)
- Garlic (2 cloves)
- Apple cider (.25 cup)
- Cider vinegar (.25 cup)
- Apples - ex. Granny Smith/Honeycrisp (2 medium - cored and cut into eighths)
- Fresh thyme (2 sprigs)
- Bay leaves (2)
- Suggested: 12-inch/30-cm skillet

Preparation Method:

1. Warm the oven to reach 350° Fahrenheit/177° Celsius.
2. Dust the meat with pepper and salt.
3. Warm the oil in the skillet using a med-high temperature setting.
4. Add meat and cook till it's evenly browned (5 min.). Scoop it into a plate.
5. Peel the potatoes - slicing them into ½-inch pieces - toss them into the skillet. Cook them using the medium temperature setting for two minutes.
6. Mince and toss in the garlic and onions. Sauté them till the onions are tender, occasionally stirring (3-5 min.). Stir in cider and vinegar.
7. Return meat and any juices to skillet. Add the remaining ingredients.
8. Move the skillet to the heated oven. Roast till the meat's internal temp is 145° Fahrenheit/63° Celsius, turning and basting meat occasionally (20-25 min.). Remove and discard thyme and bay leaves.
9. Scoop the meat onto a chopping block. Cover using a tent of foil and wait for five minutes. Slice the meat into ¼-inch slices.
10. Serve with potato mixture and, if desired, top with additional thyme.

Vegan Dishes

Gnocchi Pomodoro

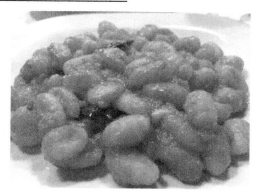

Portions Provided: 4 servings @ ¾ cup each
Time Required: 35 minutes
Nutritional Statistics (Each Portion):
- Protein Counts: 10.1 grams
- Carbohydrates: 69.4 grams
- Fat Content: 14.2 grams
- Sugars: 5.2 grams
- Dietary Fiber: 4.1 grams
- Sodium: 366.6 mg
- Calories: 448

Essential Ingredients:
- Olive oil (3 tbsp. - divided)
- Onion (1 medium)
- Garlic (2 large cloves)
- Crushed red pepper (.25 tsp.)
- Whole tomatoes -no-salt - pulsed in a food processor until chunky (1.5 cups)
- Salt (.25 tsp.)
- Butter (1 tbsp.)
- Freshly chopped basil (.25 cup)
- Shelf-stable gnocchi (500 g/17.5 oz. pkg.) or frozen cauliflower gnocchi (340 g/12 oz. pkg.)
- To Garnish: Parmesan cheese - grated

Preparation Method:
1. Warm two tablespoons of oil in a big skillet using a medium-temperature setting. Finely chop and add the onion to sauté till it's softened (5 min.).
2. Mince and add garlic and crushed red pepper - sauté it till it is also softened (1 min.).
3. Pulse the tomatoes till they're chunky and add them with salt into the skillet. Wait till boiling, and lower the temperature setting. Stir often until thickened (20 min.). Transfer the pan to a cool burner and stir in butter and basil.

4. Warm the rest of the oil (1 tbsp.) in a big nonstick skillet using a med-high temperature setting.
5. Add in the gnocchi and cook - frequently stir till it's plumped and starting to brown (5-7 min.).
6. Add the gnocchi to the tomato sauce and stir until coated. Serve with parmesan as desired.

Lasagna - Vegan-Style - Diabetic-Friendly

Portions Provided: 6 servings
Time Required: 1 hour 35 minutes
Nutritional Statistics (Each Portion):
- Protein Counts: 14.9 grams
- Carbohydrates: 42 grams
- Fat Content: 10.7 grams
- Sugars: 7.7 grams
- Dietary Fiber: 8.3 grams
- Sodium: 331.1 mg
- Calories: 324

Essential Ingredients:
- Whole-wheat lasagna noodles (230 g or 8 oz.)
- Olive oil - divided (3 tbsp.)
- Medium onion (1)
- Mushrooms (10-12 oz. or 280-340 g pkg.)
- Broccoli (2 cups)
- Garlic (3 cloves)
- Crushed tomatoes - no salt (790 g or 28 oz. can)
- Dry red wine (.25 cup)
- Ground pepper (.25 tsp.)
- Dried oregano & basil (1 tsp. each)
- Salt (.75 tsp.)
- Silken tofu (450 g or 16 oz. pkg.)
- Nutritional yeast (2 tsp.)
- To Garnish: Freshly chopped basil
- Suggested: 9x13-inch baking dish

Preparation Method:
1. Warm the oven temperature setting at 400° Fahrenheit/204° Celsius.
2. Generously spray the baking dish with a spritz of cooking oil spray.
3. Crumble and pat dry the tofu. Set it aside.
4. Prepare a big pot of water and wait for it to boil.

5. Measure and toss in the noodles and prepare per its package instructions. When ready, pour them into a colander to drain.

6. Warm oil (2 tbsp.) in a big skillet using the med-high temperature setting. Slice the mushrooms and add to the pan.

7. Chop/mince and add the onion, broccoli, and garlic - sauté them, stirring till they're softened (7-9 min.).

8. Pour in the wine, tomatoes, basil, oregano, pepper, and salt - let it simmer. Lower the temperature setting to med-low and simmer, occasionally stirring, until thickened (10 min.).

9. Stir the tofu, nutritional yeast, and the remaining one tablespoon oil in a mixing container.

10. Spread tomato sauce (1 cup) into the baking dish. Top it using ¼ of the noodles - then one cup sauce. Scoop ¼ of the tofu mixture over the top.

11. Continue to make three more layers with the rest of the noodles, sauce, and tofu mixture.

12. Cover the pan/dish with a layer of foil. Bake it until bubbling around the edges (30-40 min.).

13. Allow the lasagna to stand for ten minutes before serving. Garnish with basil, if desired.

14. Note: For Meal Prep: Prepare through step four and pop it into the fridge for up to two days. Continue with the recipe.

Roasted Tofu & Peanut Noodle Salad

Portions Provided: 5 servings
Time Required: 40 minutes
Nutritional Statistics (Each Portion):
- Protein Counts: 21.2 grams
- Carbohydrates: 41.4 grams
- Fat Content: 20.9 grams
- Sugars: 5.7 grams
- Dietary Fiber: 8.4 grams
- Sodium: 534.5 mg
- Calories: 431

Essential Ingredients:
- Lime juice (.25 cup)
- Soy sauce- l.s. (.25 cup)
- Canola oil (1 tbsp.)
- Extra-firm water-packed tofu (400-450 g/14-16-oz. pkg. - cut into 0.5-inch cubes)
- Spaghetti - whole-wheat (170 g/6 oz.)
- Smooth - natural peanut butter (.5 cup)
- Water (3 tbsp.)
- Garlic (3 cloves)
- Ginger (1 tbsp.)
- Napa cabbage (6 cups)
- Orange bell pepper (1 medium)
- Snow peas (1 cup)

Preparation Method:
1. Position rack in the lower third of the oven. Set the oven temperature to reach 450° Fahrenheit/232° Celsius.

2. Coat a big baking tray using a misting of cooking spray. Put a large pot of water on to boil for the spaghetti.

3. Combine lime juice with soy sauce and oil in a big mixing container. Stir in tofu to marinate - frequently stirring (10 min.).

4. Using a slotted spoon, transfer the tofu to the prepared baking sheet - reserve the marinade. Roast the tofu, stirring once halfway through, until golden brown (16-18 min.).

5. Prepare the spaghetti according to its package instructions and drain it into a colander. Mince the garlic and ginger. Whisk peanut butter, water (3 tbsp.), garlic, and ginger into the reserved marinade.

6. Thinly slice and add the cabbage, bell pepper, spaghetti, and snow peas - toss to coat.

7. Top with the tofu to serve.

Spaghetti Squash with Tomato Basil Sauce - Vegan-Friendly

Portions Provided: 4 servings
Time Required: 60 minutes
Nutritional Statistics (Each Portion):
- Protein Counts: 4.9 grams
- Carbohydrates: 37.2 grams
- Fat Content: 12 grams
- Sugars: 17.3 grams
- Dietary Fiber: 8.5 grams
- Sodium: 322.2 mg
- Calories: 268

Diabetic Exchanges:
- Fat: 2
- Vegetable: 7

Essential Ingredients:
- Spaghetti squash (1 medium or 4-5 lb./1.8-2.3-kg.)
- Olive oil (3 tbsp.)
- Onion (2/3 cup)
- Garlic (4 cloves)
- Vermouth/ dry red or white wine (.25 cup)
- Ripe tomatoes (910 g/approx. 4 cups/2 lb. - reserve the juices)
- Salt (.25 tsp.)
- Black pepper (.5 tsp.)
- Fresh basil leaves (8-10 torn)
- Also Needed: Rimmed baking sheet

Preparation Method:
1. Warm the oven to reach 425° Fahrenheit/218° Celsius.
2. Place a layer of parchment baking paper over the baking tray.
3. Slice the squash in half - discard its seeds. Arrange the squash halves (cut-side down) on the baking tray. Bake till it's tender when pierced with a skewer or knife (42-50 min.).
4. Meanwhile, warm oil in a big frying pan using a med-high temperature setting.
5. Chop and add onion - sautéing till it's fragrant and starting to soften (2-3 min.). Adjust the temperature setting to medium.
6. Mince and add garlic - continue cooking until golden (2 min.).
7. Dice and add tomatoes and their juices. Adjust the temperature setting to med-high.
8. Pour in vermouth, salt, and pepper. Simmer as you stir intermittently till the tomatoes begin to break down (4-5 min.).
9. Set the temperature to low to simmer for another five minutes. Transfer it from the burner and cover.
10. After the squash is cooled slightly, scrape the flesh from the shell, and mix it in with the tomato sauce and basil to serve.

Vegan Mushroom Bolognese

Portions Provided: 4 servings @ 1 ½ cup each
Time Required: 60 minutes
Nutritional Statistics (Each Portion):
- Protein Counts: 14.4 grams
- Carbohydrates: 63 grams
- Fat Content: 10.2 grams
- Sugars: 8.2 grams
- Dietary Fiber: 9.6 grams
- Sodium: 190.8mg
- Calories: 393

Essential Ingredients:
- White button mushrooms (450 g/16 oz./1 lb. divided)
- Virgin olive oil (2 tbsp.)
- Onion (.5 cup)
- Carrots (.66 or 2/3 cup)
- Celery (.66 cup)
- Salt (1 pinch)
- Unsweetened oat milk (.5 cup)
- Canned crushed tomatoes (1 cup)
- Nutmeg (.25 tsp.)
- Dry white wine (.5 cup)
- Whole-wheat pasta - ancient-grain preferred (230 g/8 oz.)
- To Garnish: Vegan Parmesan cheese

Preparation Method:
1. Load a food processor with ½ of the mushrooms - pulsing till they're roughly diced. Dice the rest of the mushrooms into ¼-inch chunks.
2. Warm oil in a big, heavy-duty pot using a medium-temperature setting. Chop and add the onion to sauté while frequently stirring till it's translucent.
3. Chop and add the carrots and celery - simmering till it's softened (3-4 min.).
4. Add all of the mushrooms with salt - simmer and stir for two to three minutes and add the oat milk. Continue to simmer while stirring until it evaporates and stir in the nutmeg.
5. Mix in the wine and cook as you stir, adding the tomatoes - wait for it to boil.
6. Adjust the temperature setting to maintain a low simmer (45 min.), stirring intermittently. (Add boiling water at ¼-cup portions if needed if it's too dry.)
7. Meanwhile, prepare a big pot of boiling water to cook the pasta per its carton's instructions.
8. Pour the pasta into a colander to drain. Serve it garnished with the sauce and dusting of parmesan to your liking.

Sides - Veggies & Rice & Other Healthy Dishes

Acorn Squash with Apples

Portions Provided: 2 servings
Time Required: 25 minutes
Nutritional Statistics (Each Portion):
- Protein Counts: 2 grams
- Carbohydrates: 40 grams
- Fat Content: 4 grams
- Sugars: 6 grams
- Dietary Fiber: 6 grams
- Sodium: 46 mg
- Calories: 204

Essential Ingredients:
- Acorn squash (1 small - 6-inches/15-cm - in diameter)
- Brown sugar (2 tbsp.)
- Granny Smith apple (1)
- Margarine - trans-fat-free (2 tsp.)

Preparation Method:
1. Peel, remove the core, and slice the apple.
2. Toss the apple and brown sugar. Set aside.
3. Poke a few holes in the squash. Pop it into the microwave for five minutes using the high-power setting.
4. Rotate the squash after three minutes.
5. Put it on the chopping block and slice it in half. Trash the seeds and load the emptied squash shell with the apple mixture.
6. Pop the container back into the microwave - continue cooking the apples until they're soft (2 min.).
7. Serve the squash with a portion of margarine.

Black Bean & Sweet Potato Rice Bowls

Portions Provided: 4 servings
Time Required: 30 minutes
Nutritional Statistics (Each Portion):
- Protein Counts: 10 grams
- Carbohydrates: 74 grams
- Fat Content: 11 grams
- Sugars: 15 grams
- Dietary Fiber: 8 grams
- Sodium: 405 mg
- Calories: 435

Essential Ingredients:
- Water (1.5 cups)
- Uncooked long grain rice (.75 cup)
- Garlic salt (.25 tsp.)
- Olive oil (3 tbsp. - divided
- Sweet potato (1 large)
- Red onion (1 medium)
- Fresh kale (4 cups)
- Black beans (15 oz./430 g can)
- Sweet chili sauce (2 tbsp./as desired)
- Optional: Lime wedges
- Optional: Garnish: More chili sauce

Preparation Method:
1. Toss the garlic salt with the rice and water in a big cooking pot or saucepan - wait for it to boil.
2. Lower the temperature setting and simmer with a lid on the pot till the water is absorbed. The rice should be tender (15-20 min.).
3. Transfer the pan from the burner and wait for about five minutes.
4. Peel and dice the potato.
5. Meanwhile, warm oil (2 tbsp.) in a skillet using the med-high temperature setting and sauté the sweet potato (8 min.).
6. Finely chop and add the onion.
7. Cook till the potato is tender (4-6 min.).
8. Remove the stems, chop, and add the kale to simmer till tender (3-4 min.).
9. Rinse and drain the beans in a colander. Fold them into the mixture to heat.
10. Gently stir in chili sauce (2 tbsp.) and rest of the oil into rice - add to the potato mixture.
11. Serve with lime wedges and another portion of the chili sauce.

Brown Rice Pilaf

Portions Provided: 6 servings @ 1¼ cups each
Time Required: 45 minutes
Nutritional Statistics (Each Portion):
- Carbohydrates: 29 grams
- Protein Counts: 5 grams
- Fat Content: 4 grams
- Sugars: 2 grams
- Dietary Fiber: 3 grams
- Sodium: 139 mg
- Calories: 172

Essential Ingredients:
- Olive oil (1 tbsp.)
- Water (3 cups)
- Brown rice (1 cup)
- Bouillon granules - chicken-flavored - l.s. (1 tsp.)
- Onion (1 small/.5 cup)
- Fresh mushrooms (.5 lb./about 2 cups)
- Ground nutmeg (.125 or ⅛ tsp.)
- Asparagus tips - cut in 1-inch pieces (.5 lb./about 2 cups)
- Finely grated Swiss cheese (2 tbsp.)
- Freshly chopped parsley (.5 cup)

Preparation Method:
1. Warm the oil in a big skillet using a medium-temperature setting.
2. Toss in the rice and sauté it till it starts browning.
3. Chop the onion and thinly slice the mushrooms.
4. Slowly add the onion, mushrooms, water, nutmeg, and bouillon granules.
5. Wait for it to boil and lower the temperature setting, place a top on the pot and let it cook for about ½ hour. Pour in water as needed.
6. Trim the asparagus into one-inch chunks and add the tips to the pot. Cover with top - cook for approximately five minutes.
7. Fold in the grated cheese with a parsley topping and enjoy it promptly for the most flavorful results.

Brussels Sprouts & Shallots

Portions Provided: 4 servings
Time Required: 25 minutes
Nutritional Statistics (Each Portion):
- Protein Counts: 5 grams
- Carbohydrates: 12 grams (Net: 4 grams)
- Fat Content: 4 grams
- Sugars: 3 grams
- Dietary Fiber: 5 grams
- Sodium: 191 mg
- Calories: 104

Essential Ingredients:
- Olive oil - divided (3 tsp.)
- Shallots (about 3 tbsp./3 sliced thin)
- Lemon zest - finely grated (.25 tsp.)
- Lemon juice - fresh squeezed (1 tbsp.)
- Salt - divided (.25 tsp.)
- Brussels sprouts (1 lb.)
- Vegetable stock/broth - no-salt (.5 cup)

- Black pepper (.25 tsp.)

Preparation Method:
1. Warm a big, nonstick skillet to warm oil (2 tsp.) using the medium temperature setting. Add and sauté the shallots until softened and lightly golden (6 min.)
2. Stir in salt (⅛ tsp.), scoop it into a bowl, and set it to the side for now.
3. Heat the rest of the oil (1 tsp.) using the medium temperature setting.
4. Trim and cut the Brussels sprouts into quarters. Add them to the pan to sauté them for three to four minutes.
5. Add the vegetable stock and wait for it to heat. Simmer with the top off of the pan until the Brussels sprouts are tender or about five to six minutes.
6. Scoop the shallots into the pan, mix in the lemon juice with zest, pepper, and the rest of the salt (⅛ tsp.).
7. Serve quickly for the best flavor results.

Bulgur & Quinoa Lunch Bowls - Meal Prep

Portions Provided: 4 servings (2 each flavor)
Time Required: 20 minutes + stand time
Nutritional Statistics (Each Portion):
Using one base and two toppings:
- Protein Counts: 8 grams
- Carbohydrates: 33 grams
- Fat Content: 20 grams
- Sugars: 8 grams
- Dietary Fiber: 10 grams
- Sodium: 0.5 mg
- Calories: 369

Essential Ingredients:
The Bulgur Base:
- Onion (1 large)
- Bulgur & quinoa/ready-mixed (150 g/5.3 oz.)
- Thyme: (2 sprigs)
- Vegetable bouillon powder (2 tsp.)
The Avocado Topping:
- Tomatoes (2)
- Avocado (1)
- Chopped basil (4 tbsp.)
- Kalamata olives (6)
- Olive oil (2 tsp.)
- Cider vinegar (2 tsp.)
- Rocket (2 big handfuls)
The Beetroot Topping:
- Chickpeas (210 g/7.4 oz. can)

- Cooked beetroot - diced (160 g/5.6 oz.)
- Tomatoes (2)
- Chopped mint (2 tbsp.)
- Ground cinnamon (2-3 pinches/to taste)
- Cumin seeds (1 tsp.)
- Cider vinegar (2 tsp.)
- Olive oil (2 tsp.)
- Orange (1 cut into segments)
- Pine nuts - toasted (2 tbsp.)

Preparation Method

1. Halve the avocado, remove the pit, and dice it. Slice the olives and tomatoes into wedges. Finely chop the onion. Dump the chickpeas into a colander and rinse - let the drain thoroughly.
2. Add the onion and bulgur mix into a pan, pour over 20 fl oz. water/600ml water and stir in the thyme and bouillon.
3. Simmer the fixings using the low-temperature setting (15 min.), leaving it to rest for about ten minutes or till the liquid is absorbed.
4. When cooled, remove the thyme and portion the bulgur into four bowls or plastic meal prep containers.
5. Toss all the fixings for the avocado topping - except for the rocket. Pile on two portions of the bulgur and top with the rocket.
6. For the beetroot topping - pile the chickpeas on top, toss the beetroot with the mint, tomato, cumin, cinnamon, vinegar, and oil.
7. Toss thoroughly, add the orange, and the remainder of the bulgur's portions, scatter with the pine nuts, and dust using a bit of the extra cinnamon.
8. Chill in the fridge till serving time
9. Tip for Prep: You can place the fixings into individual containers until serving time.

Carrots - Honey-Sage-Flavored

Portions Provided: 4 servings @ ½ cup each
Time Required: 15 minutes
Nutritional Statistics (Each Portion):

- Calories: 74
- Protein Counts: 1 gram
- Carbohydrates: 15 grams
- Fat Content: 2 grams
- Sugars: 12 grams
- Dietary Fiber: 2 grams

- Sodium: 112 mg

Essential Ingredients:

- Carrots (2 cups)
- Butter (2 tsp.)
- Honey (2 tbsp.)
- Fresh sage (1 tbsp.)
- Black pepper (.25 tsp.)
- Salt (.125 or ⅛ tsp.)

Preparation Method:

1. Slice and toss the carrots into a pot of boiling water.
2. Simmer till they're fork-tender (5 min.).
3. Drain them into a colander and set them aside.
4. Chop the sage.
5. Add the butter, toss in the carrots, pepper, sage, honey, and salt after the butter is melted.
6. Continue to sauté for approximately three minutes and serve.

Carrots with Mint

Portions Provided: 6 servings
Time Required: 25 minutes
Nutritional Statistics (Each Portion):

- Protein Counts: 1 gram
- Carbohydrates: 10 grams (Net: 2.5 grams)
- Fat Content: trace grams
- Sugars: 5 grams
- Dietary Fiber: 2.5 grams
- Sodium: 51 mg
- Calories: 44

Essential Ingredients:

- Water (6 cups)
- Baby carrots (1 lb./about 5.5 cups)
- 100% apple juice (.25 cup)
- Cornstarch (1 tbsp.)
- Ground cinnamon (.125 or ⅛ tsp.)
- Fresh mint leaves (.5 tbsp.)

Preparation Method:

1. Measure and add the water into a big saucepan.
2. Rinse and add the carrots to cook until tender (10 min.). Dump them into a colander before adding them to a serving dish.
3. Warm a pan using the medium-temperature setting to combine the juice with the cornstarch. Stir until the mixture thickens (5 min.).
4. Mince and stir in the mint and cinnamon.

5. Serve the carrots with the sauce mixture.

Celery Root

Portions Provided: 6 servings
Time Required: 25 minutes
Nutritional Statistics (Each Portion):
- Protein Counts: 2 grams
- Carbohydrates: 7 grams (Net: 4.5 grams)
- Fat Content: 2 grams
- Sugars: 1.5 grams
- Sodium: 206 mg
- Dietary Fiber: 1 gram
- Calories: 54

Essential Ingredients:
- Celery root (3 cups) or Celeriac (1) or as desired
- Vegetable broth or stock (1 cup)
- Dijon mustard (1 tsp.)
- Sour cream (.25 cup)
- Freshly snipped thyme leaves (2 tsp.)
- Black pepper and salt (.25 tsp. of each)

Preparation Method:
1. Prepare a big saucepan using the high-temperature setting to warm the stock.
2. Peel, dice, and stir in the celery root. Once boiling, adjust the temperature setting to low.
3. Place a top on the pan to simmer, occasionally stirring till the celery root is tender (10-12 min.). Scoop the celery root into a holding container and cover it so it will stay warm.
4. Raise the temperature setting under the saucepan to high. Wait for it to boil. Cook with the lid off until reduced to one tablespoon (5 min.).
5. Transfer the pan to a cool burner.
6. Stir in the pepper, salt, mustard, and sour cream. Add the thyme and celery root to the sauce.
7. Reset the heat to medium and thoroughly heat the fixings. Serve it in a warmed dish.

Creamy Low-Sodium Macaroni & Cheese

Portions Provided: 3 servings @ 1 cup each
Time Required: 30 minutes
Nutritional Statistics (Each Portion):
- Carbohydrates: 58.8 grams
- Fat Content: 14.8 grams
- Sugars: 1.2 grams
- Sodium: 123.5 mg
- Dietary Fiber: 3.3 grams
- Calories: 429

Essential Ingredients:
- Macaroni (7 oz./about 2 cups - dry)
- Unsalted butter (2 tbsp.)
- Dry mustard (.5 tsp.)
- Garlic powder (.125 or 1/8 tsp.)
- Black pepper (as desired)
- Flour (2 tbsp.)
- 1% milk (1 cup)
- Nutritional yeast (2 tbsp.)
- Mozzarella (1 oz. - grated)
- Cream cheese (28 g/1 oz.)

Preparation Method:
1. Prepare the macaroni per its package directions. Pour it into a colander to thoroughly drain it.
2. Warm a burner using a low-temperature setting. Place a pan and melt the butter.
3. Whisk the flour with the dry mustard, garlic powder, and black pepper - stir it into the melted butter. Simmer and stir till the mixture is creamy.
4. Stir in milk (¼ cup at a time), ensuring the milk is mixed thoroughly after each addition. When done, boil it for about one minute while stirring continuously.
5. Stir the mozzarella, nutritional yeast, and cream cheese into the sauce. Warm till the cheese is melted. Mix in the macaroni and enjoy promptly.

Easy Brown Rice

Portions Provided: 6 servings
Time Required: 60 minutes
Nutritional Statistics (Each Portion):
- Protein Counts: 2.3 grams
- Carbohydrates: 23.5 grams
- Fat Content: 1 gram
- Sugars: 0.2 grams
- Sodium: 4.5 mg
- Dietary Fiber: 1.1 grams
- Calories: 113
- Diabetic Starch Exchange: 1 ½

Essential Ingredients:
- Broth or water (2.5 cups)
- Brown rice (1 cup)

Preparation Method:
1. Prepare a saucepan with broth/water and the rice.

2. Wait for it to boil.
3. Once boiling, adjust the temperature setting to low and put a top on the pot. Simmer till the majority of the liquid is absorbed and it's tender (43-50 min.).
4. Wait for about five minutes before fluffing the rice using a fork.
5. Meal Prep Tip: Refrigerate cooked-cooled rice for up to three days or opt to pop it into the freezer for up to six months.

Eggplant Parmesan

Portions Provided: 6 servings @ 1.5 cups each
Time Required: 45 minutes
Nutritional Statistics (Each Portion):
- Protein Counts: 14 grams
- Carbohydrates: 28 grams
- Fat Content: 9 grams
- Sugars: 9 grams
- Dietary Fiber: 6 grams
- Sodium: 553 mg
- Calories: 241

Essential Ingredients:
- Eggplants (910 g/2 medium/about 2 lb. - total)
- Canola/olive cooking oil spray (as needed)
- Eggs (2 large)
- Water (2 tbsp.)
- Panko breadcrumbs (1 cup)
- Italian seasoning (1 tsp.)
- Parmesan cheese - grated - divided (.75 cup)
- Black pepper and salt (.5 tsp. each)
- Tomato sauce - no-salt (680 g/24 oz. jar)
- Fresh basil leaves - torn (.25 cup + extra to serve)
- Garlic (2 cloves)
- Crushed red pepper (.5 tsp.)
- Part-skim shredded mozzarella cheese (1 cup - divided)
  Also Needed:
- Baking sheets (2)
- 9x13-inch/23x33-cm baking dish

Preparation Method:
1. Position racks in the middle and lower thirds of the oven and warm it to reach 400° Fahrenheit/204° Celsius.
2. Coat the two trays and baking dish with cooking oil spray.
3. Cut the eggplants - crosswise - into ¼-inch thickness.
4. Whisk the eggs with water in a shallow bowl.
5. Toss breadcrumbs, parmesan (¼ cup), and Italian seasoning in another shallow dish.
6. Dredge the eggplant in the egg mixture - cover using the breadcrumbs, and gently press to adhere.
7. Place the eggplant on the prepared baking sheets (single-layered).
8. Generously spray both sides of the eggplant with cooking oil spray and a little pepper and salt.
9. Bake, flipping the eggplant, and switching the pans between racks halfway until the eggplant is tender and lightly browned (½ hour).
10. Mince the garlic. Combine tomato sauce, basil, garlic, and crushed red pepper in a medium mixing container.
11. Spread the sauce (½ cup) in the prepared baking dish.
12. Arrange ½ of the eggplant slices over the sauce.
13. Scoop sauce (1 cup) over the eggplant and sprinkle with parmesan (¼ cup) and mozzarella (½-cup).
14. Top with the rest of the eggplant, sauce, and cheese.
15. Bake till the top is golden (20-30 min.). Cool for five minutes. Sprinkle with more basil as desired before serving.

Fried Rice

Portions Provided: 4 servings @ 1 cup each
Time Required: 10 minutes
Nutritional Statistics (Each Portion):
- Protein Counts: 6 grams
- Carbohydrates: 31 grams
- Fat Content: 16 grams
- Dietary Fiber: 4 mg
- Sodium: 116 mg
- Calories: 279

Essential Ingredients:
- Peanut oil (3 tbsp.)
- Sesame oil (1 tbsp.)
- Cooked brown rice (2 cups)
- Green onions with tops (4)
- Carrots (3)
- Green bell pepper (.5 cup)
- Frozen peas (.5 cup)
- Egg (1)
- Soy sauce - low-sodium (2 tbsp.)

- Parsley (.25 cup)

Preparation Method:

1. Prepare a big, heavy skillet or wok to warm the oil using the med-high temperature setting.
2. Toss in the cooked rice to sauté till it's lightly golden.
3. Chop and add green onions, green pepper, carrots, and peas. Stir-fry until vegetables are tender (5 min.).
4. Make a spot in the center of the pan by pushing the veggies and rice to the sides. Break the egg into the hollow and cook, lightly scrambling till it's cooked. Stir the scrambled egg into the rice mixture.
5. Sprinkle it with sesame oil and chopped parsley.
6. Serve right away.

Garlic Mashed Potatoes

Portions Provided: 8 servings
Time Required: 30-35 minutes
Nutritional Statistics (Each Portion):

- Calories: 154
- Protein Counts: 4 grams
- Carbohydrates: 30 grams
- Fat Content: 2 grams
- Sugars: -0- grams
- Dietary Fiber: 2 grams
- Sodium: 36 mg

Essential Ingredients:

- Gold or red potatoes (3 lb./1.4 kg.)
- Fresh parsley (2 tbsp.)
- Garlic (6 cloves)
- Black pepper (.5 tsp.)
- Fat-free milk (.5 cup)
- Fat-free margarine (1 tbsp.)

Preparation Method:

1. Scrub, rinse, and chop the potatoes into big chunks. Chop the parsley.
2. Remove the skin from the garlic cloves and toss them into a pot filled with cold water. Toss in the chunks of potato and wait for it to boil.
3. Lower the temperature setting and simmer till the potatoes are fork-tender (15 min.).
4. Move the pan to a cool burner, and drain the liquid - reserving ¾ cup for the next step.
5. Pour in the reserved liquid, pepper, and olive oil into the potatoes and mash using a big fork.
6. Flavor with some pepper and parsley to serve.

Ginger-Marinated-Grilled Portobello Mushrooms

Portions Provided: 4 servings
Time Required: 1 hour 20 minutes
Nutritional Statistics (Each Portion):

- Protein Counts: 3 grams
- Fat Content: trace grams
- Carbs: 12 grams
- Dietary Fiber: 2 grams
- Sodium: 15 mg
- Calories: 60

Essential Ingredients:

- Balsamic vinegar (.25 cup)
- Pineapple juice (.5 cup)
- Fresh ginger (2 tbsp.)
- Portobello mushrooms (4 large/110 g/about 4 oz. each)
- Fresh basil (1 tbsp.)

Preparation Method:

1. Rinse and remove the mushroom stems. Chop the basil. Peel and mince the ginger.
2. Whisk the balsamic vinegar with ginger and pineapple juice.
3. Arrange the mushrooms in a glass dish (stemless side upward). Drizzle the marinade over the mushrooms and cover with foil or plastic wrap. Marinate them in the fridge - turning them once (1 hr.).
4. Prepare a broiler or grill. Lightly coat the grill rack or broiler pan using a bit of cooking oil spray.
5. Position the cooking rack four to six inches from the heat source.
6. Broil or grill the mushrooms using a medium-temperature setting - frequently flipping till tender (5 min. per side) - baste with marinade as needed.
7. Place them onto a serving platter with a dusting of basil to serve immediately.

Green Beans with Peppers & Garlic

Portions Provided: 6 servings @ ¾ cup
Time Required: 20 minutes
Nutritional Statistics (Each Portion):

- Calories: 54
- Protein Counts: 2 grams
- Carbohydrates: 7 grams
- Fat Content: 2 grams
- Sugars: 3 grams
- Dietary Fiber: 3 grams
- Sodium: 103 mg

Essential Ingredients:
- Olive oil (2 tsp.)
- Green beans (1 lb.)
- Bell pepper (1 red)
- Chili paste/pepper flakes - red (.5 tsp.)
- Garlic (1 clove)
- Sesame oil (1 tsp.)
- Salt (.5 tsp.)
- Black pepper (.25 tsp.)

Preparation Method:
1. Trim the green bean stems and mince the garlic. Deseed the pepper and chop it into thin slices.
2. Toss the green beans into a big saucepan about ¾ full of boiling water - cook for one to three minutes. They'll be crispy and a bright green.
3. Drain the greens and add them to a pan of iced water.
4. Drain again and set them to the side.
5. Warm the oil using the medium-temperature setting in a big skillet. Toss in the pepper and sauté for about one minute.
6. Combine the beans and continue sautéing for approximately one more minute. Mix in the garlic and chili paste—stirring for another minute.
7. Sprinkle them using salt and pepper with a drizzle of sesame oil.

Grilled Eggplant & Tomato Pasta - Diabetic-Friendly

Portions Provided: 4 servings @ 2 cups each
Time Required: 30 minutes
Nutritional Statistics (Each Portion):
- Protein Counts: 13.5 grams
- Carbohydrates: 62.1 grams
- Fat Content: 19.2 grams
- Sugars: 10 grams
- Dietary Fiber: 12.2 grams
- Sodium: 392.4 mg
- Calories: 449
    Diabetic Exchanges:
- Starch: 3

- Fat: 3
- Medium-Fat Protein: ½
- Vegetable 1 ½

Essential Ingredients:
- Plum tomatoes - chopped (1 lb./450 g)
- Olive oil (4 tbsp. divided)
- Freshly clipped oregano (2 tsp.)
- Garlic (1 clove)
- Black pepper & salt (.5 tsp. each)
- Red pepper - crushed (.25 tsp.)
- Eggplant (1.5 lb./680 g)
- Chopped fresh basil (.5 cup)
- Whole-wheat penne (8 oz./230 g)
- Shaved Ricotta Salat or crumbled feta cheese (.25 cup)

Preparation Method:
1. Put a big saucepan or dutch oven of water on the stovetop to boil. Warm a grill to medium-high.
2. Mince the garlic. Slice the eggplant into ½-inch pieces.
3. Toss tomatoes with three tablespoons oil, garlic, black pepper, oregano, crushed red pepper, and salt in a big mixing container.
4. Brush the eggplant with the rest of the oil (1 tbsp.).
5. Grill, flipping it once till it's tender and charred in spots, about four minutes per side. Let cool for about ten minutes.
6. Chop into small chunks and mix in with the tomatoes along with basil.
7. Meanwhile, cook pasta per its package instructions. Drain it into a colander.
8. Serve the tomato mixture on the pasta. Sprinkle it with cheese.

Lentil Medley

Portions Provided: 8 servings
Time Required: 40 minutes
Nutritional Statistics (Each Portion):
1.25 cup servings without bacon:
- Calories: 225
- Protein Counts: 10 grams
- Carbohydrates: 29 grams (Net: 13 grams)
- Fat Content: 8 grams
- Sugars: 11 grams
- Fiber: 5 grams
- Sodium: 404 mg

Essential Ingredients:
- Dried lentils (1 cup)
- Water (2 cups)

- Cucumber (1 medium)
- Fresh mushrooms (2 cups)
- Red onion (1 small)
- Soft sun-dried tomato halves**(.5 cup)
- Zucchini (1 medium)
- Rice vinegar (.5 cup)
- Minced fresh mint (.25 cup)
- Honey (2 tsp.)
- Olive oil (3 tbsp.)
- Fresh baby spinach - chopped (4 cups)
- Dried oregano & basil (1 tsp. of each)
- Crumbled feta cheese (1 cup/4 oz.)
- Optional: Bacon - cooked & crumbled (4 strips)
- **Suggested: Not packed in oil

Preparation Method:

1. Dump the lentils into a colander to thoroughly rinse and pour them into a saucepan with water. Once boiling, adjust the temperature setting and simmer with a lid on the pot until tender (20-25 min.). Pour them into a colander and rinse them using cold tap water. Empty the beans into a big mixing container.
2. Slice and toss in the mushrooms. Dice and add the cucumber, zucchini, onion, and tomatoes.
3. Whisk vinegar with the oil, honey, mint, oregano, and basil. Drizzle it over the lentil mixture and toss.
4. Add spinach, cheese, and, if desired, bacon, tossing to combine.

Marinated Portobello Mushrooms with Provolone

Portions Provided: 2 servings
Time Required: 30 minutes
Nutritional Statistics (Each Portion):
- Protein Counts: 6 grams
- Carbohydrates: 13 grams
- Fat Content: 4 grams
- Sugars: 11 grams
- Dietary Fiber: 1 gram
- Sodium: 140 mg
- Calories: 112

Essential Ingredients:
- Portobello mushrooms (2)
- Brown sugar (1 tbsp.)
- Balsamic vinegar (.5 cup)
- Dried rosemary (.25 tsp.)
- Garlic (1 tsp.)
- Provolone cheese (1 oz./.25 cup)

Preparation Method:

1. Heat a broiler or grill. Arrange the rack four inches from the heat source.
2. Spritz a glass baking dish using a spritz cooking oil spray.
3. Mince the garlic. Grate the cheese.
4. Do not immerse the mushrooms into the water when you're cleaning them. They will soak the water in like a sponge. Alternately use a paper towel or clean dampened cloth to wipe them clean.
5. Arrange the mushrooms in the dish, stemless-side (gill-side) up.
6. Whisk the vinegar with rosemary, garlic, and brown sugar - dump it over the mushrooms.
7. Let them marinate (5-10 min.).
8. Grill or broil the mushrooms till they're tender - flipping them one time (4 min. per side).
9. Sprinkle them using grated cheese - continue to cook till the cheese has melted. Serve them either solo or with a favorite entree.

Mediterranean Chickpea Quinoa Bowl - Vegetarian

Portions Provided: 4 servings @ 1 ½ cups each
Time Required: 20 minutes
Nutritional Statistics (Each Portion):
- Protein Counts: 12.7 grams
- Carbohydrates: 49.5 grams
- Fat Content: 24.8 grams
- Sugars: 2.5 grams
- Dietary Fiber: 7.7 grams
- Sodium: 646 mg
- Calories: 479
  Diabetic Exchanges:
- Starch: 2 ½
- Lean Protein: ½
- Fat: 4 ½
- Vegetable: 1 ½

Essential Ingredients:
- Roasted red peppers (200 g/7 oz. jar.)
- Slivered almonds (.25 cup)
- Olive oil - divided (4 tbsp.)
- Garlic clove (1 small)
- Paprika (1 tsp.)
- Optional: Crushed red pepper (.25 tsp.)
- Ground cumin (.5 tsp.)
- Quinoa - cooked (2 cups)
- Kalamata olives (.25 cup)

- Red onion (.25 cup)
- Chickpeas (430 g/15 oz. can)
- Cucumber (1 cup)
- Crumbled feta cheese (.25 cup)
- Fresh parsley (2 tbsp.)

Preparation Method:
1. Rinse the red peppers and mince the garlic. Finely chop the parsley.
2. Chop the olives, red onion, and cucumber.
3. Dump the beans into a colander to rinse thoroughly.
4. Place peppers, almonds, oil (2 tbsp.), garlic, paprika, cumin, and crushed red pepper in a mini food processor.
5. Puree till it's incorporated and smooth.
6. Combine the quinoa with the olives, red onion, and the remaining oil (2 tbsp.) in a medium mixing bowl.
7. To serve, portion the quinoa mixture into four bowls and top with equal amounts of chickpeas, cucumber, and red pepper sauce. Sprinkle with feta and parsley.
8. Meal Prep Tip: Put a lid on each of the bowls and put the sauce into an individual small container to add at serving time.

Mushroom Stroganoff

Portions Provided: 2 servings **Time Required**: 30 minutes

Nutritional Statistics (Each Portion):
- Protein Counts: 11 grams
- Carbohydrates: 50 grams
- Fat Content: 9 grams
- Sugars: 8 grams
- Dietary Fiber: 4 grams
- Sodium: 0.7 mg
- Calories: 329

Essential Ingredients:
- Olive oil (2 tsp.)- Onion (1)
- Paprika (1 tbsp.)
- Garlic cloves (2)
- Mixed mushrooms (300 g/10.6 oz.)
- Beef or vegetable stock - l.s. (150 ml/5 fl. oz.)
- Worcestershire sauce/vegetarian alternative (1 tbsp.)
- Sour cream - low-fat (3 tbsp.)
- Parsley (1 small bunch)
- Cooked wild rice (250 g/8.8 oz. pouch)

Preparation Method:
1. Chop the onion, mushrooms, and parsley. Mince the garlic

2. Warm the oil in a big non-stick frying pan and soften the onion (5 min.).
3. Toss in the paprika and garlic and sauté (1 min.).
4. Mix in the mushrooms and cook using a high-temperature setting, often stirring (5 min.).
5. Pour in the stock and Worcestershire sauce. Wait for it to boil and bubble for five minutes until the sauce thickens - extinguish the heat and stir through the sour cream and most of the parsley.
6. Be sure the pan is removed from the heat.
7. Heat the wild rice and stir through the rest of the chopped parsley and serve with the stroganoff.

Pea & Spinach Carbonara - Vegetarian

Portions Provided: 4 servings
Time Required: 20 minutes
Nutritional Statistics (Each Portion):
- Protein Counts: 20.2 grams
- Carbohydrates: 54.1 grams
- Fat Content: 14.5 grams
- Sugars: 2.5 grams
- Dietary Fiber: 8.2 grams
- Sodium: 586.4 mg
- Calories: 430
  Diabetic Exchanges:
- Medium-Fat Protein: ½
- High-Fat Protein: ½
- Vegetable: 1
- Fat: 1
- Starch: 3

Essential Ingredients:
- Olive oil (1.5 tbsp.)
- Panko breadcrumbs - whole-wheat suggested (.5 cup)
- Garlic (1 small clove)
- Parmesan cheese - grated (8 tbsp. divided)
- Fresh parsley - finely chopped (3 tbsp.)
- Large eggs: Yolks (3) + Whole (1)
- Salt (.25 tsp.)
- Black pepper (.5 tsp.)
- Fresh tagliatelle or linguine (260 g/9 oz. pkg.)
- Baby spinach (8 cups)
- Peas (1 cup - fresh or frozen)

Preparation Method:
1. Pour water (10 cups) into a big soup pot - wait for it to boil using a high-temperature setting.

2. Prepare a big skillet to warm the oil using a med-high temperature setting.

3. Mince and add the breadcrumbs and garlic - sauté them till they're toasted (2 min.). Toss them into a mixing container and two tablespoons of parmesan and parsley. Set to the side for now.

4. Whisk the rest of the parmesan (6 tbsp.), all of the eggs, pepper, and salt in a big mixing container

5. Simmer the pasta in a pot of boiling water, occasionally stirring (1 min.).

6. Add peas and spinach - cooking until the pasta is tender (1 min.).

7. Reserve ¼ cup of the cooking water. Drain and toss it into a big mixing container.

8. Gently mix the reserved cooking water into the egg mixture. Slowly combine the mixture with the pasta.

9. Serve topped with the breadcrumb mix.

Potato Salad

Portions Provided: 8 servings @ ¾ cup each
Time Required: 15-20 minutes
Nutritional Statistics (Each Portion):
- Protein Counts: 2 grams
- Carbohydrates: 14 grams
- Fat Content: 1 gram
- Sugars: 2 grams
- Dietary Fiber: 2 grams
- Sodium: 120 mg
- Calories: 77

Essential Ingredients:
- Potatoes (1 lb.)
- Carrot (.5 cup/1 large)
- Celery (.5 cup/2 ribs)
- Yellow onion (1 cup/1 large)
- Black pepper (1 tsp.)
- Minced dill (2 tbsp.)
- Vinegar - red wine (2 tbsp.)
- Low-calorie mayonnaise (.25 cup)
- Dijon mustard (1 tbsp.)

Preparation Method:
1. Dice the carrot, onion, and celery.
2. Dice and boil or steam the potatoes (approx. 10 min.).
3. Toss each of the fixings into a serving dish.
4. Thoroughly combine and serve.

Rice Noodles & Spring Veggies

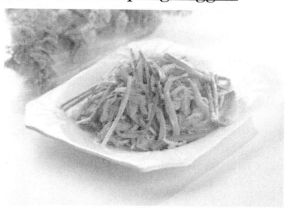

Portions Provided: 6 servings @ 1½ cups each
Total Time Required: 20 minutes
Nutritional Statistics (Each Portion):
- Protein Counts: 4 grams
- Carbohydrates: 37 grams
- Fiber: 1 gram
- Fat Content: 5 grams
- Sodium: 222 mg
- Calories: 201

Essential Ingredients:
- Rice noodles (8 oz./230 g pkg.)
- Peanut & sesame oil (1 tbsp. each)
- Garlic (2 cloves)
- Fresh ginger (1 tbsp.)
- Soy sauce - l.s. (2 tbsp.)
- Broccoli florets (1 cup)
- Scallions (2)
- Bean sprouts (1 cup - fresh)
- Cherry tomatoes (8)
- Fresh spinach (1 cup)
- Optional: Crushed red chili flakes (to taste)

Preparation Method:
1. Prepare a big pot with water (¾ full) - wait for it to boil.
2. Once boiling, toss in the noodles to cook till tender (6 min. or per its pkg. instructions).
3. Empty the noodles into a colander. Thoroughly rinse with cold tap water.
4. Warm each type of oil in a big skillet using a medium-temperature setting.
5. Mince and toss in the ginger and garlic - stir-frying till they're fragrant.
6. Chop and mix in the broccoli and soy sauce - continue to cook (3 min.).
7. Slice the tomatoes into halves. Chop the spinach and scallions.

8. Add the rest of the veggies and cooked noodles - tossing till they're thoroughly warmed.

9. Serve the noodles garnished with a portion of the red chili flakes.

Roasted Chickpea & Sweet Potato Pitas

Portions Provided: 6 servings - 2 pita halves
Time Required: 30 minutes
Nutritional Statistics (Each Portion):
- Calories: 462
- Protein Counts: 14 grams
- Carbohydrates: 72 grams
- Fat Content: 15 grams
- Sugars: 13 grams
- Dietary Fiber: 12 grams
- Sodium: 662 mg

Essential Ingredients:
- Lemon juice (1 tbsp.)
- Sweet potatoes (2 medium/about 1.25 lb./570 g)
- Chickpeas or garbanzo beans (2 cans @ 15 oz./430 g each)
- Red onion (1 medium)
- Canola oil - divided (3 tbsp.)
- Garlic cloves (2)
- Greek yogurt - plain (1 cup)
- Arugula or baby spinach (2 cups)
- Whole-wheat pita pocket halves - warmed (12)
- Ground cumin (1 tsp.)
- Minced fresh cilantro (.25 cup)
- Garam masala (2 tsp.)
- Salt - divided (.5 tsp.)
- Suggested Pan Size: 15x10x1-inch/38x25x3-cm

Preparation Method:
1. Warm the oven to reach 400° Fahrenheit or 204° Celsius.
2. Peel and cube the potatoes. Add them into a big microwave-safe container. Microwave them covered, using the high setting for five minutes.
3. Rinse and drain the beans. Chop the onion.
4. Stir in chickpeas and onions - toss with oil (2 tbsp.), garam masala, and 1/4 teaspoon salt.
5. Spread it into the pan. Roast until potatoes are tender (15 min.). Cool slightly.
6. Mince and add the garlic and remaining oil in a microwave-safe bowl. Prepare it using the high setting until the garlic is lightly browned (1-1.5 min.).

7. Stir in yogurt, lemon juice, cumin, and the rest of the salt.

8. Toss potato mixture with arugula. Spoon into pita.

9. Top with sauce and cilantro and serve.

Sheet Pan Roasted Root Veggies

Portions Provided: 8 servings @ 1 cup each
Time Required: 50 minutes
Nutritional Statistics (Each Portion):
- Protein Counts: 1.5 grams
- Carbohydrates: 15.2 grams
- Fat Content: 5.5 grams
- Fiber: 3.4 grams
- Sugars: 5.7 grams
- Sodium: 202.5mg
- Calories: 112
-

Essential Ingredients:
- Sweet potato (1 medium)
- Parsnips (2 medium)
- Carrots (2 large)
- Beets (2 medium)
- Red onion (1 medium)
- Olive oil (3 tbsp.)
- Apple cider/balsamic vinegar (1.5 tbsp.)
- Fresh herbs - ex. - Rosemary, thyme, sage, etc. (1 tbsp.)
- Kosher salt and black pepper (.5 tsp. each)

Preparation Method:
1. Position the racks in the upper and lower thirds of the oven.
2. Set the oven temperature at 425° Fahrenheit/218° Celsius.
3. Cover two big baking trays using a sheet of parchment baking paper.
4. Peel and slice carrots and parsnips into 1/2-inch-thick slices on a diagonal, then cut into half-moons.
5. Cut sweet potato into 3/4-inch cubes. Peel and slice beets and onion into 1/2-inch-thick wedges (12 cups raw vegetables total).
6. Toss the veggies with oil, vinegar, herbs, salt, and pepper in a large bowl until well coated.
7. Portion them onto the baking trays - scattering them into a single layer.
8. Roast the veggies, rotating the pans in the oven from the top to the bottom levels about halfway through its cooking cycle till they're fork-tender (30-40 min.).

Spicy Roasted Broccoli

Portions Provided: 8 servings @ 1 cup each
Time Required: 30 minutes
Nutritional Statistics (Each Portion):
- Protein Counts: 2 grams
- Fat Content: 11 grams
- Carbohydrates: 5 grams
- Sodium: 301 mg
- Calories: 86

Essential Ingredients:
- Broccoli (1.25 lb./about 8 cups) broccoli
- Salt-free seasoning blend (.5 tsp.)
- Olive oil (4 tbsp. divided)
- Black pepper (.25 tsp.)
- Garlic (4 cloves)

Preparation Method:
1. Use a sharp knife and discard the large stems, and cut the broccoli into two-inch pieces.
2. Warm the oven to 450° Fahrenheit/232° Celsius.
3. Mix the olive oil and broccoli in a mixing container. Sprinkle with pepper and seasoning. Move it to a baking tray (with a rim). Set a timer and bake (15 min.).
4. Meanwhile, mince and add the garlic with the pepper, seasoning blend, and olive oil in a separate mixing container.
5. After the broccoli is done, sprinkle the oil mixture over the broccoli while shaking the pan.
6. Place back into the oven for another eight to ten additional minutes before serving.

Spicy Snow Peas

Portions Provided: 6 servings @ 1 cup each
Time Required: 7-10 minutes
Nutritional Statistics (Each Portion):
- Protein Counts: 3 grams
- Carbohydrates: 13 grams
- Fat Content: 1 gram
- Sugars: 4 grams
- Dietary Fiber: 2 grams
- Sodium: 222 mg
- Calories: 73

Essential Ingredients:
- Snow peas (1 lb./approx. 7 cups)
- Rice vinegar (4 tbsp.)
- Soy sauce - red. sod. (3 tbsp.)
- Sesame oil (1 tsp.)
- Brown sugar (2 tbsp.)
- Cornstarch (1 tbsp.)
- Chinese five-spice powder (.5 tsp.)
- Garlic (1 clove)
- Optional: Red pepper

Preparation Method:
1. Wash and trim the strings and stems from the peas.
2. Chop the garlic and red pepper.
3. Prepare a big saucepan of water (3/4 full). Once boiling, toss in the peas, and lower the temperature setting to simmer (2 min.).
4. Drain the peas into a colander and submerge them into a container of iced water to stop the cooking process. Leave them in the colander to drain - setting it to the side.
5. Whisk the soy sauce with the vinegar, cornstarch, brown sugar, and 5-spice powder in a mixing container - stirring till it's all incorporated.
6. Prepare a big skillet to warm the oil using the medium-temperature setting. Fold in the peas and garlic.
7. Raise the temperature to high - stir often. Stir in the soy sauce mixture to simmer till it's thickened (1-2 min.).
8. Sprinkle with crushed red pepper and serve immediately.

Steak Fries

Portions Provided: 4 servings - 6 wedges each
Time Required: 45 minutes
Nutritional Statistics (Each Portion):
- Protein Counts: 1.6 grams
- Fat Content: 2.4 grams
- Fiber: 1.5 grams
- Total Carbs: 13.7 grams
- Sugars: 1.1 grams
- Sodium: 160.8 mg
- Calories: 80

Essential Ingredients:
- Red/yellow potatoes/a mix (3 large/about 12 oz. total)
- Olive oil (2 tsp.)
- Thyme & rosemary - dried & crushed (.25 tsp. each)
- Black pepper (.125 or 1/8 to .25 tsp.)
- Salt (.25 tsp.)

Preparation Method:

1. Set the oven temperature to 450° Fahrenheit/232° Celsius.
2. Cut each potato into eight wedges.
3. Whisk the olive oil with rosemary, thyme, pepper, and salt.
4. Mix in the potato wedges - tossing to coat.
5. Spread the wedges - single-layered - in a shallow roasting pan.
6. Bake until they are crispy, flipping them once (30-35 min.).
7. Serve them in four portions.

Stuffed Potatoes with Salsa & Beans - Diabetic Approved

Portions Provided: 4 servings
Time Required: 25 minutes
Nutritional Statistics (Each Portion):

- Protein Counts: 9.2 grams
- Carbohydrates: 56.7 grams
- Fat Content: 8 grams
- Sugars: 5 grams
- Dietary Fiber: 11 grams
- Sodium: 421.7 mg
- Calories: 324
  Diabetic Exchanges:
- Lean Protein: ½
- Fat: 1 ½
- Starch: 2

Essential Ingredients:

- Russet potatoes (4 medium)
- Fresh salsa (.5 cup)
- Ripe avocado (1 sliced)
- Pinto beans (15 oz. or 430 g can)
- Chopped pickled jalapeños (4 tsp.)

Preparation Method:

1. Rinse, drain, and lightly mash the beans. Chop the jalapeños.
2. Poke each of the potatoes using a skewer or fork.
3. Microwave on using the medium setting. Turn the potatoes once or twice until they're softened (approx. 20 min.). Alternatively, bake the potatoes at 425° Fahrenheit/218° Celsius till they're tender (45 min. to 1 hr.).
4. Place them on a cutting block to cool slightly.

5. Make a lengthwise cut to open the potato - not cutting it all the way through. Tightly pinch each of the potatoes' ends to expose the flesh.
6. Garnish them using jalapeños, beans, salsa, and avocado. Serve piping hot.

Warm Rice & Pintos

Portions Provided: 4 servings
Time Required: 30 minutes
Nutritional Statistics (Each Portion):

- Calories: 331
- Protein Counts: grams
- Carbohydrates: 50 grams
- Sugars: 5 grams
- Fat Content: 8 grams
- Dietary Fiber: 9 grams
- Sodium: 465 mg

Essential Ingredients:

- Small onion (1)
- Garlic cloves (2 minced)
- Frozen corn (1 cup)
- Chili powder (1.5 tsp.)
- Olive oil (1 tbsp.)
- Pinto beans (430 g or 15 oz. can)
- Green chilies (110 g or 4 oz. can)
- Salsa (.5 cup)
- Chopped fresh cilantro (.25 cup)
- Ground cumin (1.5 tsp.)
- Ready-to-serve brown rice (8.8 oz./250 g pkg.)
- Romaine - quartered lengthwise through the core (1 bunch)
- Finely shredded cheddar cheese (.25 cup)

Preparation Method:

1. Prepare a big skillet to warm the oil using the med-high temperature setting. Empty the beans into a colander to thoroughly rinse and drain.
2. Chop and mix in the corn and onion. Simmer and stir until the onion is tender (4-5 min.). Mix in and stir the chili powder, garlic, and cumin (1 min.).
3. Add beans, rice, chopped green chilies, salsa, and cilantro - heat through, stirring occasionally. Serve over romaine wedges. Sprinkle it with cheese.

Snacks

Air-Fried Crispy Chickpeas

Portions Provided: 4 servings @ ¼ cup each
Time Required: 20 minutes
Nutritional Statistics (Each Portion):
- Protein Counts: 4.7 grams
- Carbohydrates: 14.1 grams
- Fat Content: 5.8 grams
- Dietary Fiber: 3.4 grams
- Sodium: 85.8 mg
- Calories: 132

Essential Ingredients:
- Unsalted chickpeas, rinsed and drained (15 oz. can)
- Toasted sesame oil (1.5 tbsp.)
- Smoked paprika (.25 tsp.)
- Salt (.125 tsp. or 1/8 tsp.)
- Crushed red pepper (.25 tsp.)
- Cooking oil spray (as needed)
- Lime (2 wedges)

Preparation Method:
1. Warm the Air Fryer to reach 400° Fahrenheit/204° Celsius.
2. Rinse and thoroughly drain the chickpeas and toss them with the oil in a medium mixing container.
3. Sprinkle it with paprika, crushed red pepper, and salt.
4. Pour the mixture into an Air Fryer basket and coat with a spritz of cooking oil spray.
5. Air-fry them until they're nicely browned (12-14 min.), occasionally shaking the basket.
6. Squeeze lime wedges over the chickpeas and serve.

Almond & Apricot Biscotti

Portions Provided: 24 servings
Time Required: 55-60 minutes
Nutritional Statistics (Each Portion):
- Protein Counts: 2 grams
- Carbohydrates: 12 grams
- Fat Content: 2 grams
- Sugars: 6 grams
- Dietary Fiber: 1 gram
- Sodium: 17 mg
- Calories: 75

Essential Ingredients:
- Baking powder (1 tsp.)
- A. P. flour (.75 cup)
- Flour - whole-wheat/meal (.75 cup)
- Brown sugar (.25 cup - tightly packed)
- Eggs (2)
- 1 % milk - l.f. (2 tbsp.)
- Canola oil (2 tbsp.)
- Almond extract (.5 tsp.)
- Almonds (.25 cup)
- Dried apricots (.66 or 2/3 cup)
- Dark honey (2 tbsp.)

Preparation Method:
1. Set the oven temperature at 350° Fahrenheit/177° Celsius. Prepare a nonstick baking tray or spritz a similar pan with a cooking oil spray.
2. Whisk each variety of flour with baking powder and brown sugar.
3. Whisk the eggs with milk, honey, almond extract, and canola oil.
4. Thoroughly mix the fixings till the dough is just starting to form.
5. Chop and mix in the almonds and apricots.
6. Flour your hands and toss till the dough is incorporated fully.
7. Arrange the dough on a long sheet of plastic wrap - shaping it by hand into a flattened log (12x3-inches and one-inch high). Remove the plastic wrap to invert the dough onto a baking tray.
8. Bake until lightly browned (20-25 min.). Move it to another baking sheet to cool for ten minutes.
9. Place the cooled dough on a cutting board. Use a serrated knife to cut crosswise on the diagonal into 24 slices (½ -inch wide). Place them on the baking tray (cut side downwards).
10. Pop the pan back into the oven to bake it till it's crispy (15-20 min.).

11. Put the pan onto a wire rack to thoroughly cool the biscotti.
12. Keep it in a closed container for freshness, and enjoy it anytime!

Almond Chai Granola

Portions Provided: 8 cups @ ½ cup each
Time Required: 1 hour 40 minutes + chilling time

Nutritional Statistics (Each Portion):
- Protein Counts: 6 grams
- Carbohydrates: 29 grams
- Fat Content: 16 grams
- Sugars: 16 grams
- Dietary Fiber: 4 grams
- Sodium: 130 mg
- Calories: 272

Essential Ingredients:
- Chai tea bags (2)
- Boiling water (.25 cup)
- Quick-cooking oats (3 cups)
- Almonds -coarsely chopped (2 cups)
- Sweetened shredded coconut (1 cup)
- Honey (.5 cup)
- Olive oil (.25 cup)
- Sugar (.33 cup)
- Vanilla extract (2 tsp.)
- Ground nutmeg & cinnamon (.75 tsp. each)
- Salt (.75 tsp.)
- Ground cardamom (.25 tsp.)
- Suggested: 15x10-inch/38x25-cm rimmed pan

Preparation Method:
1. Warm the oven to 250° Fahrenheit/121° Celsius.
2. Steep the tea bags in boiling water for five minutes.
3. Meanwhile, coarsely chop the almonds and toss them with the oats and coconut.
4. Discard the tea bags - stir the remaining fixings into the tea. Pour the tea mixture over the oat mix - thoroughly stirring to coat. Spread evenly in a greased pan.
5. Bake till it's nicely browned, stirring every 20 minutes (1.25 hrs.). Cool thoroughly without stirring, and store in an airtight container.

Almond - Fruit Bites

Portions Provided: 4 dozen servings
Time Required: 40-45 minutes + chilling time
Nutritional Statistics (Each Portion):
- Protein Counts: 2 grams
- Carbohydrates: 10 grams (Net: 1 gram)
- Fat Content: 5 grams
- Sugars: 7 grams
- Dietary Fiber: 2 grams
- Sodium: 15 mg
- Calories: 86

Essential Ingredients:
- Sliced almonds - divided (3.75 cups)
- Dried apricots (2 cups)
- Dried cherries/cranberries (1 cup)
- Pistachios - toasted (1 cup)
- Almond extract (.25 tsp.)
- Honey (.25 cup)

Preparation Method:
1. Pour almonds (1 ¼ cups) into a food processor. Pulse till the nuts are finely chopped - move to a shallow bowl and reserve for coating.
2. Toss the remainder of the almonds into the food processor (2.5 cups) and pulse until they are finely chopped. Add the extract.
3. While processing, gradually add honey. Empty it into a big mixing container - fold in the apricots and cherries.
4. Divide the mixture into six portions. Shape them into ½-inch-thick rolls.
5. Wrap it in plastic and pop it into the fridge until firm, about one hour.
6. Unwrap and cut rolls into 1.5-inch pieces. Roll half of them in the reserved almonds, pressing gently to adhere.
7. Roll the remaining half in pistachios. If desired, wrap individually in waxed paper, twisting ends to close.
8. Store them in airtight containers, layered between waxed paper if unwrapped.

Almonds with a Spicy Kick

Portions Provided: 2.5 cups @ ¼ cup portions
Time Required: 40 minutes + cooling time
Nutritional Statistics (Each Portion):
- Protein Counts: 8 grams
- Carbohydrates: 9 grams (Net: 2 grams)
- Fat Content: 20 grams
- Sugars: 3 grams

- Dietary Fiber: 4 grams
- Sodium: 293 mg
- Calories: 230

Essential Ingredients:

- Sugar (1 tbsp.)
- Ground cinnamon (.5 tsp.)
- Cayenne pepper (.25 tsp.)
- Paprika (1 tsp.)
- Kosher salt (1.5 tsp.)
- Ground coriander and cumin (.5 tsp. each)
  ****
- Unchilled egg white (1)
- Unblanched almonds (2.5 cups)
- Also Needed: 15x10x1-inches/38x25x1-cm baking pan

Preparation Method:

1. Warm the oven to reach 325° Fahrenheit/163° Celsius.
2. Grease the baking pan with a spritz of oil spray.
3. Sift or whisk the first seven ingredients (up to the line ***).
4. Use another container to whisk the egg white till it's foamy.
5. Add almonds and toss to cover. Sprinkle them using the spice mixture, tossing more to coat. Scatter the mix in a single layer onto the greased pan.
6. Set a timer to bake for ½ hour, mixing it at ten-minute intervals.
7. Spread them onto waxed paper until the almonds are thoroughly cooled before storing them.

Ambrosia with Coconut & Toasted Almonds

Portions Provided: 8 servings
Time Required: 30 minutes
Nutritional Statistics (Each Portion):

- Protein Counts: 3 grams
- Carbohydrates: 30 grams
- Fat Content: 5 grams
- Sugars: 21 grams
- Dietary Fiber: 6 grams
- Sodium: 2 mg
- Calories: 177

Essential Ingredients:

- Slivered almonds (.5 cup)
- Shredded coconut - unsweetened (.5 cup)
- Oranges (5)
- Pineapple (1 small/approx. 3 cups)
- Red apples (2)
- Banana (1)
- Cream sherry (2 tbsp.)
- Fresh mint leaves for garnish

Preparation Method:

1. Warm the oven to 325° Fahrenheit/163° Celsius.
2. Scatter the almonds on a baking sheet tray to toast intermittently, stirring till they are fragrant and golden (10 min.). Immediately move them onto a plate for cooling.
3. Pour the coconut onto the baking tray and toast, often stirring till browned (10 min.) - toss them promptly onto a plate to cool.
4. Core and cube the apples. Peel and cube the pineapple and slice the banana in half - slicing it crosswise. Break the oranges apart.
5. Toss the pineapple with apples, oranges, sherry, and bananas - gently mixing and tossing.
6. Portion the fruit mix into serving dishes/bowls.
7. Garnish them using the toasty coconut and almonds with a sprinkle of mint. Enjoy the delicious treat promptly.

Apples & Dip

Portions Provided: 8 servings
Time Required: 6-7 minutes
Nutritional Statistics (Each Portion):

- Protein Counts: 6 grams
- Fat Content: 2 grams
- Carbohydrates: 19 grams
- Sugars: 15 grams
- Dietary Fiber: 2.5 grams
- Sodium: 202 mg
- Calories: 118

Essential Ingredients:

- Unchilled fat-free cream cheese (230 g/8 oz.)
- Brown sugar (2 tbsp.)
- Vanilla (1.5 tsp.)
- Chopped unsalted peanuts (2 tbsp.)
- Apples (4 medium or 8 small)
- Orange juice (.5 cup)

Preparation Method:

1. Put the cream cheese on the countertop about five minutes before prep time.
2. Whisk the brown sugar with the vanilla and cream cheese till it's smooth. Fold in the peanuts. Core and slice the apples.

3. Slice and add the apples into another container with a spritz of orange juice to prevent browning.
4. Drain the apples and serve with a portion of the dip.

Apricot & Almond Crisp

Portions Provided: 6 servings @ ½ cup each
Time Required: 30 minutes
Nutritional Statistics (Each Portion):
- Protein Counts: 3 grams
- Carbohydrates: 17 grams
- Fat Content: 6 grams
- Added Sugars: 6 grams
- Dietary Fiber: 3 grams
- Sodium: 1 mg
- Calories: 134

Essential Ingredients:
- Olive oil (1 tsp.)
- Apricots (1 lb.)
- Almonds - chopped (.5 cup)
- Oats - certified gluten-free (1 tbsp.)
- Anise seeds (1 tsp.)
- Honey (2 tbsp.)

Preparation Steps:
1. Set the oven temperature to 350° Fahrenheit/177° Celsius.
2. Brush olive oil in a nine-inch glass pie dish. Slice the apricots into halves and remove the pits. Put them into a pie dish.
3. Chop the almonds and sprinkle them over the apricots with anise seeds and oats on top with a drizzle of honey.
4. Bake till the topping is golden, and apricots are bubbly hot (25 min.). Serve warm.

Apricot & Soy Nut Trail Mix

Portions Provided: 5 cups @ ¼ cup each
Time Required: 5-6 minutes
Nutritional Statistics (Each Portion):
- Protein Counts: 11 grams
- Carbohydrates: 18 grams (Net: 7 grams)
- Fat Content: 11 grams
- Sugars: 8 grams
- Fiber: 3 grams
- Sodium: 4 mg
- Calories: 198

Essential Ingredients:
- *1 cup each*:

- Chopped dried - apricots
- Roasted soy nuts
- Raisins
- Pumpkin seeds
- Shelled - roasted pistachios

Preparation Method:
1. Simply toss each of the fixings listed into a large bowl.
2. Scoop out portions (¼-cup each) and pour them into a zip-top plastic snack bag.

Artichokes Alla Romana

Portions Provided: 8 servings
Time Required: 1 hour 15 minutes
Nutritional Statistics (Each Portion):
- Protein Counts: 6 grams
- Carbohydrates: 18 grams
- Fat Content: 3 grams
- Sugars: 2 grams
- Dietary Fiber: 5 grams
- Sodium: 179 mg
- Calories: 123

Essential Ingredients:
- Fresh breadcrumbs - whole-wheat preferably (2 cups)
- Olive oil (1 tbsp.)
- Globe artichokes (4 large)
- Shallot (1 tbsp.)
- Lemons (2 halved)
- Grated parmesan cheese (.33 cup)
- Garlic (3 cloves)
- Fresh oregano (1 tsp.)
- Lemon zest (1 tbsp.)
- Fresh parsley - Italian flat-leaf (2 tbsp.)
- Black pepper (.25 tsp.)
- Chicken/vegetable stock - l.s. (1 cup + 2-4 tbsp.)
- Dry white wine (1 cup)

Preparation Method:
1. Warm the oven to reach 400° Fahrenheit/204° Celsius.
2. You can make the recipe easier by mincing the garlic and shallot. Chop the oregano and parsley.
3. Toss the breadcrumbs and olive oil in a mixing container. Scatter the crumbs in a shallow baking tray to bake - stir halfway through the cycle till the crumbs are nicely browned as desired (10 min.). Set aside to cool.

4. Prepare one artichoke at a time by discarding any tough outer leaves and trimming the stem flush with the base. Discard the top 1/3 of the leaves using a serrated knife, and trim off any remaining thorns with a pair of kitchen scissors.

5. Use a lemon half to rub the cut edges to avoid discoloration. Separate the inner leaves - discarding the small leaves in the middle. Scoop out the fuzzies while squeezing a bit of lemon juice into the cavity. Trim the rest of the artichokes using the identical process.

6. Toss the breadcrumbs with the lemon zest, parsley, garlic, parmesan, and pepper in a big mixing container. Add stock (2-4 tbsp.), one tablespoon at a time, using just enough to make the stuffing clump.

7. Mound about 2/3 of the stuffing in the middle of the artichokes.

8. Begin at the base, spreading the leaves open and spooning a rounded teaspoon of stuffing near each leaf base.

9. Use a Dutch oven with a tight-fitting lid to combine one cup stock with the shallot, wine, and oregano. Once boiling, lower the temperature setting to low. Place the artichokes in the liquid - single-layered (stem-end down). Put the lid on the pot to simmer till the outer leaves are nicely tender (45 min.). Add water as needed.

10. Scoop the artichokes onto a rack and allow for cooling. Slice each artichoke into quarters and serve.

Baked Apples with Cherries & Almonds

Portions Provided: 6 servings
Time Required: 70 minutes
Nutritional Statistics (Each Portion):
- Protein Counts: 2 grams
- Carbohydrates: 39 grams (Net: 3 grams)
- Fat Content: 4 grams
- Sugars: 31 grams
- Dietary Fiber: 5 grams
- Sodium: 7 mg
- Calories: 200

Essential Ingredients:
- Almonds (3 tbsp.)
- Dried cherries (.33 cup)
- Wheat germ (1 tbsp.)

- Brown sugar - tightly packed (1 tbsp.)
- Ground nutmeg (.125 tsp.)
- Small Golden Delicious apples (1.75 lb./6/790 g)
- Water (.25 cup)
- Dark honey (2 tbsp.)
- Ground cinnamon (.5 tsp.)
- Apple juice (.5 cup)
- Canola/walnut oil (2 tsp.)

Preparation Method:
1. Warm the to reach 350° Fahrenheit/177° Celsius.

2. Coarsely chop the cherries and almonds - toss them with the brown sugar, wheat germ, cinnamon, and nutmeg till they are incorporated.

3. Leave the apples unpeeled if desired, or remove the peeling using a vegetable peeler. Make it fancy - skip every other row. Start at the stem end, core each apple, stopping at about ¾ inches from the apple's bottom.

4. Portion the prepared cherry mix over the apples.

5. Carefully place them in a cast-iron skillet or small baking dish. Be sure to place them sitting upright.

6. Empty the water and apple juice into the pan. Sprinkle it using the oil and honey over the apples. Tightly cover the pan using a sheet of foil.

7. Bake until the apples are tender (50 min.- 1 hr.). Serve the apples with a drizzle of pan juices.

8. Serve them as desired - hot or cold.

Berries Marinated in Balsamic Vinegar

Portions Provided: 2 servings @ ¾ cup
Time Required: 20 minutes
Nutritional Statistics (Each Portion):
- Protein Counts: 2 grams
- Carbohydrates: 33 grams
- Fat Content: 4 grams
- Added Sugars: 8 grams
- Dietary Fiber: 4 grams
- Sodium: 56 mg
- Calories: 176

Essential Ingredients:
- Brown sugar (2 tbsp.)
- Balsamic vinegar (.25 cup)
- Vanilla extract (1 tsp.)

- Raspberries - blueberries & strawberries (.5 cup each)
- Shortbread biscuits (2)

Preparation Method:
1. Whisk the balsamic vinegar with brown sugar and vanilla.
2. Rinse, slice, and add all of the berries.
3. Pour the balsamic vinegar mixture over the berries and wait for them to marinate (10-15 min.).
4. Drain the marinade and serve promptly, or pop it into the fridge.
5. Portion the berries into two serving dishes.
6. Serve with a shortbread biscuit on the side.

Cinnamon-Raisin Oatmeal Cookies

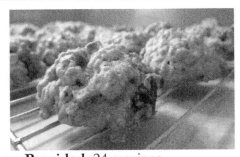

Portions Provided: 24 servings
Time Required: 1 hour 15 minutes
Nutritional Statistics (Each Portion):
- Protein Counts: 1.5 grams
- Carbohydrates: 14.5 grams
- Fat Content: 3.3 grams
- Sugars: 7.8 grams
- Dietary Fiber: 1 gram
- Sodium: 74.2 mg
- Calories: 91

Essential Ingredients:
- White flour - whole-wheat (1 cup)
- Ground cinnamon (1 tsp.)
- Salt (.5 tsp.)
- Light brown sugar - tightly packed (.66 or 2/3 cup)
- Baking powder (1 tsp.)
- Melted - unsalted butter (6 tbsp.)
- Vanilla extract (1.5 tsp.)
- Egg (1 large)
- Oats - suggested - Old-fashioned rolled (1 cup)
- Raisins (.5 cup)

Preparation Method:
1. Set the oven temperature to 350° Fahrenheit/177° Celsius.
2. Lightly spray a baking tray using a tiny bit of cooking oil spray.

3. Whisk flour with the baking powder, cinnamon, and salt in a medium-sized mixing container. Whisk the egg with the sugar, butter, and vanilla in a big mixing container.
4. Toss the flour mixture with the oats and raisins. Stir the mixture using a wooden spoon till it's thoroughly combined.
5. Drop batter (level tablespoon each) onto the baking tray, making one dozen cookies for each batch.
6. Bake till they are nicely browned on the bottom (12-14 min.)
7. Let cool on the baking sheet for five minutes before transferring to a wire rack to thoroughly cool. Continue with the rest of the batter.

Crispy Potato Skins

Portions Provided: 2 servings - 2 pieces each
Time Required: 1 hour 15 minutes
Nutritional Statistics (Each Portion):
- Protein Counts: 2 grams
- Carbohydrates: 10 grams
- Fat Content: trace grams
- Sugars: 1 gram
- Dietary Fiber: 4 grams
- Sodium: 12 mg Calories: 50

Essential Ingredients:
- Russet potatoes (2 medium)
- Cooking spray - butter-flavored (as desired)
- Black pepper (.125 or 1/8 tsp.)
- Fresh rosemary (1 tbsp.)

Preparation Method:
1. Heat the oven to 375° Fahrenheit/191° Celsius.
2. Wash the potatoes and pierce with a fork. Pop them into the oven and bake until the skins are crispy (1 hr.).
3. Slice the potatoes in half and remove the pulp, leaving about 1/8-inch of the potato flesh attached.
4. Spray the inside of each potato skin with cooking spray.
5. Mince and press in the pepper and rosemary. Pop them back into the oven to bake (5-10 min.). Serve immediately.

Fresh Tomato Crostini

Portions Provided: 4 servings
Time Required: 40 minutes
Nutritional Statistics (Each Portion):
- Protein Counts: 3 grams
- Carbohydrates: 16 grams
- Fat Content: 3.5 grams
- Dietary Fiber: 1 gram
- Sodium: 176 mg
- Calories: 107

Essential Ingredients:
- Olive oil (2 tsp.)
- Plum tomatoes (4)
- Fresh basil (.25 cup)
- Garlic (1 clove)
- Black pepper
- Crusty Italian peasant bread (.25 lb./110 g)

Preparation Method:
1. Chop the tomatoes, garlic, and basil.
2. Whisk and combine tomatoes with pepper, basil, oil, and garlic in a mixing container.
3. Cover and let stand for ½ hour.
4. Slice the bread into four slices and toast it.
5. Portion the tomato mixture with any juices over the toast and serve as desired.

Fruit Compote & Yogurt Ala Mode

Portions Provided: 8 servings
Time Required: 30 minutes
Nutritional Statistics (Each Portion):
- Protein Counts: 5 grams
- Carbohydrates: 47 grams
- Fat Content: trace grams
- Sugars: 33 grams
- Dietary Fiber: 5 grams
- Sodium: 68 mg
- Calories: 208

Essential Ingredients:
- Water (1.25 cups)
- Unsweetened orange juice (.5 cup)
- Mixed dried fruit (12 oz./340 g pkg.)
- Ground ginger & nutmeg (.25 tsp.)
- Cinnamon (1 tsp.)
- Fat-free vanilla frozen yogurt (4 cups)

Preparation Method:
1. Dice the larger chunks of fruit.
2. Combine water with the dried fruit, orange juice, nutmeg, cinnamon, and ginger in a saucepan using a medium-temperature setting. Gently stir and simmer for ten minutes with a top on the pan.
3. Discard the top and let it simmer using a low-temperature setting for another ten minutes or till the fruit is softened.
4. Serve warm or cold in bowls with vanilla frozen yogurt.

Fruit Kebabs

Portions Provided: 2 servings
Time Required: 10 minutes
Nutritional Statistics (Each Portion):
- Protein Counts: 4 grams
- Carbs: 39 grams
- Fat Content: 2 grams
- Sugars: 6 grams
- Dietary Fiber: 4 grams
- Sodium: 53 mg
- Calories: 190

Essential Ingredients:
- Sugar-free - low-fat yogurt - lemon flavored (6 oz./170 g)
- Fresh lime juice & zest (1 tsp. each)
- Kiwi (1)
- Strawberries (4)
- Banana (half of 1)
- Red grapes (4)
- Pineapple (4 chunks @ .5-inch/1-cm each)
- Wooden skewers (4)

Preparation Method:
1. Whisk the yogurt with the lime zest and juice. Pop it into the fridge for now.
2. Peel and quarter the kiwi and cut the banana into four (½-inch) chunks.
3. Thread the mixture of fruit onto each skewer. Continue till all skewers are loaded.
4. Enjoy it with the lemon-lime dip.

Fruit & Nut Bar

Portions Provided: 24 servings
Time Required: 25 minutes + cooling time
Nutritional Statistics (Each Portion):
- Protein Counts: 2 grams
- Carbs: 11 grams (Net: 3 grams)
- Fat Content: 2 grams
- Sugars: 6 grams
- Dietary Fiber: 2 grams
- Sodium: 4 mg
- Calories: 70

Essential Ingredients:
- Quinoa flour (.5 cup)
- Cornstarch (2 tbsp.)

- Oats (.5 cup)
- Chopped dried figs (5)
- Chopped dried apricots (5 apricot halves)
  Rest of the Fixings @ .25 cup each:
- Flaxseed flour
- Chopped almonds
- Wheat germ
- Honey
- Chopped dried pineapple

Preparation Method:
1. Cover a baking tray using a layer of parchment.
2. Combine each of the fixings until unincorporated.
3. Press the mixture into the pan to a thickness of half an inch.
4. Set a timer to bake the bar at 300° Fahrenheit/149° Celsius for 20 minutes.
5. Cool thoroughly and cut into 24 pieces.

Fruit Salsa & Sweet Chips

Portions Provided: 8 servings
Time Required: varies @ 2-3 hours
Nutritional Statistics (Each Portion):
Eight chips + 1/3 cup of salsa:
- Protein Counts: 2 grams
- Carbohydrates: 24 grams
- Fat Content: trace grams
- Sugars: 8 grams
- Dietary Fiber: 10 grams
- Sodium: 181 mg
- Calories: 105

Essential Ingredients:
   The Crisps:
- Tortillas - f.f. & whole-wheat (8)
- Cinnamon (.5 tbsp.)
- Sugar (1 tbsp.)
   The Salsa:
- Fresh fruit ex. - oranges, apples, kiwi, grapes, strawberries, etc. (3 cups)
- Jam - any flavor - sugar-free (2 tbsp.)
- Orange juice (2 tbsp.)
- Honey/agave nectar (1 tbsp.)

Preparation Method:
1. Warm the oven to reach 350° Fahrenheit/177° Celsius.
2. Slice each of the tortillas into eight wedges. Lay the pieces on two baking sheets - not touching. Lightly spritz using a cooking oil spray.
3. Whisk the sugar with the cinnamon. Sprinkle evenly over the tortilla wedges. Bake in the heated oven until the pieces are crisp (10-12 min.).
4. Put them onto a cooling rack. Chop the fruit into cubes and toss them into a mixing container.
5. In a separate container, mix the jam with orange juice and honey. Pour and mix it into the diced fruit. Cover the bowl and place it into the fridge to chill (2-3 hrs.).

Peanut Butter Energy Balls - G.F. & Diabetic-Friendly

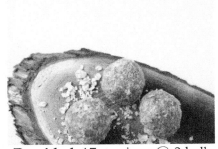

Portions Provided: 17 servings @ 2 balls each
Time Required: 20 minutes
Nutritional Statistics (Each Portion):
- Protein Counts: 4.4 grams
- Carbohydrates: 18.2 grams
- Fat Content: 9.2 grams
- Sugars: 9.7 grams
- Dietary Fiber: 2.1 grams
- Sodium: 47.7 mg
- Calories: 174

Essential Ingredients:
- Rolled oats (2 cups)
- Natural peanut/favorite nut butter (1 cup)
- Honey (.5 cup)
- Mini chocolate chips (.25 cup)
- Unsweetened shredded coconut (.25 cup)

Preparation Method:
1. Combine oats with nut butter, chocolate chips, honey, and coconut in a mixing container.
2. Roll the mixture into balls (1 tbsp. each). Store in the fridge for up to five days or in the freezer to enjoy for about three months.

Rainbow Ice Pops

Portions Provided: 6 servings

Time Required: 5-6 minutes
Nutritional Statistics (Each Portion):
- Protein Counts: 0.5 grams
- Carbohydrates: 14 grams
- Fat Content: trace of grams
- Sugars: 11 grams
- Dietary Fiber: 1 gram
- Sodium: 6 mg
- Calories: 60

Essential Ingredients:
- 100% apple juice/another favorite (2 cups)
- Watermelon (1.5 cups)
- Blueberries (.5 cups)
- Cantaloupe (1.5 cups)
- Strawberries (1.5 cups)
- Paper cups (6 @ 6-8 oz. each)
- Craft sticks (6)

Preparation Method:
1. Mix up all of the fruit and divide it into each of the cups.
2. Empty 1/3 cup of juice into each cup.
3. Put the cups into the freezer—about one hour—until they are partially frozen.
4. Place the stick in the middle of the cup and freeze until solid.
5. Pop one out of the freezer anytime for a delicious snack or dessert.

Spicy-Sweet Snack Mix

Portions Provided: 12 servings
Time Required: 60 minutes
Nutritional Statistics (Each Portion):
- Protein Counts: 5 grams
- Fat Content: 2 grams
- Carbohydrates: 39 grams
- Sugars: 3 grams
- Dietary Fiber:5 grams
- Sodium: 218 mg
- Calories: 194

Essential Ingredients:
- Garbanzos (2 cans @ 430 g/15 oz. each)
- Dried pineapple chunks (1 cup)
- Garlic powder (1 tsp.)
- Wheat squares cereal (2 cups)
- Chili powder (.5 tsp.)
- Raisins (1 cup)
- Worcestershire sauce (2 tbsp.)
- Honey (2 tbsp.)
  Also Needed:
- 15.5-inch by 10.5-inch or 39 by 7-cm baking tray
- Cooking spray - butter-flavored
- Suggested: Cast-iron skillet

Preparation Method:
1. Heat the oven to reach 350° Fahrenheit/177° Celsius.
2. Lightly spritz a baking tray using cooking oil spray.
3. Dump and rinse the beans into a colander, drain, and pat dry.
4. Generously spritz the skillet using the cooking oil spray.
5. Pour the beans into the skillet. Cook them using a medium temperature setting, frequently stirring till the beans begin to brown (10 min.).
6. Empty the garbanzos into the baking tray. Lightly spritz the beans using a cooking oil spray. Set a timer to bake until they're crispy (20 min.), stirring as needed.
7. Lightly spritz a roasting pan using the cooking oil spray. Measure and add the raisins, pineapple, and cereal into the pan. Lastly, stir the garbanzos.
8. Use a big glass measuring cup to whisk the honey with the Worcestershire sauce and spices. Pour it over the mix and gently toss it. Lightly spray it using the cooking oil spray.
9. Bake the snack for 10 to 15 minutes, tossing it during mid-cycle.
10. Transfer the pan to the countertop to cool. Store it in a tightly closed container.

Strawberry-Chocolate Greek Yogurt Bark

Portions Provided: 32 servings
Time Required: 3 hours 10 minutes
Nutritional Statistics (Each Portion):
- Protein Counts: 2 grams
- Carbohydrates: 4 grams
- Fat Content: 1.3 grams
- Sugars: 3.5 grams
- Dietary Fiber: 0.2 grams
- Sodium: 7.6 mg
- Calories: 34

Essential Ingredients:
- Greek yogurt - Whole-milk - plain (3 cups)
- Vanilla extract (1 tsp.)
- Pure maple syrup/honey (.25 cup)
- Sliced strawberries (1.5 cups)
- Mini chocolate chips (.25 cup)

Preparation Method:

1. Cover a rimmed baking tray using a layer of parchment baking paper.
2. Stir yogurt with the honey/syrup and vanilla in a mixing container. Spread on the prepared baking sheet into a rectangle (10-by-15-inch).
3. Slice and scatter the strawberries on top and sprinkle them with chocolate chips.
4. Freeze till they are firm (minimum of 3 hrs.).
5. Break the 'bark' into 32 portions (1.75x2.5-inch pieces).

Sandwiches

Baked Falafel Sandwiches with Yogurt-Tahini Sauce

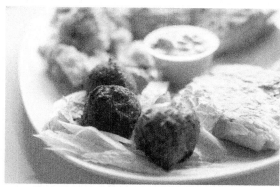

Portions Provided: 6 servings
Time Required: 55 minutes to 1 hr.
Nutritional Statistics (Each Portion):
- Protein Counts: 18 grams
- Carbohydrates: 64.6 grams
- Fat Content: 7.7 grams
- Dietary Fiber: 14.7 grams
- Sodium: 535 mg
- Calories: 388

Essential Ingredients:
The Sauce:
- Greek yogurt - whole milk & plain (1 cup)
- Lemon juice (1 tbsp. - fresh)
- Sesame seed paste - Tahini (1 tbsp.)
The Falafel:
- Water (.75 cup)
- Uncooked bulgur (.25 cup)
- Cooked chickpeas/garbanzo beans (3 cups)
- Freshly chopped cilantro & green onions (.5 cup each)
- Water (.33 to .5 cup)
- A.P. flour (2 tbsp.)
- Ground cumin (1 tbsp.)
- Baking powder (1 tsp.)
- Crushed red pepper (.25 - 0.5 tsp.)
- Salt (.75 tsp.)
- Garlic (3 cloves)
Remaining Ingredients:
- Mediterranean-Style white flatbreads (6 each @ 79 g/2.8 oz.)
- Sliced tomato (12 @ ¼-inch-thickness)
- Optional: Freshly chopped cilantro (to taste)
- Cooking spray (as needed)

Preparation Method:
1. Whisk the first three ingredients (juice, yogurt & tahini), stirring with a whisk until blended to make the sauce. Cover with foil, plastic, or a top to chill until ready to serve.
2. To prepare falafel, boil the water (¾ cup) in a saucepan and toss in the bulgur. Transfer the pan to a cool burner and wait for ½ hour till it's tender. Drain it into a colander and set it aside.
3. Warm the oven to 425° Fahrenheit/218° Celsius.
4. Combine the chickpeas and the next nine fixings for the falafel (through the garlic) in a food processor. Pulse the mixture about ten times or till it's thoroughly blended and smooth (it will be wet).
5. Scoop the chickpea mixture into a big mixing container and fold in the bulgur.
6. Portion the mixture into 12 servings (¼ cup of each), shaping each portion into a ¼-inch-thick patty.
7. Arrange the prepared patties on a baking tray coated with cooking oil spray.
8. Bake them until browned (10 min. per side.). Spread about 2.5 tablespoons of sauce onto each flatbread.
9. Top each flatbread with two falafel patties, two tomato slices, and chopped cilantro as desired.

Buffalo Chicken Salad

Portions Provided: 4 servings
Time Required: 50-55 minutes
Nutritional Statistics (Each Portion):
- Calories: 300
- Protein Counts: 31 grams
- Carbohydrates: 26 grams
- Sodium: 367mg

Essential Ingredients:
- Chicken breasts (3- 4 oz./85-110 g)
- Low-cal mayo (.25 cup)
- White wine vinegar (.25 cup)
- Whole chipotle peppers (2)
- Celery (2 stalks)
- Small onion (1 @ approx. ½ cup)
- Carrots (2)
- Root vegetable (rutabaga) thinly sliced (.5 cup)
- Whole-grain tortillas (2 @ 12-inch/30-cm - in diameter)
- Spinach (4 oz./110 g - cut in strips)

163

Preparation Method:

1. Dice the celery and onion. Peel and cut the carrots into matchsticks. Thinly slice the rutabaga. (You can use some leftover chicken if desired.)
2. Grill or bake the chicken at 375° Fahrenheit/191° Celsius to reach an internal temp of 165° Fahrenheit/74° Celsius (20 min. each side). Wait for it to cool and cube.
3. Using a blender, puree the wine vinegar with the peppers and mayonnaise.
4. Combine each of the fixings in a mixing container—omit the tortillas and spinach.
5. Put a two-ounce portion of the spinach, divide the mixture on each tortilla, wrap, and serve.

Chicken & Cherry Lettuce Wraps

Portions Provided: 4 servings
Time Required: 25 minutes
Nutritional Statistics (Each Portion):

- Calories: 257
- Protein Counts: 21 grams
- Total Carbs: 22 grams (Net: 3 grams)
- Fat Content: 10 grams
- Sugars: 15 grams
- Dietary Fiber: 4 grams
- Sodium: 381 mg

Essential Ingredients:

- Chicken breasts (.75 lb./340 g)
- Ground ginger (1 tsp.)
- Carrots (1.5 cups)
- Pitted fresh sweet cherries (1.25 cups)
- Green onions (4)
- Almonds (.33 cup)
- Pepper & salt (.25 tsp. of each)
- Rice vinegar (2 tbsp.)
- Honey (1 tbsp.)
- Teriyaki sauce - l.s. (2 tbsp.)
- Olive oil (2 tsp.)
- Bibb or Boston lettuce leaves (8)

Preparation Method:

1. Trim and cube the chicken into ¾-inch cubes (making sure all fat is removed). Sprinkle it with ginger, salt, and pepper.
2. Use the medium-high temperature setting to warm a skillet. Heat the oil.
3. Add chicken to the heated pan to cook. Stir until no longer pink (3-5 min.).
4. Remove from heat.

5. Shred the carrots and coarsely chop the cherries, onions, and almonds and stir them.
6. Whisk the vinegar with honey and teriyaki sauce, fold it into the chicken mixture and portion the mixture into the leaves of lettuce; fold the lettuce over the filling and serve.

Spinach Wrap & Tuna Salad

Portions Provided: 4 servings
Time Required: 5-6 minutes
Nutritional Statistics (Each Portion):

- Calories: 194
- Protein Counts: 17 grams
- Carbohydrates: 27 grams
- Fat Content: 3 grams
- Sugars: 1 gram
- Dietary Fiber: 4 grams
- Sodium: 450 mg

Essential Ingredients:

- Light tuna - packed in water (64-oz./1800 g - pouch)
- Small red onion (.25 cup/half 0f 1)
- Medium cucumber (half of 1)
- Dill weed (.5 tsp.)
- Celery (2 ribs)
- Juice (1 lemon)
- Olive oil (2 tbsp.)
- Seasoning blend - Salt-free (.5 tsp.)
- Freshly cracked pepper (.25 tsp.)
- 100 % Whole-wheat bread (8 slices)
- Baby spinach leaves (1 cup)

Preparation Method:

1. Peel, deseed, and dice the onion, celery, and cucumber.
2. Mix the tuna, onion, cucumber, dill weed, and celery.
3. Lightly drizzle the olive oil and lemon juice —stir.
4. Use the pepper and seasoning blend to flavor the mixture.
5. Make the sandwich using ¼ of the spinach leaves and ½ cup of the tuna salad.
6. Note: Enjoy it if kept in the fridge for three days.

Turkey Wrap

Portions Provided: 4 servings
Time Required: 10-15 minutes
Nutritional Statistics (Each Portion):
- Calories: 226
- Protein Counts: 28 grams
- Carbohydrates: 15 grams
- Fat Content: 6 grams
- Sugars: -0- grams
- Dietary Fiber: 4 grams
- Sodium: 253 mg

Essential Ingredients:
- Avocado (.25 cup)
- Low-sodium sliced deli turkey (12 oz./340 g)
- Salsa (.25 cup)
- Whole wheat tortillas (2 @ 12-inches/30-cm each)
- Green cabbage (1 cup)
- Tomatoes (.5 cup)
- Carrots (.5 cup)

Preparation Method:
1. Mash the salsa and avocado and set to the side.
2. Thinly slice the carrots and tomatoes. Shred the cabbage.
3. Spread the salsa over the tortillas - adding the turkey tomatoes, cabbage, and carrots.
4. Add them running lengthwise down the tortilla. Roll it up and cut it in halves

Veggie & Hummus Sandwich - Vegan & Diabetic Friendly

Portions Provided: 1 serving
Time Required: 10 minutes
Nutritional Statistics (Each Portion):
- Calories: 325
- Protein Counts: 12.8 grams
- Carbohydrates: 39.7 grams
- Fat Content: 14.3 grams
- Sugars: 6.8 grams
- Dietary Fiber: 12.1 grams
- Sodium: 407 mg
  Diabetic Exchanges:
- Carbohydrate: ½
- Lean Protein: ½
- Vegetable: 1
- Starch: 1 ½
- Fat: 2

Essential Ingredients:
- Whole-grain bread (2 slices)
- Hummus (3 tbsp.)
- Avocado (¼ of 1)
- Mixed salad greens (.5 cup)
- Red bell pepper (¼ of 1 medium)
- Cucumber (.25 cup)
- Carrot (.25 cup)

Preparation Method:
1. Mash the avocado and rinse the greens. Slice the cucumber, bell pepper, and carrot. Shred the carrot.
2. Spread one slice of bread with hummus and the other with avocado.
3. Fill the sandwich with greens, cucumber, bell pepper, and carrot. Slice in half to serve.
4. Meal Prep Tip: Put the sandwich in the fridge for up to four hours.

Delicious Desserts

Apple Dumplings

Portions Provided: 8 servings
Time Required: 2 hours 40 minutes
Nutritional Statistics (Each Portion):
- Protein Counts: 3 grams
- Carbohydrates: grams
- Fat Content: 2.5 grams
- Added Sugars: 5 grams
- Dietary Fiber: 6 grams
- Sodium: 14 mg
- Calories: 178

Essential Ingredients:
- Honey (1 tsp.)
- Butter (1 tbsp.)
- Buckwheat flour (2 tbsp.)
- Flour - whole-wheat (1 cup)
- Rolled oats (2 tbsp.)
- Apple liquor/Brandy (2 tbsp.)
  The Filling:
- Nutmeg (1 tsp.)
- Honey (2 tbsp.)
- Tart apples (6 large)
- Zest - 1 lemon

Preparation Method:
1. Set the oven temperature to 350° Fahrenheit/177° Celsius.
2. Combine the butter with honey, oats, and all the flour in a food processor. Mix it several times till the mixture is a fine meal.
3. Mix in the brandy. Mix several times till the mixture begins shaping into a ball. Scoop the dough from the food processor, wrap it tightly in plastic, and pop it into the fridge (2 hrs.).
4. Thinly slice the apples and toss with the honey, nutmeg, and lemon zest. Set them aside for now.
5. Roll the dough into ¼-inch thickness - using a tiny bit of flour on the working surface. Cut it into eight-inch circles.
6. Lightly coat an eight-cup muffin tin using a spritz of cooking oil spray.
7. Lay a circle of dough over each cup. Fill it with the apple mixture. Fold over each of the sides - pinching the tops to seal.

8. Set a timer to bake for ½ hour until it's nicely browned.

Apple-Berry Cobbler

Portions Provided: 6 servings @ 2/3 or .66 cup each
Time Required: 45 minutes
Nutritional Statistics (Each Portion):
- Protein Counts: 3 grams
- Carbohydrates: 31 grams
- Fat Content: trace grams
- Added Sugars: 7 grams
- Dietary Fiber: 4 grams
- Sodium: 111 mg
- Calories: 136

Essential Ingredients:
  The Filling:
- Fresh blueberries & raspberries (1 cup of each)
- Apples (2 cups)
- Lemon zest (1 tsp.)
- Turbinado - brown sugar (2 tbsp.)
- Cinnamon (.5 tsp.)
- Cornstarch (1.5 tbsp.)
- Lemon juice (2 tsp.)
  The Topping:
- Soy milk (.25 cup)
- Salt (.25 tsp.)
- Large egg white (1)
- Vanilla (.5 tsp.)
- Turbinado or brown sugar (1.5 tbsp.)
- Pastry flour - whole-wheat (.75 cup)
- Also Needed: Oven-proof ramekins (6)

Preparation Method:
1. Warm the oven in advance to reach 350° Fahrenheit/177° Celsius.
2. Lightly spray the ramekins using a spritz of cooking oil spray.
3. Chop the apples and prepare the lemon (zest and juice).
4. Toss the raspberries with cinnamon, apples, blueberries, lemon zest, sugar, and lemon juice. Mix in the cornstarch and stir till it liquifies. Place it to the side for now.
5. In another container, whisk the egg white with the sugar, soy milk, vanilla, salt, and pastry flour. Stir till it's thoroughly mixed.

6. Scoop the berry mixture into the ramekins. Scoop a portion of the topping over each. Arrange the ramekins on a big baking sheet - put the tray into the oven.
7. Bake till the topping is golden brown (½ hour). Enjoy it piping hot.

Apple & Blueberry Cobbler

Portions Provided: 8 servings
Time Required: 45 minutes
Nutritional Statistics (Each Portion):
- Protein Counts: 4 grams
- Carbohydrates: 38 grams
- Fat Content: 6 grams
- Added Sugars: 6 grams
- Dietary Fiber: 4 grams
- Sodium: 202 mg
- Calories: 222

Essential Ingredients:
- Apples (2 large)
- Lemon juice (1 tbsp.)
- Cornstarch (2 tbsp.)
- Ground cinnamon (1 tsp.)
- Sugar (2 tbsp.)
- Fresh/frozen blueberries (12 oz./340 g)
  For the Topping:
- Whole-wheat & A. P. flour (.75 cup of each)
- Baking powder (1.5 tsp.)
- Sugar (2 tbsp.)
- Salt (.25 tsp.)
- Cold trans-free margarine - cut into chunks (4 tbsp.)
- Fat-free milk (.5 cup)
- Vanilla extract (1 tsp.)

Preparation Method:
1. Set the oven temperature to 400° Fahrenheit/204° Celsius.
2. Lightly coat a nine-inch square baking dish with cooking spray.
3. Peel, core, thinly slice the apple and toss it into a big mixing container. Sprinkle them with lemon juice.
4. Whisk the sugar, cornstarch, and cinnamon in a mixing container. Scoop the mixture with the apples and gently toss to cover. Fold in the blueberries.
5. Spread the mixture into the baking dish. Place it to the side for now.
6. Use a separate big mixing container to combine each type of flour with the salt, sugar, and baking powder.

7. Cut the chilled margarine into the fry components till it's coarsely crumbled. Fold in the vanilla and milk - mixing just until a moist dough forms.
8. Generously flour a working surface - knead the bread dough till it's smooth and manageable (6-8 times).
9. Roll the prepared dough into a rectangle (½-inch thickness). Use a cookie cutter to cut out shapes - gathering the scraps and roll out to make more cuts.
10. Place the dough pieces over the apple-blueberry mixture till the top is covered. Bake till the apples are deliciously tender and the topping is golden (30 min.).
11. Serve it piping hot.

Apple Pie

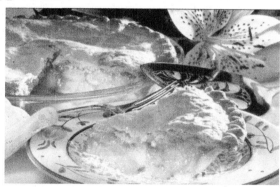

Portions Provided: 8 servings
Time Required: 70 minutes
Nutritional Statistics (Each Portion):
- Protein Counts: 4 grams
- Carbohydrates: 29 grams
- Sodium: 2 mg
- Calories: 204

Essential Ingredients:
The Crust:
- Water (1 tbsp.)
- Dry rolled oats (1 cup)
- Ground almonds (.25 cup)
- Brown sugar (2 tbsp. - tightly packed)
- Pastry flour - whole-wheat (.25 cup)
- Canola oil (3 tbsp.)
The Filling:
- Frozen apple juice concentrate (.33 cup)
- Tart apples (6 cups/approximately 4 large)
- Cinnamon (1 tsp.)
- Quick-cooking tapioca (2 tbsp.)

Preparation Method:

1. Peel and slice the apples.
2. Set the oven temperature to 425° Fahrenheit/218° Celsius.
3. Mix the dry fixings in one bowl and the dry in another.
4. Combine the two to form the dough.
5. Blend until the dough sticks together. You may need more or less water.
6. Push the prepared dough into a nine-inch pie plate. Set to the side.
7. Mix each of the fixings. Let it stand for about fifteen minutes.
8. Stir and place into the pie crust.
9. Bake for 15 minutes at 425° Fahrenheit - reduce the heat for the last 40 minutes at 350° Fahrenheit/177° Celsius. At the end of the baking time, let the apple pie cool for 15-20 minutes.
10. Slice and serve.

Banana Splits

Portions Provided: 4 servings
Time Required: 10 minutes
Nutritional Statistics (Each Portion):
- Protein Counts: 17 grams
- Carbohydrates: 61 grams
- Fat Content: 6 grams
- Sugars: 38 grams
- Dietary Fiber: 9 grams
- Sodium: 88 mg
- Calories: 340

Essential Ingredients:
- Peaches (2 small)
- Fresh raspberries (1 cup)
- Bananas (4 small)
- Greek yogurt - f.f. - vanilla-flavored (2 cups)
- Honey (2 tbsp.)
- Granola without raisins (.5 cup)
- Sliced almonds - toasted (2 tbsp.)
- Sunflower kernels (2 tbsp.)

Preparation Method:
1. Slice the peaches. Peel and slice the bananas into halves (lengthwise).
2. Portion the bananas among four shallow dishes.
3. Top with remaining fixings and serve.

Blueberry Cheesecake

Portions Provided: 8 servings
Time Required: 15 minutes & 2 hours chilling time
Nutritional Statistics (Each Portion):
- Protein Counts: 6 grams
- Carbohydrates: 35 grams
- Fat Content: 7 grams
- Sugars: 14 grams
- Dietary Fiber: 1.5 grams
- Sodium: 532 mg
- Calories: 346

Essential Ingredients:
- Non-fat milk (2 cups)
- Whipped dessert topping - f.f. (1 container)
- Sugar - & fat-free cheesecake pudding mix (2 pkg.)
- Blueberries/favorite fruit (2 cups)

Preparation Method:
1. Mix both packages of pudding with the milk (the mixture will be thick).
2. Pour ½ of the pudding mix into the graham cracker shell. Spread out.
3. Scoop one cup of blueberries over the top of the pudding, pressing it into pudding.
4. Mix half of the whipped dessert topping into the remaining pudding mixture. Pour it over the tops of the blueberries. Spread it out and smooth.
5. Spread the remainder of the whipped topping and blueberries over the pie. Refrigerate for two hours or until set.

Carrot & Spice Quick Bread

Portions Provided: 17 servings @ ½-inch slices
Time Required: 60 minutes
Nutritional Statistics (Each Portion):
- Protein Counts: 2 grams
- Carbohydrates: 15 grams
- Fat Content: 5 grams
- Added Sugars: 6 grams
- Dietary Fiber: 1 gram
- Sodium: 82 mg
- Calories: 110

Essential Ingredients:
- *Sifted A. P. flour (.5 cup)*
- *Flour - whole-wheat (1 cup)*
- *Baking soda (.5 tsp.)*
- *Ground cinnamon (.5 tsp.)*
- *Bak. powder (2 tsp.)*
- *Ground ginger (.25 tsp.)*
- Unchilled trans- margarine, softened (.33 cup)

- Brown sugar - tightly packed (.25 cup + 2 tbsp.)
- Skim milk (.33 cup)
- Vanilla extract (1 tsp.)
- Orange juice - unsweetened (2 tbsp.)
- Egg whites (2) or egg substitute (equivalent to 1 egg) beaten
- Orange rind - grated (1 tsp.)
- Carrots (1.5 cups)
- Golden raisins (2 tbsp.)
- Walnuts (1 tbsp.)
- Also Needed: 2 - 1/2-x-4.5-x-8.5-inch loaf pan

Preparation Method:

1. Warm the oven till it reaches 375° Fahrenheit/191° Celsius.
2. Spray the pans using a spritz of cooking oil spray.
3. Whisk the first six dry fixings (*in italics*) in a mixing container and set it to the side for now.
4. Using a mixer or stirring vigorously by hand to cream the margarine and sugar in a big mixing container. Mix in milk, egg, orange juice, vanilla, and orange rind.
5. Chop the walnuts. Lastly, shred and mix in the carrots, walnuts, and raisins. Add reserved dry fixings and thoroughly combine.
6. Scoop the batter into a loaf pan. Bake till a wooden pick inserted in the center comes out clean (45 min.). Cool in the pan for ten minutes.
7. Transfer it to a cooling rack to cool thoroughly.

Chocolate Cake

Portions Provided: 12 servings
Time Required: 55 minutes
Nutritional Statistics (Each Portion):

- Protein Counts: 4 grams
- Carbohydrates: 24 grams
- Fat Content: 6 grams
- Sugars: 13 grams
- Dietary Fiber: 3 grams
- Sodium: 168 mg
- Calories: 150

Essential Ingredients:

The Cake:
- Pastry flour - whole-wheat (1.5 cups)
- Kosher salt (.25 tsp.)
- Baking soda (1 tsp.)
- Water (2 tbsp.)
- Chia seeds (2 tsp.)
- Dark chocolate - unsweetened (2 oz./56 g)
- Roasted mashed yam (2 tbsp.)
- Butter - unsalted - softened (2 tbsp.)
- Brown sugar (.25 cup)
- Applesauce - unsweetened (.25 cup)
- Honey (.25 cup)
- Vanilla (1.5 tsp.)
- Greek yogurt - plain fat-free (.5 cup)
- Boiling water (.5 cup)
  For Topping:
- Dark chocolate bar (2 oz./56 g melted)
- Optional: Cinnamon (2 tsp.)
- Optional: Thinly sliced strawberries (12 oz./340 g)
- Also Needed: Nine-inch round cake pan

Preparation Method:

1. Set the oven temperature at 375° Fahrenheit/191° Celsius.
2. Spray the cake pan with a tiny bit of cooking oil spray and flour lightly.
3. Sift the flour with the salt and baking soda in a mixing container- place it to the side for now.
4. Combine the chia seeds with water in a mixing container and wait for a few minutes for the mixture to gel.
5. Melt the unsweetened dark chocolate and wait for it to cool slightly.
6. Mix the butter with applesauce, brown sugar, yams, and honey (2 min.).
7. Add chia gel - beat for another two minutes.
8. Mix in vanilla and then the chocolate. Slowly fold in ½ of the flour mixture and ½ of the yogurt.
9. Continue using the rest of the yogurt and the rest of the flour mixture. Carefully mix in the boiling water and empty the batter into the cake pan.
10. Set a timer to bake it for about 20 minutes. Test the cake using a toothpick — it should come out wet but not gooey. Don't over-bake.
11. Cool it in the pan on a baker cooling rack (20 min.). Transfer the cake from the pan and slice it into twelve pieces.
12. Melt the chocolate bar and drizzle it over the cake. Plate it with a garnish of strawberries and cinnamon to serve.

Chocolate Peanut Butter Vegetarian Energy Bars

Portions Provided: 16 servings
Time Required: 1 hour 25 minutes
Nutritional Statistics (Each Portion):
- Protein Counts: 5.4 grams
- Carbohydrates: 17.4 grams
- Fat Content: 12.7 grams
- Sugars: 11.1 grams
- Dietary Fiber: 2.7 grams
- Sodium: 90 mg
  Diabetic Exchanges:
- Other Carbohydrate: ½
- Fruit: ½
- Fat: 3

Essential Ingredients:
- Medjool dates - chopped (.75 cup)
- Natural peanut butter - creamy (1 cup)
- Rolled oats (.5 cup)
- Salt (.25 tsp.)
- Unsalted dry-roasted peanuts - chopped (.5 cup)
- Chocolate chips - bittersweet (.75 cup)
- Suggested Pan: 8-inch/20-cm square

Preparation Method:
1. Beforehand, soak the dates in a mixing container with boiling water for ten minutes. Drain, and save the soaking water.
2. Meanwhile, cover the baking tray using a layer of parchment baking paper, overlapping two sides. Lightly spray the parchment using a spritz of cooking oil spray.
3. Combine the oats with the soaked dates, peanut butter, and salt in a food processor, pulsing till the tips are finely chopped, and starting to clump. If the mixture seems dry, add a tiny bit of the reserved soaking water (1 tbsp. at a time).
4. Scoop the mixture to the medium bowl and fold in the peanuts. Spread the mixture evenly and firmly into the prepared pan.
5. Put the chips of chocolate into a microwave-safe bowl - cook using the medium-temperature setting (50%) till melted (2-3 min.). Spread the chocolate over the oat mixture.
6. Pop them in the fridge to chill (1 hr.).
7. Use the overhanging parchment to remove it from the pan. Slice it into 16 squares.
8. Meal Prep Tip: Pop them in the fridge to enjoy for up to seven days.

Cran-Fruit Coffee Cake with Crumb Topping

Portions Provided: 10 servings
Time Required: 55 minutes
Nutritional Statistics (Each Portion):
- Protein Counts: 4 grams
- Carbohydrates: 50 grams
- Fat Content: 9 grams
- Sugars: 31 grams
- Dietary Fiber: 3 grams
- Sodium: 198 mg
- Calories: 281

Essential Ingredients:
- Whole-wheat flour (.25 cup)
- Brown sugar - firmly packed (.5 cup)
- Pecans (.25 cup)
- Trans-free margarine (2 tbsp. melted)
  For the Cake:
- Whole-wheat flour (.75 cup)
- Plain flour (.75 cup)
- Bak. powder (1.5 tsp.)
- Sugar (.75 cup)
- Bak. soda (.25 tsp.)
- Vanilla (1.25 tsp.)
- Fat-free sour cream (8 oz.)
- Egg whites (2)
- Margarine (4 tbsp.)
- Dried fruits: Ex: Raisins, apples, pineapple, or apricots (.5 cup)
- Fresh cranberries (1 cup)

Preparation Method:
1. Set the oven temperature to 350° Fahrenheit/177° Celsius.
2. Lightly spray the baking pan using a tiny bit of cooking oil spray.
3. Chop the nuts, cranberries, and dried fruit.
4. Prepare the topping by mixing the brown sugar with the flour and pecans in a mixing container. Fold/work in the margarine after it's melted till the mixture is crumbly. Set aside.
5. Sift the flour with the baking powder, sugar, and baking soda.
6. In another container, whisk the vanilla with the egg whites, margarine, and sour cream using an electric mixer (med-low speed) till it's thoroughly incorporated (2 min.). Combine the flour mixture with the sour cream mixture till it's smooth.

170

7. Dump ½ of the batter into the pan. Top it off using the fruit, spreading the rest of the batter over the fruit. Sprinkle with topping.
8. Bake till it's done (45 min.).
9. Cut the coffee cake into ten wedges and enjoy it warm.

Creamy Fruit Dessert

Portions Provided: 4 servings
Time Required: 10 minutes + chilling time
Nutritional Statistics (Each Portion):
- Protein Counts: 6 grams
- Carbohydrates: 41 grams (Net: 1 gram)
- Fat Content: 2 grams
- Dietary Fiber: 2 grams
- Sugars: 38grams
- Sodium: 241 mg
- Calories: 206

Essential Ingredients:
- Fat-free cream cheese - softened (4 oz./110 g)
- Plain fat-free yogurt (.5 cup)
- Sugar (1 tsp.)
- Water-packed sliced peaches - drained (14.5 oz. can/410 g)
- Mandarin oranges - drained (15 oz./430 g can)
- Water-packed pineapple chunks - drained (8 oz./230 g can)
- Toasted shredded coconut (4 tbsp.)
- Vanilla extract (.5 tsp.)

Preparation Method:
1. Blend the yogurt with the sugar, vanilla, and cream cheese using an electric mixer's high-speed setting till it's creamy.
2. Drain the canned fruit and combine the peaches with the oranges and pineapple.
3. Mix in the cream cheese mixture. Put a layer of foil over the container and pop it into the fridge until it's well-chilled.
4. Serve it with a portion of shredded coconut.

Easy Peach Cobbler Dump Cake

Portions Provided: 12 servings
Time Required: 55 minutes
Nutritional Statistics (Each Portion):
- Protein Counts: 2.8 grams
- Carbohydrates: 39.5 grams
- Fat Content: 5.2 grams
- Sugars: 23.1 grams
- Dietary Fiber: 1.3 grams
- Sodium: 30.8 mg
- Calories: 211

Essential Ingredients:
- Frozen sliced peaches (16 oz. pkg./3 cups)
- Salt (.125 or 1/8 tsp.)
- Lemon juice (1 tbsp.)
- Whole milk (.75 cup)
- Light brown sugar (3 tbsp.)
- Organic yellow cake mix (1 box/15.85 to 18 oz.)
- Grapeseed or canola oil (.25 cup)
- Suggested: 13-by-9-inch glass baking dish

Preparation Method:
1. Thaw the peaches.
2. Warm the oven to reach 350° Fahrenheit/177° Celsius.
3. Lightly mist the baking dish using a cooking oil spray.
4. Toss the peaches with the salt and brown sugar in a saucepan - wait for it to boil using a medium-temperature setting.
5. Transfer the pan from the burner and stir in lemon juice. Transfer to the prepared baking dish.
6. Whisk the cake mix with the milk and oil in a mixing container.
7. Dump the batter over the peach mixture, spreading to cover the peaches as much as possible.
8. Bake the cake until it's a nice brown as desired (28-30 min.). Cool for 15 minutes before serving.

Flourless Honey-Almond Cake

Portions Provided: 10 servings
Time Required: 2 hours
Nutritional Statistics (Each Portion):
- Protein Counts: 7.6 grams
- Carbohydrates: 22 grams
- Fat Content: 13.8 grams
- Sugars: 17.4 grams
- Sodium: 208.3 mg
- Dietary Fiber:2.9 grams
- Calories: 235

Essential Ingredients:
The Cake:
- Whole almonds - toasted 1.5 cups)
- Unchilled eggs (4 large - separated)
- Honey (.5 cup)
- Vanilla extract (1 tsp.)
- Salt (.5 tsp.)
- Baking soda (.5 tsp.)
Topping Ingredients:

- Honey (2 tbsp.)
- Sliced almonds, toasted (.25 cup)
- Also Needed: 9-inch/23-cm springform pan

Preparation Method:

1. Warm the oven to reach 350° Fahrenheit/177° Celsius.
2. Coat the baking pan using a bit of cooking oil spray.
3. Cover the pan's bottom using a sheet of parchment baking paper and lightly spray the paper.
4. Finely grind the whole almonds in a food processor (1.75 cups ground).
5. Beat four egg yolks, baking soda, honey, vanilla, and salt in a big mixing container using an electric mixer (or use a paddle attachment on a stand mixer) using a medium-speed setting till it's incorporated.
6. Mix in the ground almonds and mix using the low-setting till combined.
7. Beat four egg whites in another big mixing container using the electric mixer (use clean beaters on a hand-held mixer or the whisk attachment on a stand mixer) using the medium speed setting till it's foamy white and doubled in volume - but not stiff enough to hold peaks (1-2 min. depending on the type of mixer).
8. Gently fold the egg whites into the nut mixture till they're "just" combined. Scrape the batter into the prepared pan and bake until the cake is a nice brown as desired (25-28 min.)
9. Cool the cake in the pan for ten minutes. Run a butter knife around the edge of the pan to remove the side ring - thoroughly cool. Move the cake to a serving platter and drizzle the top with honey and a sprinkle of sliced almonds.

Fruit Cake

Portions Provided: 12 servings
Time Required: 2 hours - varies
Nutritional Statistics (Each Portion):

- Protein Counts: 5 grams
- Carbohydrates: 41 grams
- Fat Content: 5 grams
- Sugars: 25 grams
- Dietary Fiber: 5 grams
- Sodium: 117 mg

- Calories: 229

Essential Ingredients:

- Assorted chopped dried fruit - currants, cherries, figs, or dates (2 cups)
- Unsweetened applesauce (.5 cup)
- Crushed pineapple packed in juice - drained (.5 cup)
- Zest and juice (1 medium orange + 1 lemon)
- Apple juice - unsweetened (.5 cup)
- Pure vanilla extract (2 tbsp.)
- Sugar (.25 cup)
- Flour - whole-wheat (1 cup)
- Flaxseed flour (.25 cup)
- Rolled oats (.5 cup)
- Baking soda & powder (.5 tsp. each)
- Egg (1)
- Chopped/crushed walnuts (.5 cup)

Preparation Method:

1. Toss the dried fruit with the applesauce, fruit zests and juices, pineapple, and vanilla. Let the mixture soak for 15 to 20 minutes.
2. Cover the bottom of a 9x4-inch pan using a layer of parchment baking paper.
3. Warm the oven temperature to reach 325° Fahrenheit/163° Celsius.
4. Whisk the sugar with oats, baking powder, flour (all), and baking soda.
5. Combine the fruit and liquid mixture to the dry fixings and stir to combine.
6. Whisk and mix in the egg and walnuts - stirring to combine.
7. Pour mixture into a loaf pan - bake till a wooden toothpick inserted in the middle comes out clean (1 hr.).
8. Wait for about ½ hour for the fruit cake before removing it from the pan.

Glazed Chocolate-Pumpkin Bundt Cake

Portions Provided: 1 serving
Time Required: 3 hours 30 minutes
Nutritional Statistics (Each Portion):

- Protein Counts: 3.8 grams
- Carbohydrates: 46.8 grams
- Fat Content: 5.1 grams
- Sugars: 33.2 grams
- Dietary Fiber: 3.4 grams
- Sodium: 237.2 mg
- Calories: 236

Essential Ingredients:
The Cake:
- A.P. flour (1 cup)
- Salt (.25 tsp.)
- Granulated sugar (1 cup)
- Pastry flour - whole-wheat (.75 cup)
- Cocoa powder - not Dutch-process - unsweetened (.75 cup)
- Baking soda and powder (1.5 tsp. each)
- Pumpkin pie spice (1 tsp.)
- Buttermilk - nonfat (1 cup)
- Pumpkin puree - unsweetened (15-oz./430 g can)
- Dark brown sugar, packed (.75 cup)
- Large eggs - Unchilled (2 @ 1 whole + 1 white)
- Canola oil (.25 cup)
- Vanilla extract (1 tbsp.)
- Light corn syrup (.25 cup)
Glaze & Garnish:
- Packed confectioners' sugar (.5 cup)
- Nonfat buttermilk (1 tbsp.)
- Toasted chopped nuts or mini chocolate chips (2 tbsp.)
- Suggested: 12-cup Bundt pan

Preparation Method:
1. Warm the oven to 350° Fahrenheit/177° Celsius.
2. Cover the pan using a cooking oil spray. Whisk each type of flour with baking powder, cocoa, baking soda, granulated sugar, salt, and pumpkin spice in a mixing container.
3. Blend the pumpkin puree with one cup of buttermilk and brown sugar in a big mixing container using an electric mixer on a low-speed setting.
4. Mix in all of the eggs, then the corn syrup, oil, and vanilla. Slowly add the dry fixings, mixing till just combined.
5. Dump the batter into the prepared pan.
6. Bake the cake until a wooden skewer inserted in the center comes out with only a few moist crumbs attached (1-1.25 hrs.). Cool it on a wire rack (15 min.). Transfer it from the pan and let it thoroughly cool (2 hrs.).
7. Combine the confectioners' sugar and buttermilk (1 tbsp.) in a mixing dish, stirring until thoroughly smooth.
8. Arrange the cake on a serving plate, drizzle the glaze over the top, and garnish chocolate chips or nuts while the glaze is still moist.

Grilled Pineapple with Chili-Lime

Portions Provided: 6 servings
Time Required: 15 minutes
Nutritional Statistics (Each Portion):
- Protein Counts: 1 gram
- Carbohydrates: 20 grams (Net: 2 grams)
- Fat Content: 2 grams
- Sugars: 17 grams
- Dietary Fiber: 1 gram
- Sodium: 35 mg
- Calories: 97

Essential Ingredients:
- Lime juice (1 tbsp.)
- Fresh pineapple (1)
- Honey/agave nectar (1 tbsp.)
- Olive oil (1 tbsp.)
- Salt (1 dash)
- Chili powder (1.5 tsp.)
- Brown sugar (3 tbsp.)

Preparation Method:
1. Peel pineapple, removing any eyes from fruit. Cut lengthwise into six wedges; remove the core.
2. Whisk the rest of the fixings until blended. Brush pineapple with half of the glaze; reserve the remaining mixture for basting.
3. Grill the pineapple with the lid on using the medium temperature setting. You can also choose to broil it until it's lightly browned (2-4 min. per side), occasionally basting with the reserved glaze.

Grapefruit- Lime & Mint Yogurt Parfait

Portions Provided: 6 servings
Time Required: 15 minutes
Nutritional Statistics (Each Portion):
- Protein Counts: 10 grams
- Carbohydrates: 39 grams (Net: -0- grams)
- Fat Content: 3 grams
- Sugars: 36 grams
- Dietary Fiber: 3 grams
- Sodium: 115 mg
- Calories: 207

Essential Ingredients:
- Plain yogurt - reduced-fat (4 cups)
- Red grapefruit (4 large)
- Lime juice (2 tbsp.)
- Zest of lime (2 tsp.)
- Honey (3 tbsp.)
- Fresh mint leaves

Preparation Method:

1. Remove a thin slice from each grapefruit's bottom and top. Stand the fruit upright on a cutting board.
2. Discard the peel and outer membrane from the grapefruit. Slice along the membrane of each segment to dislodge the fruit.
3. Combine the yogurt with lime juice and zest.
4. Layer ½ of the grapefruit and half of the yogurt mixture into six parfait glasses. Make another set of layers.
5. Drizzle with honey and top with freshly torn mint.
6. Serve and enjoy!

Lemon Pudding Cakes

Portions Provided: 6 servings
Time Required: 55 minutes
Nutritional Statistics (Each Portion):
- Protein Counts: 4 grams
- Carbohydrates: 34 grams
- Fat Content: 4 grams
- Sugars: 28 grams
- Dietary Fiber: 2 grams
- Sodium: 124 mg
- Calories: 174

Essential Ingredients:
- Eggs (2)
- Salt (.25 tsp.)
- Sugar (.75 cup)
- Fresh lemon juice (.33 cup)
- Skim milk (1 cup)
- A. P. flour (3 tbsp.)
- Finely grated lemon peel (1 tbsp.)
- Butter (1 tbsp.)

Preparation Method:

1. Warm the oven temperature to reach 350° Fahrenheit/177° Celsius.
2. Coat six (six-ounce) custard cups with a tiny bit of cooking oil spray.
3. Separate the egg whites and yolks into two separate mixing containers.
4. Use a stand/electric mixer using a high-speed setting to beat the egg whites with the salt. Gradually mix in sugar (¼ cup) - beat till the sugar is thoroughly incorporated and stiff peaks are created.
5. Melt the butter. Whisk the egg yolks with the sugar (½ cup) till it's thoroughly blended. Pour in milk, flour, lemon peel,

lemon juice, and butter. Mix until it's creamy smooth (2-3 min.).
6. Gently fold the egg whites into the egg yolk mixture until just combined. Place ½ cup of the mixture into each custard cup. Set the cups in a baking pan (13x9-inches) and place them in the oven.
7. Fill the baking pan with boiling water till the water reaches halfway up the custard cups' sides.
8. Bake until pudding tops are golden and firm (40-45 min.).
9. Transfer the tray to the countertop and cool the custard cups on a wire rack.

Mixed Berry Pie

Portions Provided: 6 servings
Time Required: 10-15 minutes
Nutritional Statistics (Each Portion):
- Protein Counts: 2 grams
- Carbohydrates: 20 grams
- Fat Content: 5 grams
- Sugars: 8 grams
- Dietary Fiber: 2 grams
- Sodium: 169 mg
- Calories: 133

Essential Ingredients:
- Instant vanilla pudding -fat-free - sugar-free - made with fat-free milk (.5 cup)
- Sliced strawberries (.75 cup/12-15 medium strawberries)
- Raspberries (.75 cup)
- Graham cracker pie crusts (6 single-serve - tart-size)
- Light whipped topping (6 tbsp.)
- To Garnish: Mint leaves (6)

Preparation Method:

1. Make the pudding according to the instructions on the package.
2. Toss the berries in a mixing container.
3. Divide the pudding among the pie crusts (about 4 tsp. each).
4. Add about two tablespoons of the berry mix to each pie - top each with one tablespoon whipped topping. Garnish with mint leaves.
5. Serve immediately or place in the refrigerator until ready to serve.

Peach Tart

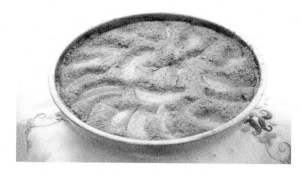

Portions Provided: 8 servings
Time Required: 70 minutes + cooling time
Nutritional Statistics (Each Portion):
- Protein Counts: 4 grams
- Carbohydrates: 36 grams (Net: 12 grams)
- Fat Content: 8 grams
- Sugars: 21 grams
- Dietary Fiber: 3 grams
- Sodium: 46 mg
- Calories: 222

Essential Ingredients:
- Ground nutmeg (.25 tsp.)
- A. P. flour (1 cup)
- Unchilled butter (.25 cup)
- Sugar (3 tbsp.)
  The Filling:
- Peaches (910 g/2 lb./about 7 medium)
- Sugar (.33 cup)
- A. P. flour (2 tbsp.)
- Ground cinnamon (.25 tsp.)
- Almond extract (.125 or 1/8 tsp.)
- Sliced almonds (.25 cup)
- Whipped cream - optional
- Suggested: One tart pan (9-inch - fluted - removable bottom)

Preparation Method:
1. Warm the oven to 375° Fahrenheit/191° Celsius.
2. Cream the butter with the nutmeg and sugar till it's fluffy (5-7 min.). Beat in flour until blended (mixture will be dry).
3. Push the mixture into the bottom and up sides of an ungreased tart pan.
4. Put the pan onto a baking tray. Bake on a middle oven rack until lightly browned (10-12 min.). Cool on a wire rack.
5. Peel and slice the peaches. Toss them with sugar, flour, cinnamon, and extract - add to the crust. Sprinkle with almonds.

6. Bake the tart on a lower oven rack until it's golden brown and peaches are tender (40-45 min.).
7. Cool them on a wire rack and serve with a portion of whipped cream

Peaches & Cream

Portions Provided: 2 servings
Time Required: 45 minutes
Nutritional Statistics (Each Portion):
- Protein Counts: 5 grams
- Carbs: 48 grams
- Fat Content: 1 gram
- Sugars: 21 grams
- Dietary Fiber: 4 grams
- Sodium: 105 mg
- Calories: 221

Essential Ingredients:
- Low-fat granola (.33 cup)
- Cinnamon (.125 or 1/8 tsp.)
- Peaches (2 medium)
- Vanilla ice cream - f.f. (1 cup)

Preparation Method:
1. Peel and thinly slice the peaches.
2. Spritz a small baking container using some cooking oil spray.
3. Warm the oven to 350° Fahrenheit/177° Celsius.
4. Put the peaches into the dish and sprinkle using the granola and cinnamon.
5. Bake till the fruit is bubbly (30 min.).
6. Cool it down for about five or ten minutes.
7. Add the ice cream and serve.

Poached Citrusy Pears

Portions Provided: 4 servings
Time Required: 35 minutes
Nutritional Statistics (Each Portion):
- Protein Counts: 1 gram
- Carbohydrates: 34 grams
- Fat Content: 0.5 grams
- Dietary Fiber: 2 grams
- Sodium: 9 mg
- Calories: 140

Essential Ingredients:
- Apple juice (.25 cup)
- Orange juice (1 cup)
- Ground nutmeg & cinnamon (1 tsp. each)
- Fresh raspberries (.5 cup)
- Pears (4 whole)

- Orange zest (2 tbsp.)

Preparation Method:

1. Remove the peel from the pears - leave the stems connected. Use a coring tool to remove the core from the bottom/base. Put in a shallow baking dish.
2. Use the medium-temperature setting to blend the juices, nutmeg, and cinnamon - stirring till it's evenly mixed.
3. Do not boil, but simmer for thirty minutes, turning the pears often.
4. Take them from the dish; garnish with the orange zest and raspberries.

Rhubarb & Almond Crumble Tart

Portions Provided: 10 servings
Time Required: 2 hours
Nutritional Statistics (Each Portion):

- Protein Counts: 7 grams
- Carbohydrates: 65 grams
- Fat Content: 30 grams
- Sugars: 39 grams
- Dietary Fiber: 3 grams
- Sodium: 0.42 grams
- Calories: 545

Essential Ingredients:

- Short crust pastry (13.2 oz./375 g pack)
- Plain flour (as needed)
- Rhubarb (750 g/26.5 oz.)
- Golden caster sugar (140 g/4.9 oz.)
- Juice (1 large orange)
  Topping Ingredients:
- Cold butter - diced (4.9 oz./140 g)
- Ground cinnamon (25 tsp.)
- Ground almond (3.5 oz./100 g)
- Plain flour (4.9 oz./140 g)
- Light muscovado sugar (175 g/6.2 oz.)
- Flaked almonds (1 handful)

Preparation Method:

1. Heat oven to 392° Fahrenheit/200° Celsius.
2. Roll the pastry onto a lightly floured surface, then line a 23cm tart tin with it. Chill in the refrigerator.
3. Slice the rhubarb into thumb-sized chunks and add it to the roasting tray with the sugar and juice. Toss and cover with foil to bake for 30-40 minutes. Tip into a sieve over a bowl, then reserve the syrup.
4. Meanwhile, press a sheet of baking paper into the tart case, add the beans - bake for

20 minutes. Remove beans and paper and bake for an additional ten minutes.

5. Combine the topping ingredients, except the almonds, till they're crumbly.
6. When the case is cooked, adjust the oven setting to 356° Fahrenheit/180° Celsius.
7. Spoon the rhubarb over the case and crumble the topping. Scatter with almonds to bake (20 min.).
8. Cool the tart slightly and serve with the rhubarb syrup and a bit of crème fraîche.

Rice - Fruity Pudding

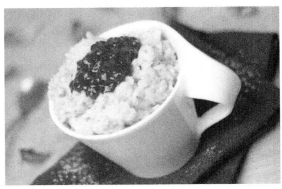

Portions Provided: 8 servings @ ½ cup each
Time Required: 45 minutes
Nutritional Statistics (Each Portion):

- Protein Counts: 17 grams
- Carbohydrates: 48 grams
- Added Sugars: 9 grams
- Dietary Fiber: 1 gram
- Sodium: 193 mg
- Calories: 257

Essential Ingredients:

- Water (2 cups)
- Brown rice - Long-grain (1 cup)
- Evaporated milk - f.f. (4 cups)
- Brown sugar (.5 cup)
- Lemon zest (.5 tsp.)
- Egg whites (6)
- Vanilla extract (1 tsp.)
- Crushed pineapple (.25 cup)
- Dried apricots, chopped (.25 cup)
- Raisins (.25 cup)

Preparation Method:

1. Warm the oven till it reaches 325° Fahrenheit/163° Celsius.
2. Prepare a saucepan with two cups of water, wait for it to boil.

3. Pour in the rice and simmer (10 min.). Dump it into a colander and drain thoroughly.

4. Pour the evaporated milk and brown sugar into the pan and cook till it's heated.

5. Add the lemon zest, cooked rice, and vanilla extract. Simmer using a low-temperature setting till the mixture is thick and the rice is tender (½ hr.). Move it to a cool burner to cool. Whisk the egg whites in a mixing container and empty them into the rice mixture.

6. Chop the apricots and add with the pineapple and raisins - stirring till well blended.

7. Lightly coat a baking dish using a spritz of cooking oil spray. Spoon the pudding and fruit mixture into the baking dish.

8. Bake till the pudding is set (20 min.). Serve warm or cold.

Rice - Mango Pudding

Portions Provided: 4 servings
Time Required: 60 minutes
Nutritional Statistics (Each Portion):
- Protein Counts: 6 grams
- Carbohydrates: 58 grams
- Fat Content: 3 grams
- Sugars: 20 grams
- Dietary Fiber: 3 grams
- Sodium: 176 mg
- Calories: 275

Essential Ingredients:
- Water (2 cups)
- Salt (.25 tsp.)
- Uncooked brown rice - long-grain (1 cup)
- Ripe mango (1 medium)
- Vanilla soy milk (1 cup)
- Ground cinnamon (.5 tsp.)
- Sugar (2 tbsp.)
- Vanilla extract (1 tsp.)
- Optional: Chopped - peeled mango

Preparation Method:
1. Warm a big, heavy saucepan of water - add salt and wait for it to boil.
2. Mix in the rice.
3. Lower the temperature and place a top on the pan. Simmer till the water has dissipated and the rice is tender (35-40 min.).

4. Peel, seed, and slice the mango. Mash it using a potato masher or fork.

5. Combine the milk with sugar, cinnamon, and mashed mango into the rice.

6. Simmer it with the top *off* on low until the liquid is almost absorbed - occasionally stirring (for 10-15 min.).

7. Transfer the pan to a cool burner and mix in the vanilla. Serve warm or cold with chopped mango as desired.

Delicious Beverage Options

Blueberry-Lavender Lemonade

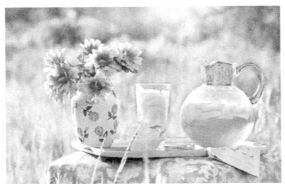

Portions Provided: 16 servings
Time Required: 15 minutes
Nutritional Statistics (Each Portion):

- Protein Counts: -0- grams
- Carbohydrates: 8 grams
- Fat Content: -0- grams
- Sugars: 7 grams
- Sodium: 7 mg
- Calories: 33

Essential Ingredients:

- Dried lavender flowers (1 tbsp.)
- Water (2 cups)
- Blueberries (16 oz./450 pkg.)
- Granulated sugar (.25 cup)
- Lemon juice (1 cup)
- Splenda sweetener (2 tbsp.)
- To Finish: Water - cold
- Ice (4 cups)

Preparation Method:

1. Use a one-gallon pitcher, add the ice.
2. Boil water (2 cups) in a saucepan. Measure and mix in the blueberries, sugar, and lavender to the pan. Boil for five minutes until the blueberries have popped and the sugar has liquified.
3. Strain the blueberry mixture over the pitcher of ice and discard the strained fruit mix.
4. Mix in the lemon juice and Splenda. Fill it to the top with cold water. Stir thoroughly and serve.

Blackberry Iced Tea with Ginger & Cinnamon

Portions Provided: 6 servings @ 1 cup + ice
Time Required: 20 minutes
Nutritional Statistics (Each Portion):

- Protein Counts: trace grams
- Carbohydrates: 6 grams
- Fat Content: -0- grams
- Sugars: 5 grams
- Dietary Fiber: trace grams
- Sodium: 3 mg
- Calories: 25

Essential Ingredients:

- Water (6 cups)
- Blackberry herbal tea bags (12)
- Minced fresh ginger (1 tbsp.)
- Cinnamon sticks (8 @ 3-inch-long)
- Unsweetened cranberry juice (1 cup)
- Sugar substitute (as desired)
- Ice cubes (crushed)

Preparation Method:

1. Prepare a big saucepan to warm the water to just before boiling.
2. Add tea bags, ginger, and two cinnamon sticks.
3. Move the pan from the burner for it to steep (15 min.).
4. Pass the mixture through a fine-mesh sieve, placed over a pitcher.
5. Add the juice and sweetener to your liking. Pop it into the fridge till it's chilled and very cold.
6. To serve, fill six tall glasses with crushed ice.
7. Pour the tea over the ice and garnish it with cinnamon sticks and enjoy it promptly.

Chocolate-Peanut Butter Protein Shake

Portions Provided: 1 serving
Time Required: 5 minutes
Nutritional Statistics (Each Portion):
- Protein Counts: 26.1 grams
- Carbohydrates: 41.3 grams
- Fat Content: 15.9 grams
- Sugars: 19.9 grams
- Dietary Fiber: 9.9 grams
- Sodium: 121.6 mg
- Calories: 402

Essential Ingredients:
- Soy milk - Unsweetened - vanilla (1 cup)
- Sliced frozen banana (.75 cup)
- Reduced-fat plain Greek yogurt (.5 cup)
- Cocoa powder (1 tbsp.)
- Peanut butter - organic (1 tbsp.)

Preparation Method:
1. Slice the banana.
2. Combine cocoa powder with milk, yogurt, banana, and peanut butter in a blender -mix to your liking.
3. Serve in a chilled mug.

Cookies & Cream Shake

Portions Provided: 3 servings
Time Required: 5 minutes
Nutritional Statistics (Each Portion):
- Protein Counts: 9 grams
- Carbs: 52 grams
- Fat Content: 3 grams
- Sugars: 29 grams
- Dietary Fiber: 11.5 grams
- Sodium: 224 mg
- Calories: 270

Essential Ingredients:
- Vanilla soy/soya milk - chilled (1.33 cups)
- Fat-free vanilla ice cream (3 cups)
- Chocolate wafer cookies (6 crushed)

Preparation Method:
1. Mix the ice cream with the milk in a blender till it's frothy and smooth.
2. Add in the cookies a few at a time, pulsing till thoroughly blended as desired. Pour them into chilled mugs and serve.

Cranberry Spritzer

Portions Provided: 10 servings
Time Required: 6 minutes

Nutritional Statistics (Each Portion):
- Protein Counts: trace grams
- Carbohydrates: 24 grams
- Fat Content: trace grams
- Sugars: 10 grams
- Dietary Fiber: trace grams
- Sodium: 9 mg
- Calories: 100

Essential Ingredients:
- Seltzer water (1 quart)
- Sugar (.25 cup)
- Fresh lemon juice (.5 cup)
- Raspberry sherbet (1 cup)
- Cranberry juice - low-cal (1 quart)
- Lemon or lime (10 wedges)

Preparation Method:
1. Use chilled cranberry juice, carbonated water, and lemon juice to fill a large pitcher.
2. Mix in the sugar and sherbet.
3. Pour the drink into frosty glasses with a wedge of lime or lemon.
4. Serve and enjoy it!

Ginger-Cinnamon & Blackberry Iced Tea

Portions Provided: 6 servings
Time Required: 15 minutes + chilling time
Nutritional Statistics (Each Portion):
1 cup portion + ice:
- Protein Counts: trace grams
- Carbohydrates: 6 grams
- Fat Content: -o- grams
- Dietary Fiber: trace grams
- Sodium: 3 mg Calories: 25

Essential Ingredients:
- Cinnamon sticks (8 @ 3-inches-long)
- Fresh ginger (1 tbsp.)
- Water (6 cups)
- Blackberry herbal tea bags (12)
- Fresh ginger (1 tbsp.)
- Cranberry juice - unsweetened (1 cup)
- Sugar substitute (as desired)
- Crushed ice cubes

Preparation Method:
1. Use a big saucepan and heat water - just before boiling. Mince the ginger.
2. Add tea bags, two cinnamon sticks, and ginger. Transfer the pan to a cool burner and cover it with a top to steep (15 min.).
3. Empty the mixture into a fine-mesh sieve while over a serving pitcher.

4. Mix in the sweetener and juice as desired. Chill it in the fridge.
5. To serve, add crushed ice to glasses.
6. Pour the tea over the ice and garnish it with cinnamon sticks. Enjoy it right away for the best results.

Iced Latte

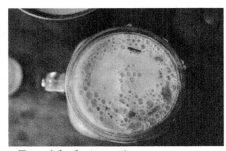

Portions Provided: 4 servings
Time Required: 5-8 minutes
Nutritional Statistics (Each Portion):
- Protein Counts: 3 grams
- Carbohydrates: 18 grams
- Fat Content: trace grams
- Sugars: 11 grams
- Dietary Fiber: -0- grams
- Sodium: 82 mg
- Calories: 84

Essential Ingredients:
- Brewed decaffeinated espresso coffee - cooled (2 cups)
- Milk - f.f. (1.5 cups)
- Golden brown sugar (2 tbsp.)
- Sugar-free almond syrup (2 tbsp.)
- Ice cubes (as desired)
- Whipped topping - f.f. (1 cup)
- Ground espresso beans (1 tsp.)

Preparation Method:
1. In a pitcher, combine the espresso, brown sugar, milk, and syrup. Stir to mix evenly. Refrigerate until cold.
2. Fill four chilled glasses with ice cubes. Pour coffee over ice.
3. Add whipped topping (¼ cup) to each drink and sprinkle with ground espresso beans.

Island Chiller

Portions Provided: 16 servings
Time Required: 5 minutes + freezing time
Nutritional Statistics (Each Portion):
- Protein Counts: 1 gram
- Carbohydrates: 19 grams

- Fat Content: -0- grams
- Sugars: 15 grams
- Dietary Fiber: 2 grams
- Sodium: 2 mg
- Calories: 80

Essential Ingredients:
- Frozen strawberries - unsweetened (2 pkg. @ 280 g/10 oz. each)
- Crushed pineapple with juice (1.5 cups/850 g/about 30 oz.)
- Orange juice with pulp (3 cups)
- Chilled carbonated water (2 quarts)
- Fresh strawberries (16)

Preparation Method:
1. Load a blender with the pineapple with juice, frozen berries, and orange juice. Mix till it's frothy smooth
2. Pour the mixture into ice cube trays to freeze.
3. To serve, add three cubes into a tall glass. Fill it with carbonated water (½ cup). Wait until the mixture becomes slushy. Garnish with a strawberry to serve.

Minty-Lime Iced Tea

Portions Provided: 1 serving
Time Required: 5-6 minutes
Nutritional Statistics (Each Portion):
- Protein Counts: -0- grams
- Carbohydrates: 4 grams
- Fat Content: -0- grams
- Sodium: 9 mg
- Calories: 16

Essential Ingredients:
- Unsweetened tea (1 cup)
- Fresh mint leaves (2 tbsp +1 sprig for garnish)
- Lime juice concentrate (2 tbsp.)
- Ice cubes (5-6)
- Sugar substitute (as desired)

Preparation Method:
1. Brew the tea and cool it.
2. Use a blender to combine the tea with mint leaves, lime juice, and ice cubes.
3. Blend till it's creamy smooth.
4. Mix in sweetener to your liking.
5. Serve in a chilled glass with a sprig of mint as desired.

Mock Champagne

Portions Provided: 4 servings @ 5 ounces or 2/3 cup **Time Required**: 5 minutes

Nutritional Statistics (Each Portion):
- Protein Counts: trace grams
- Carbohydrates: 14 grams
- Sodium: 4 mg
- Calories: 55

Essential Ingredients:
- Apple juice or apple cider (2 cups - unsweetened)
- Fresh lemon juice (1.5 tsp.)
- Lemon-flavored sparkling water (2 cups)

Preparation Method:
1. Chill a wine/champagne glass.
2. Combine each of the fixings and serve. (Simple as that!)

Non-Alcoholic Margarita

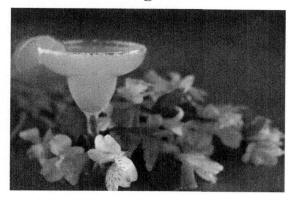

Portions Provided: 2 servings
Time Required: 10 minutes
Nutritional Statistics (Each Portion):
- Protein Counts: trace grams
- Carbohydrates: 17 grams
- Fat Content: -0- grams
- Sugars: 13 grams
- Dietary Fiber: trace grams
- Sodium: 2 mg
- Calories: 68

Essential Ingredients:
- *The Syrup*:
- Sugar (.5 cup)
- Water (.5 cup)
- *Margaritas*:
- Ice (2 cups)
- Fresh lime juice (.5 cup)
- Simple syrup (3 tbsp.)
- To Garnish: Cut fresh fruit

Preparation Method:
1. Use a small saucepan to heat sugar and water. Stir until the sugar is liquified.
2. Remove from the burner and chill.
Load a blender with ice, juice, and simple syrup.
3. Blend till it's creamy - pour into a chilled mug and garnish the rim with cut fruit.

Strawberry-Banana Milkshake

Portions Provided: 2 servings
Time Required: 6-7 minutes
Nutritional Statistics (Each Portion):
- Protein Counts: 6 grams
- Carbohydrates: 40 grams
- Fat Content: 1 gram
- Added Sugars: 17 grams
- Dietary Fiber: 8 grams
- Sodium: 117 mg
- Calories: 183

Essential Ingredients:
- Frozen strawberries (6)
- Banana (1 medium)
- Soy milk (.5 cup)
- Vanilla frozen yogurt - f.f. (1 cup)
- Strawberries (2 fresh)

Preparation Method:
1. Chop the frozen berries and slice the fresh strawberries.
2. Load a blender to combine the frozen strawberries, soy milk, banana, and frozen yogurt.
3. Mix till it's creamy smooth.
4. Pour into tall, frosty glasses and garnish using fresh strawberry slices.
5. Serve right away for the most flavorful results.

Strawberry Mockarita

Portions Provided: 6 servings
Time Required: 5-7 minutes
Nutritional Statistics (Each Portion):
- Protein Counts: 1 gram
- Carbohydrates: 16 grams
- Fat Content: -0- grams
- Sugars: 13 grams
- Dietary Fiber: 2 grams
- Sodium: 3 mg
- Calories: 64

Essential Ingredients:
- Sliced strawberries (4 cups)
- Lime juice (.25 cup)

- Sugar (.25 cup)
- Water (2 cups)
- Ice (2 cups)

Preparation Method:
1. Toss each of the fixings into a blender.
2. Mix till incorporated and smooth to serve.
3. Enjoy!

Tropical Hurricane Punch

Portions Provided: 6 servings
Time Required: 10 minutes
Nutritional Statistics (Each Portion):
- Protein Counts: 1 gram
- Carbohydrates: 15 grams
- Fat Content: trace grams
- Sugars: 12 grams
- Dietary Fiber: 2 grams
- Sodium: 6 mg
- Calories: 64

Essential Ingredients:
- Juice (about 2 tbsp./1 lemon)
- Cranberry juice (8 oz./230 g)
- Chopped pineapple (1.5 cups)
- Citrus fruit (2 cups)
- Ice (1 cup ice + extra for serving)

Preparation Method:
1. Toss each of the fixings (omitting the ice) and puree until it's smooth.
2. Add one cup of ice and continue to pure until it's creamy.
3. Serve over ice as desired, garnished with a couple of chunks of pineapple or orange slices and enjoy!

Watermelon-Cranberry Agua Fresca

Portions Provided: 6 servings @ ¾ cup each
Time Required: 8-10 minutes
Nutritional Statistics (Each Portion):
- Protein Counts: 1 gram
- Carbohydrates: 20 grams
- Fat Content: -0- grams
- Sugars: 16 grams
- Dietary Fiber: 1 gram
- Sodium: 9 mg
- Calories: 84

Essential Ingredients:
- Seedless watermelon (2.5 lb./about 7 cups)
- Fruit-sweetened cranberry juice/nectar (1 cup)
- Fresh lime juice (.25 cup)
- Lime (1 @ 6 slices)

Preparation Method:
1. Remove the rind from the watermelon and dice the fruit.
2. Place the melon in a food processor or blender, mixing till it's creamy and smooth to your liking.
3. Pass the puree through a fine-mesh sieve placed over a bowl to eliminate the pulp and clarify the juice. Empty the juice into a large pitcher.
4. Add the cranberry and lime juices, stirring thoroughly
5. Refrigerate till it's chilled. Pour into tall cold glasses - garnish each with a slice of lime and enjoy!

Chapter 4:
Six-Week Meal Plan

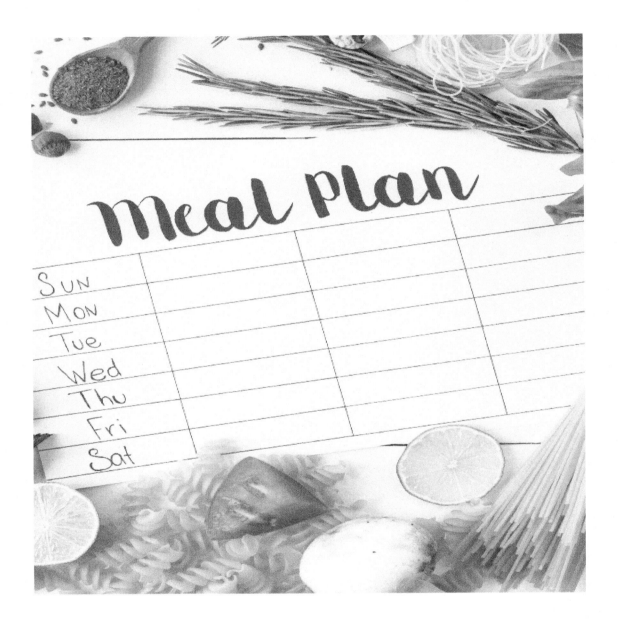

How to Save Money with Shopping Lists & Meal Plans

The best way to save money is to follow a few simple guidelines. As with any diet plan, it begins with the food purchased. Before you take the trip to the market, consider some of these tips:

- Prepare an essential food shopping list. You have six weeks shown below - realizing many items are already included in a general shopping list.

- Have a snack before you head to the grocery store. You won't be as tempted to purchase unhealthy junk food.

Remain Focused

- Always read the ingredient panels. Keep in mind; you have many hidden components. Typically, low sodium foods will have five percent of your daily values or less of sodium for each serving.

- Fresh foods also often have more health-promoting vitamins, fiber, and minerals - versus all the prepackaged goodies.

Tweak Your Cooking Habits

Make your meals more flavorful without additional fats or salt using spices, herbs, flavored vinegar, peppers, onions, garlic/garlic powder, ginger, lemon, or sodium-free bouillon.

Take Time & Wash Away Harmful Components. Get in the habit of rinsing away the excess salt if you used canned foods such as veggies and beans.

Prepare casseroles and stews and casseroles with only 2/3 of the meat the recipe calls for and add extra veggies, tofu, whole-wheat pasta, bulgur, or brown rice. You'll see that many are included in your meal plan and array of new recipes. Experiment using spices and substitutions.

Now, let's take a look at your meal plan! Keep in mind; you can exchange any of the suggested items in the plan as long as they maintain the same net carbs. Each of the items also shows its mg of sodium to help maintain your blood pressure. As you see, I tried to maintain an average of 1500 mg sodium daily.

Meal Plans & Shopping Lists - Six Weeks

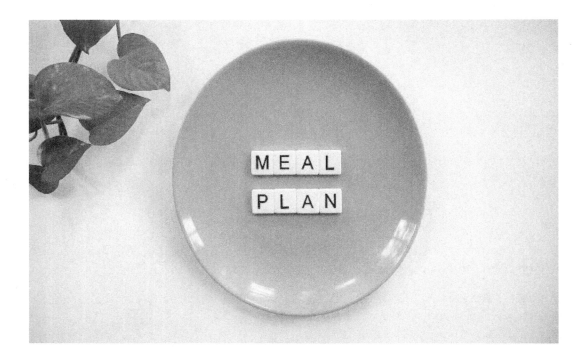

Keep in mind your list will vary somewhat from the actual ingredients, but they are very close. For example, some recipes call for 1% milk, and others ask for low-fat (l.f.).

You have a list of most used items and another for each week of the diet plan included.

Basic Food Items - Six Weeks

These items are general pantry items used weekly in various recipes:

- Table salt
- Kosher salt
- Black pepper
- Black peppercorns - whole
- Granulated sugar
- Sugar substitute blend equivalent to .75 cup sugar (.75 cup)
- Splenda (2 individual packets)
- Raw sugar (1 cup)
- Light brown sugar + Brown sugar Turbinado or brown sugar
- Cocoa powder - unsweetened (.25 cup)
- **Ground spices**
- Cayenne pepper
- New Mexico chili powder/your favorite
- Old Bay Seasoning blend
- Anise seeds

- Bay leaf (6)
- Cumin seeds
- Curry powder
- Dill
- Dried oregano
- Dried sage
- Cardamom
- Cloves
- Coriander
- Cinnamon
- Coriander
- Cumin
- Ginger
- Ground nutmeg (.125 or ⅛ tsp.) + Grated nutmeg (.25 tsp.)
- Turmeric
- Garam masala

- Garlic powder
- Herb seasoning blend - salt-free rb & Garlic seasoning salt
- Jamaican jerk seasoning
- Lemon-pepper seasoning
- Onion powder
- Paprika + Smoked paprika
- Parsley flakes (1.5 tbsp.)
- Red pepper - crushed (.25 tsp.)
- Jamaican jerk seasoning (1 tbsp.)
- Tarragon (1 tsp./to your liking)
- Thyme (.5 tsp.)

Note for one recipe: This recipe is used two times:
Flour: 0.5 cup x 2 each:

- Amaranth flour x2
- Tapioca flour x2
- Millet flour x2
- **Other Flour**
- All-purpose (A. P.)
- Brown rice
- Buckwheat
- Flaxseed
- Whole-wheat
- Pastry flour - whole-wheat
- Quinoa flour

- Baking powder + No-sodium baking powder
- Baking soda
- Cornstarch
-
- Wheat germ
- Yellow cornmeal

- Honey or agave nectar
- Vanilla extract
  Oils Suggested:
- Avocado
- Canola
- Grapeseed
- Olive
- Peanut
- Sesame
- Toasted sesame
- Vegetable
- Reduced-fat balsamic vinaigrette

Vinegar

- Apple cider
- Balsamic
- Cider vinegar
- Red-wine
- Rice
- Rice vinegar - unseasoned
- Sherry
- White wine vinegar
- Honey/agave nectar (1 tbsp.)
- Maple syrup + Pure maple syrup/honey
- Dark honey (1 tbsp.)
- Barbecue sauce
- Low-cal mayo
- Dijon mustard
- No-salt-added ketchup
- Soy sauce - reduced-sodium
- Spicy brown mustard
- Mayonnaise

Week One - Meal Plan

Breakfasts	Snack time	Lunchtime	Snack time	Dinnertime
Day 1 Chocolate Smoothie with Banana & Avocado 102 mg	Baked Brie Envelopes 133 mg	Chilean Lentil Stew with Salsa Verde 454.7 mg	Banana Splits 88 mg	Cabbage Lo Mein 551.7 mg
Day 2 Apple Corn Muffins 127 mg	Citrus Salad 11 mg	Crispy Oven-Fried Fish Tacos 472.3 mg	Apple Pie 2 mg	Irish Pork Roast with Roasted Root Vegetables 327 mg
Day 3 White Cheddar - Black Bean Frittata 378 mg	Almond - Fruit Bites 15 mg	Chicken Fajitas - Party Pack 380 mg	Leftover Apple Pie 2 mg	Roasted Salmon with Olives - Garlic & Tomatoes 545 mg
Day 4 Baked Banana-Nut Oatmeal Cups 165.6 mg	Ginger Carrot and Turmeric Smoothie 112 mg	Philly Cheesesteak Stuffed Peppers 465	Grapefruit-Lime & Mint Yogurt Parfait 115 mg	Chicken Stir-Fry with Basil - Eggplant & Ginger 395 mg
Day 5 Berry Muesli 45 mg	Turkey Wrap 253 mg	Garlic Shrimp & Spinach 444 mg	Peach Tart 46 mg	Easy Low-Sodium Chicken Breast + Carrots - Honey-Sage 182 mg
Day 6 Buckwheat Pancakes 150 mg	High-Protein Strawberry Smoothie 141 mg	Chicken-Spaghetti Squash Bake 494 mg	Leftover Peach Tart 46 mg	Skillet Steak with Mushroom Sauce 356 mg
Day 7 Quick-Cooking Oats - Vegan 152.4 mg	Chicken & Cherry Lettuce Wraps 381 mg	Veggie-Filled Meat Sauce with Zucchini Noodles 334 mg	Peaches & Cream 105 mg	Shrimp Orzo & Feta 307 mg

Week One: Ingredient Shopping List

You will be using these items during week one, along with the original listing of ingredients.

Optional Toppings:
- Fresh cilantro
- Sliced ripe olives
- Additional salsa
- Pico de Gallo (as desired)

The Pantry

- Sparkling water (.5 cup)
- Yellow cornmeal (.5 cup)
- Low-fat - whole-wheat (12 tortillas @ 8-inch each)
- Corn tortillas (8)
- Whole wheat tortillas (2 @ 12-inches each)
- Mediterranean-Style white flatbreads (6 each @ 79 g/2.8 oz.
- Dry whole-wheat breadcrumbs (.75 cup)
- Whole-grain cereal flakes (1 cup)
- Low-fat granola (.33 cup)
- Granola without raisins (.5 cup)
- Uncooked bulgur (.25 cup)
- Lo mein noodles (8 oz. pkg.)
- Uncooked whole-wheat orzo pasta (1.25 cups)
  Oats:
- Quick-cooking (.5 cup)
- Rolled (4 cups)
- Old-fashioned (1 cup)
- Dried fruit: Apricots - raisins or dates (.5 cup)
- Dried apricots (2 cups)
- Dried cherries/cranberries (1 cup)
- Quick-cooking tapioca (2 tbsp.)
- Ground almonds (.25 cup)
- Sliced almonds (4cups) (2 tbsp.) (.33 cup)
- Toasted chopped pecans (.5 cup)
- Pine nuts (2 tbsp.)
- Pistachios - toasted (1 cup)
- Toasted walnuts (.25 cup)
- Sunflower kernels (2 tbsp.)
- Honey (4 tbsp.) + Honey or cane or brown sugar (1-2 tsp.)
- Maple syrup/organic brown sugar/coconut sugar/stevia (1 tbsp.
- Chile-garlic sauce (1 tsp.)
- Salsa (.75 cup)
- Cooked chickpeas/garbanzo beans (3 cups)
- Canned black beans (1 cup)
- Tomato paste (2 tbsp.)
- Tomato sauce - no salt (1 cup)
- Condensed cream of mushroom soup - ex. Campbell's 25% Less-Sodium (2 - 10 oz. cans)
- French green lentils (1.5 cups)
- Unsalted chicken broth (.75 cup)
- Vegetable/chicken broth - l.s. or water (4 cups)

Refrigerated
- Puff pastry dough (1 sheet)
- Salsa (.25 cup)
- Coleslaw mix (3 cups)

- Sour cream - fat-free (.5 cup)
- Low-fat cottage cheese -low-salt (.5 cup)
- Butter (.25 cup) (2 tsp.)
- Large eggs (15)
- Whipped cream - optional
- Fat-free milk (.5 cup) (.75 cup)
- Milk - l.f. (2.5 cups) + (1 fl. oz./2 tbsp.)
- 1% milk (1.25 cup)
- Almond milk - unsweetened (1 cup or 240 ml.)
- Vanilla soy milk (2 cups)
- Fruit yogurt (1 cup)
- Greek yogurt - f.f. vanilla (2 cups)
- Plain yogurt - reduced-fat (4 cups) +Plain whole-milk Greek yogurt (1 cup)
- Provolone cheese (4 slices)
- Brie cheese (170 g/6 oz.)
- Crumbled feta cheese (.5 cup)
- Shredded white cheddar cheese (.5 cup)
- Cheddar cheese - low-fat - shredded (.5 cup)
- Shredded extra-sharp Cheddar cheese (.5 cup)
- Tahini/sesame seed paste (1 tbsp.)

Meats

- Cod (1 lb.)
- Uncooked shrimp (1 lb./21-30 count) (1.25 lb./26-30-count per lb.)
- Chicken breasts (2 pounded to even thickness @ 0.5-inch) (4.25 lb.) (12 oz.)
- Low-sodium sliced deli turkey (12 oz.)
- Beef top sirloin steak (12 oz. - 1-inch thick)
- Top round steak (12 oz. or 340 g)

Frozen

- Frozen apple juice concentrate (1/3 cup)
- Vanilla ice cream - f.f. (1 cup)
- Corn kernels (.5 cup)
- Broccoli rabe (6 oz.)
- Sliced fresh mushrooms (3 cups)
- Frozen peas (2 cups)
- Frozen blueberries (.5 cup)
- Fresh/frozen strawberries (1 cup)

Fruit

- Tart apples (6 cups/approximately 4 large)
- Apple (1) (.5 cup)
- Avocado (1 ½) + (.25 cup)
- Bananas Small (1) Medium (1) (.75 cup) (4 large + more for sweetness as desired)
- Pitted fresh sweet cherries (1.25 cups)
- Cranberries - frozen/fresh (.5 cup)
- Orange (4)
- Lime juice (2 tbsp.) Zest of lime (2 tsp.) Lime juice (2 tbsp./1 large)
- Lemon: Juice (.25 cup) (4 tbsp.) + Fresh lemon zest (2.5 tsp.)
- Frozen or fresh pineapple (1 cup or 140 g)
- Fresh ginger (.5 tbsp.)

- Fresh sliced strawberries (3 cups)
- Fresh mint leaves
- Peaches (11)
- Fresh raspberries (1 cup)
- Red grapefruit (5 large)

Veggies

- Bell peppers (2 large) +
- Green sweet bell pepper (half of 1) +
- Red bell pepper (1.5) +
- Sweet green and red bell peppers (.33 cup of each)
- Red bell pepper (.5 cup)
- Broccoli florets (7 cups)
- Carrots (6.5 cups)
- Fresh cilantro (2 tbsp.) 1 pinch Fresh cilantro/green onions (.5 cup each) + Green onions (4)
- Fennel (1 bulb)/Celery (4-6 stalks) = (1.25 cups total)
- Garlic (23 cloves)

- Ginger (3 tbsp.)
- Bibb or Boston lettuce leaves (8)
- Green cabbage (1 cup) + Napa cabbage (4.5 cups/half of 1 head)
- Italian parsley (1 cup)
- Mushrooms (23 oz.)
- Onion (1 medium) + Large onion (2)
- Green onions (3)
- Scallions (1 bunch)
- Shallot (5 tbsp./1 large divided)
- Snow peas (1 cup)
- Spaghetti squash (1 medium/3 lb.)
- Spinach (1 lb.)
- Spring greens (4 cups)
- Tomatoes (.5 cup) + Sliced tomato (12 @ ¼-inch-thickness)
  Medium tomatoes (2)

Week Two - Meal Plan

Breakfasts	Snack time	Lunchtime	Snack time	Dinnertime
Day 1 Cantaloupe Dash Smoothie <Trace mg	Almond Chai Granola 130 mg	Chopped Superfood Salad with Salmon & Creamy Garlic Dressing 357 mg	Lemon Pudding Cakes 124 mg	Chicken - Spring Pea & Farro Risotto with Lemon 575 mg
Day2 Asparagus Omelet Tortilla Wrap 444 mg	Rice - Mango Pudding 176 mg	Shrimp Scampi Zoodles 530 mg	Leftover Rice - Mango Pudding 176 mg	Beef Stroganoff 193 mg
Day 3 Blueberry Low-Sodium Pancakes 113 mg	Spinach Wrap & Tuna Salad 450 mg	Garden Vegetable Beef Soup 621 mg	Leftover Lemon Pudding Cakes 124 mg	Lasagna - Vegan-Style 331 mg
Day 4 Roasted Portobello Mushrooms Florentine 472 mg	Whole-Grain Banana Bread 150 mg	Chimichurri Meal-Prep Noodle Bowls 377 mg	Leftover Whole-Grain Banana Bread 150 mg	Lemon-Thyme Roasted Chicken with Fingerlings 307 mg
Day 5 Peanut Butter & Chia Berry Jam English Muffin 287 mg	Spicy-Sweet Snack Mix 218 mg	Mushroom-Swiss Turkey Burgers 504 mg	Creamy Fruit Dessert 241 mg	Low-Sodium Dash Meatloaf+ Green Beans with Peppers & Garlic 183 mg
Day 6 Spinach & Mushroom Quiche 442.5 mg	Fruit Kebabs 53 mg	Ginger Chicken Noodle Soup 267 mg	Blueberry Cheesecake 532 mg	Roasted Salmon +Potato Salad 2700 mg
Day 7 Overnight Oats with Fruit 53 mg	Spicy- sweet Snack Mix 218 mg	Cobb Salad Thai-Style 472 mg	Leftover Blueberry Cheesecake 532 mg	Orange Rosemary Roasted Chicken+ Garlic Mashed Potatoes 131 mg

Week Two - Ingredient Shopping List

The Pantry

- Chai tea bags (2)
- Oats Old-fashioned (.33 cup)
- Oats Quick-cooking (3 cups)
- Silken tofu (450 g or 16 oz. pkg.)
- Wheat squares cereal (2 cups)
- English muffin - Whole-wheat suggested (1 toasted)
- 100 % Whole-wheat bread (8 slices)
- Whole wheat tortilla (1 @ 8 inches - warmed)
- Dried soba noodles (3 oz./85 g)
- Yolkless egg noodles (4 cups - uncooked)
- Whole-wheat lasagna noodles (230 g or 8 oz.)
- Zucchini noodles (3 medium zucchini/8 cups)
- Whole-grain spaghetti (110 g/4 oz.)
- Uncooked brown rice - long-grain (1 cup)
- Chia seeds (2 tsp.)
- Unsalted peanuts (.5 cup)
- Walnuts (2 tbsp.)
- Sunflower seeds - toasted (.5 cup)
- Almonds -coarsely chopped (2 cups)
- Toasted shredded coconut (4 tbsp.)
- Sweetened shredded coconut (1 cup)
- Sugar- & fat-free cheesecake pudding mix (2 pkg.)
- Panko breadcrumbs (.75 cup)
- Flour: ½ cup of each:
  - Quinoa
  - Millet
  - Rice
  - Tapioca
  - Amaranth - brown
- Lemon-pepper seasoning- salt-free (.5 tsp.)
- Seasoning blend - Salt-free (.5 tsp.)
- Raw sugar (.5 cup)
- Vanilla extract (.5 tsp.) Vanilla extract (4 tsp.)
- Asian toasted sesame salad dressing (.75 cup)
- Natural - organic peanut butter (2 tsp.)
- Peanut butter (2 tbsp. creamy)
- Garbanzos (2 cans @ 15 oz. each)
- Undiluted cream of mushroom soup - fat-free (half of 1 small can)
- Chicken broth or stock - l.s. (5 cups)
- Reduced-sodium beef broth (4 cans @ 14.5 oz. each)
- Tomato paste (.25 cup)
- Diced tomatoes - undrained (14.5 oz. can)
- Crushed tomatoes - no salt (28 oz. can)
- Light tuna - packed in water (64-oz. pouch)
- Water-packed sliced peaches (14.5 oz. can/410 g)
- Mandarin oranges (15 oz./430 g can)
- Water-packed pineapple chunks (8 oz./230 g can)
- Dry white wine (.33 cup)
- Dry red wine (.25 cup)

Refrigerated

- Large eggs (17)
- Heavy cream (.25 cup)
- Whipped dessert topping - f.f. (1 container)
- Oat milk (1 cup)
- Soy milk - vanilla-flavored (1 cup)
- Plain soya/soy milk (1 cup)
- Whole milk (.25 cup)
- Skim milk (1 cup)
- Fat-free milk (.5 cup) (4 tbsp.)
- Non-fat milk (2.5 cups)
- Cream cheese - f.f. (4 oz./110 g)
- Sour cream - f.f. (.5 cup)
- Yogurt - plain & f.f. (1 cup + 3 tbsp.)
- Nonfat vanilla Greek yogurt (5.5 oz. carton)
- Sugar-free - low-fat yogurt - lemon flavored (6 oz.)
- Parmesan cheese - grated (.25 cup) (4 tbsp. + 3 tsp.)
- Gruyère cheese - shredded (1.5 cups)
- Crumbled feta cheese (.5 cup)
- Swiss cheese (4 slices)
- Fat-free margarine (1 tbsp.)
- Butter (4 tbsp.)
- Light butter with canola oil (4 tsp.)

Meat

- Lean ground turkey (1 lb.)
- Boneless beef round steak (.5 lb.)
- 90% lean ground beef (3 lb.)
- Raw shrimp (1 lb.)
- Peeled cooked shrimp (340 g/12 oz.)
- Wild salmon fillets (1 lb. + 4 @ 6 oz. each)
- Shredded rotisserie chicken (2 cups)
- Chicken legs & thighs (3 @ 8 oz. each)
- Chicken breast halves (6 @ 8 oz. each) (4 small @ 1-1.25 lb. total) (1 lb./450 g)

Frozen

- Frozen cantaloupe (2.5 cups)
- Frozen banana (1 sliced)
- Mixed frozen berries - unsweetened (.5 cup)

Fruit

- Dried pineapple chunks (1 cup)
- Raisins (1 cup)
- Lemon juice (2 cups)
- Lemon (7)
- Fresh orange juice (.33 cup)
- Medium ripe avocado (1)
- Kiwi (1)
- Strawberries (4)
- Banana (half of 1) Mashed banana (2 cups)
- Blueberries/favorite fruit (2 cups)
- Red grapes (4)
- Assorted fresh fruit (.5 cup)
- Ripe mango (1 medium)
- Pineapple chunks (4 chunk @ .5-inch each)

Veggies

- Semi-pearled farro (6 tbsp.)
- Shelled edamame (1 cup)
- Fresh asparagus spears (4)
- Red bell pepper (1)

- Broccoli (4 cups)
- Red cabbage (2 cups) + Shredded cabbage (1.5 cups)
- Medium carrot (2) + 10 oz. pkg. + (2 cups) + 1 large
- Celery (6 ribs)
- Medium cucumber (1/2)
- Garlic (32 cloves)
- Fresh ginger (1 tbsp.)
- Fresh or frozen cut green beans (.5 cup) + Green beans (1 lb.)
- Curly kale (8 cups)
- Romaine - torn (1 bunch)
- Portobello mushrooms (2 large) + Portobello caps (8)
- Mushrooms (10-12 oz.) + (1.25 cups)
- Fresh mixed wild mushrooms - ex. -button - shiitake - crimini or oyster mushrooms (8 oz.)
- Green onion (1)
- Small red onion (.25 cup/half 0f 1)
- Yellow onion (4 large)
- Shallots (.25 cup)
- Sweet onion (2 cups)
- Sweet red pepper (1 medium)

- Fresh/frozen-thawed peas (.25 cup)
- Fresh snow peas - halved (1 cup)
- Fingerling potatoes or tiny new red or white potatoes (1 lb.)
- Gold or red potatoes (4 lb.)
- Red potato (about 5 oz./1 medium)
- Baby arugula (3 cups)
- Baby spinach leaves (10 cups)
- Tomato (1 small)
- Medium zucchini (7)
- Chopped mint (2 tbsp.)
- Freshly chopped basil x 2
- Chili paste/red pepper flakes (.5 tsp.)
- Fresh dill (.25 cup) (2 tbsp.) (.5 tsp.)
- Fresh cilantro/coriander (.25 cup) Fresh cilantro leaves (.25 cup)
- Fresh oregano (3 tbsp.)
- Fresh flat-leaf parsley (2.25 cups) + (4.5 tbsp.)
- Fresh rosemary (3 tsp.)
- Fresh thyme (1 tbsp. + 1 tsp. + garnishes)

Week Three - Meal Plan

Breakfasts	Snack time	Lunchtime	Snack time	Dinnertime
Day 1 Chocolate Berry Dash Smoothie* 55 mg	Apples & Dip 202 mg	Asparagus Soup 401 mg	Chocolate Cake 168 mg	Chicken Cutlets with Sun-Dried Tomato Cream Sauce 250 mg
Day 2 Pecan - Rhubarb Muffins 190 mg	Artichokes Alla Romana 179 mg	Asian Vegetable Salad 168 mg	Leftover Chocolate Cake 168 mg	Baked Parchment-Packed Tuna Steaks & Veggies with Sauce 511.6 mg
Day 3 Leftover Pecan - Rhubarb Muffins 190 mg	Almonds with a Spicy Kick 293 mg	Curried Cream of Tomato Soup with Apples 89 mg	Grilled Pineapple with Chili-Lime 35 mg	Beef & Bean Sloppy Joes 537.5 mg
Day 4 Baked Oatmeal 105 mg	Fruit Compote & Yogurt Ala Mode 68 mg	Baby Beet & Orange Salad 135 mg	Apple-Berry Cobbler 111 mg	Chicken & Spinach Skillet Pasta with Lemon & Parmesan 499.2 mg
Day 5 Spinach & Avocado Smoothie - Gluten-Free 237.9 mg	Almond & Apricot Biscotti 17 mg	Chicken Chili Verde - 569.6 mg	Carrot & Spice Quick Bread 82 mg	Broiled Sea Bass 77 mg
Day 6 Roasted Portobello Mushrooms Florentine 472 mg	Ambrosia with Coconut & Toasted Almonds 2 mg	Winter Kale & Quinoa Salad with Avocado 252.6 mg	Leftover Carrot & Spice Quick Bread 82 mg	Brown Sugar Pork Tenderloin Stir-Fry 502 mg
Day 7 Raspberry Peach Puff Pancake 173 mg	Berries Marinated in Balsamic Vinegar 56 mg	Turkey Medallions with Tomato Salad 458 mg	Poached Citrusy Pears 9 mg	Sesame-Garlic Beef & Broccoli with Whole-Wheat Noodles 335.6 mg

Week Three - Ingredient Shopping List

The Pantry

- Dry white wine (2 cups)
- Cream sherry (2 tbsp.)
- Dark honey (1 tbsp.)
- Organic cocoa powder (2 tbsp.)
- Unsweetened dark chocolate (2 oz.)
- Dark chocolate bar (2 oz. melted)
- Pink salmon - deboned (6 oz. can/pouch)
- Fresh breadcrumbs - whole-wheat (2 cups) + Panko breadcrumbs (1 cup)
- Hamburger buns - whole wheat (4)
- Shortbread biscuits (2)
- Oats - certified gluten-free (1 tbsp.)
- Uncooked rolled oats (3 cups)
- Rolled oats - gluten-free (.5 cup)
- Uncooked steel-cut oats (.25 cup)
- Uncooked pearl barley (.5 cup)
- Uncooked red wheat berries (.5 cup)
- Flaxseed (2 tbsp.)
- Long-grain brown rice - uncooked (1 and 2/3 cup) +Uncooked brown rice (1 cup)
- Ready-to-serve brown rice (8.8 oz. pkg.)
- Wild rice - cooked (.5 cup)
- G. F. penne pasta/whole-wheat penne pasta (8 oz.)
- Linguine - whole-wheat preferred (6 oz.)
- Cooked quinoa (1 cup)
- Uncooked quinoa (3 tbsp.)
- Pepitas (2 tbsp.)
- Anise seeds (1 tsp.)
- Chia seeds (1 tbsp.)
- Fennel seeds (3 tsp.)
- Pumpkin seeds (1 cup)
- Toasted sesame seeds (1 tsp.)
- Almonds (4 cups)
- Cashews (3.5 tbsp.)
- Shelled - roasted pistachios (1 cup)
- Roasted soy nuts (1 cup)
- Unsalted peanuts (2 tbsp.)
- Pecans (2 tbsp.)
- Walnuts (1 cup)
- Golden raisins (2 tbsp.)
- Raisins (1 cup)
- Evaporated skim milk (12 oz. can)
- Natural salted peanut or almond butter - crunchy or creamy (2 tbsp.)
- Mixed dried fruit (12 oz. pkg.)
- Dried cherries (.33 cup)
- Dried figs (6/about 1 cup)
- Dried apricots (1.66 or 1 - 2/3 cup)
- Sun-dried tomatoes - oil-packed & slivered (.5 cup + 1 tbsp.)

- Canned tomatoes No-salt-added - drained (3 cups)
- Diced tomatoes - no-salt (14 oz. can)
- Tomato puree - canned - no-salt (.75 cup)
- Chopped green chilies (4 oz. can)

- No-salt-added cream-style corn (14.75 oz. can)
- No-salt-added pinto beans - divided (3 - 15 oz. cans)
- Low-sodium chickpeas (15 oz. can)
- Garbanzo beans - l.s. (15 oz. can)
- Black beans - low-sodium (15 oz. or 430 g can) (1.75 cups)
- Unsalted prepared white beans (1 cup) or White beans (½ of a 15.5 oz. can) 1 % milk (2 cups)
- Unsalted chicken stock (4 cups)
- Vegetable stock - l.s. (2 cups)
- Chicken broth - l.s. (15 oz. can) (9 cups) (.25 cup)
- Vegetable/chicken broth - l.s. (6 cups)
- Chicken/vegetable broth - reduced-sodium (6 cups)
- Chicken/vegetable stock - l.s. (1 cup + 2-4 tbsp.)
- Blue cheese dressing (approx. 1 small 12 oz. bottle/as desired)
- Applesauce - unsweetened (1 cup)

Refrigerated

- Large eggs (20)
- Egg whites (2) or egg substitute (equivalent to 1 egg) beaten
- Unsalted butter (2 tbsp.)
- Butter (2 tbsp.) (2 tsp.)
- Unchilled trans margarine (.33 cup)
- Parmesan cheese - grated - (1 cup)
- Finely shredded cheddar cheese (.25 cup)
- Blue cheese (.25 cup) + (5 oz. container)
- Crumbled goat or feta cheese (.25 cup)
- Gruyère cheese - shredded (1.5 cups)
- Reduced-fat cream cheese (1 tbsp.) (8 oz.)
- Sour cream (6 tbsp.)
- 1 % milk - l.f. (2 tbsp.)
- Skim milk (1.33 cup)
- Soy milk (.25 cup)
- Fat-free milk (2.5 cups)
- Whole milk (.25 cup)
- Unsweetened plain almond/coconut/soy/hemp milk (.5 cup)
- Chilled light vanilla soy milk (1 cup)
- Heavy cream (.5 cup) + Half-and-Half (.25 cup)
- Vanilla yogurt (.25 cup)
- Plain yogurt - nonfat (1.5 cup)
- Fat-free lemon yogurt (.5 cup)
- Apple juice (.75 cup)
- Unsweetened orange juice (2 tbsp.) + (3 cups)
- Orange juice - Calcium-fortified (1.75 cups)
- Orange zest (1 tsp.)
- Medium peaches (2)
- Soft/silken tofu (.33 cup)
- Prepared salsa verde (2 cups)

Meat

- Cooked bacon (5 slices)
- Beef sirloin steak (1 lb.) + Beef - top sirloin steak (1 lb. @ ¾-inch thickness)
- 90% lean ground beef (340 g/12 oz.)
- Tuna (1.25 lb.)

- Uncooked shrimp - 26-30 per pound (1 lb.)
- White sea bass fillets (2 @ 4 oz. each)
- Turkey breast tenderloins (20 oz./570 g pkg.)
- Chicken breast or thighs (1 lb.) +Chicken thighs (2.5 lb.)

Frozen

- Fat-free vanilla frozen yogurt (4 cups)
- Banana (1)
- Blueberries (.25 cup)
- Corn (4 cups)
- Country-style hash browns with green peppers & onions (2.5 cups)
- Peas (1 cup)
- Peas & carrots (1 cup)

Fruit

- Red apples (10) (3.5 cups) (4 medium or 8 small)
- Small Golden Delicious apples (1.75 lb./
- Apricots (1 lb.)
- Avocados (3 + ¼ of 1)
- Banana (2 cups) + Banana (2)
- Fresh blueberries & raspberries (1 cup of each) + Fresh raspberries (.5 cup)
- Fresh Cantaloupe or other melon chunks (.5 cup)
- Shredded coconut - unsweetened (.5 cup)
- Lemons (7-8) + Lime juice (3 tbsp.)
- Fresh mint leaves for (2) garnish recipes
- Medium nectarines (2)
- Oranges (11)
- Pears (4 whole)
- Fresh pineapple (1) + chunks (1 cup) + Pineapple (1 small/approx. 3 cups)
- Fresh raspberries (1 cup)
- Fresh strawberries (3.5 cups) (12 oz.)
- Blueberries & strawberries (.5 cup each)
- Berries - such as blueberries or blackberries (.5 cup)

Veggies

- Fresh asparagus (2 lb. or 910 g)
- Roasted mashed yam (2 tbsp.)
- Globe artichokes (4 large)
- Fresh tarragon (1 tbsp.)
- Baby beets with greens (2 bunches/about 1 cup greens & 4 cups of beets)
- Napa cabbage (1.5 cups or ¼ of 1 head)

- Mixed salad greens (8 cups - torn)
- Bok choy (1.5 cups)
- Romaine (2 bunches or 20 cups)
- Iceberg lettuce (1 head) + 6 leaves
- Broccoli florets (4 cups)
- Carrots (5 cups) + (4 medium)
- Celery (3 ribs) + (3.5 cup)
- Cucumber (1)
- Fennel bulb (1 large/about 2 lb.)
- Garlic cloves (28) + (4 tbsp.)
- Green beans (1 lb.)
- Medium green pepper (1)
- Kale (5.5 cups) + Baby kale (1.5 cups)
- Red cabbage (1 cup)
- Portobello mushrooms (2 large)
- Fresh mixed wild mushrooms - ex. -button - shiitake - crimini or oyster mushrooms (8 oz.)
- Red onion (2 cup) + (2 large)
- Sweet onion (1.5 cups)
- Yellow onion (6 cups) (4 medium)
- Onion (2-3 large)
- Yellow onion (2 small
- Green onions (diced)
- Julienned red bell pepper (.5 cup) + Poblano peppers (2 cups/2 large)
- Rhubarb (1.25 cups)
- Scallion (1)
- Shallot (1 tbsp.) + (.5 cup)
- Snow peas (1.5 cups)
- Spinach (15.5 cups) + Fresh baby spinach (about 10 cups)
- Potatoes: Yukon Gold (1 lb. + 2 cups) + Russet (2 large)
- Sweet potato (1 small/1.5 cups)
- Diced fresh tomatoes (3 cups)
- Medium tomatoes (3)
- Grape tomatoes (1 cup)
- Roma tomatoes (4)
- Fresh Italian parsley - flat-leaf (2 tbsp.) (1 tbsp.) (.33 cup)

Fresh Spices
- Oregano (1 tsp.)
- Basil (1 tbsp.)
- Cilantro (2 cups)
- Parsley (3 tbsp.)
- Thyme leaves (1 tbsp. + garnishes)
- Basil (.25 cup)

Week Four -Meal Plan

Breakfasts	Snack time	Lunchtime	Snack time	Dinnertime
Day 1 Fresh Fruit Smoothie 7 mg	Apricot & Almond Crisp 1 mg	Chickpea & Potato Curry 532.8 mg	Chocolate Peanut Butter Energy Bars 90 mg	Baked Cod 220 mg
Day 2 Apple Corn Muffins 127 mg	Fruit Kebabs 53 mg	Balsamic Bean Salad with Vinaigrette 174mg	Cran-Fruit Coffee Cake with Crumb Topping 198 mg	Beef & Blue Cheese Penne with Pesto 434 mg
Day 3 Spinach & Mushroom Quiche 442.5 mg	Artichoke Dip Raw veggies 130 mg	Cream of Wild Rice Soup 180 mg	Leftover Chocolate Peanut Butter Energy Bars 90 mg	Creamy Chicken & Mushrooms 329.2 mg
Day 4 Baked Oatmeal 105 mg	Rainbow Ice Pops 6 mg	Salad Skewer Wedges 401 mg	Cran-Fruit Coffee Cake with Crumb Topping 198 mg	Pork Carnitas - Slow-Cooked 377 mg
Day 5 Leftover Apple Corn Muffins* 127 mg	Baked Apples with Cherries & Almonds 7 mg	Warm Rice & Pintos Salad - Diabetic-Friendly 465 mg	Peaches & Cream* 105 mg	Lasagna - Vegan-Style* 322.2 mg
Day 6 Whole Grain Banana Pancakes 146 mg	Cantaloupe Dash Smoothie <trace mg	Ginger Chicken Noodle Soup* 535 mg	Rice - Fruity Pudding 193 mg	Pork Tenderloin with Apple-Thyme Sweet Potatoes 257.1 mg
Day 7 Asparagus Omelet Tortilla Wrap 444 mg	Apricot & Soy Nut Trail Mix 4 mg	Shrimp & Nectarine Salad 448 mg	Leftover Rice - Fruity Pudding 193 mg	Paella with Chicken Leeks & Tarragon 182 mg

Week Four - Ingredient Shopping List

The Pantry

- Dry white wine (.5 cup)
- Vermouth/ dry red or white wine (.25 cup)
- Evaporated milk - f.f. (4 cups)
- Whole wheat tortilla (1 @ 8 inches
- Crispy corn tortillas (12 - 16-inch)
- Low-fat granola (.33 cup)
- Uncooked rolled oats (3 cups)
- Unsalted prepared white beans (1 cup) or White beans (½ of a 15.5 oz. can) 1 % milk (2 cups)
- Medjool dates (.75 cup)
- Organic creamy peanut butter (1 cup)
- Bittersweet chocolate chips (.75 cup)
- Rolled oats (.5 cup)
- Oats - certified gluten-free (1 cup)
- Wild rice - cooked (.5 cup)
- Long-grain brown rice (1 + 2/3 cup)
- Ready-to-serve brown rice (8.8 oz. pkg.)
- Penne pasta - whole-wheat (2 cups - uncooked
- Blue cheese dressing (approx. 1 small 12 oz. bottle/as desired)
- Fennel seeds - crushed (1 tsp.)
- Pumpkin seeds (1 cup)
- Almonds (6 tbsp.) + (.5 cup)
- Chopped unsalted dry-roasted peanuts (.5 cup)
- Pecans (.25 cup)
- Roasted pistachios (1 cup)
- Roasted soy nuts (1 cup)
- Walnuts (.25 cup)
- Dried fruits: Ex: Raisins, apples, pineapple, or apricots (.5 cup)
- Chopped dried figs (5)
- Raisins (1.25 cup)
- Dried cherries (.33 cup)
- Chopped dried apricots (5 apricot halves) + (.25 cup)
- Artichoke hearts in water (15.5 oz. can)
- Black beans - low-sodium (15 oz. or 430 g can)
- Garbanzo beans - l.s. (15 oz. can)
- Low-sodium chickpeas (15 oz. can)
- Pinto beans (15 oz. can)
- Unsalted white beans (1 cup or ½ of a 15.5-oz. can)
- Diced tomatoes - no-salt (14 oz. can)
- Chopped green chilies (4 oz. can)
- Chicken/vegetable broth - reduced-sodium (6 cups)
- Vegetable stock - l.s. (2 cups)
- Chicken broth - l.s. (2 cans @14 oz. each)
- Unsalted chicken broth - fat-free (2 cups)
- Crushed pineapple (.25 cup)
- Unsweetened applesauce (.5 cup)

Refrigerated

- Eggs (23)
- Egg substitute or egg whites (.75 cup)
- Butter (1 tsp.)
- Trans-free margarine (6 tbsp.)
- Blue cheese crumbles (140 g/5 oz. container)
- Finely shredded cheddar cheese (.25 cup)

- Gorgonzola cheese (.25 cup)
- Gruyère cheese - shredded (1.5 cups)
- Parmesan cheese - grated (2 tbsp.)
- Half-&-Half (1 cup)
- Whole milk (.25 cup)
- Milk – fat free (1 tbsp. + .75 cup)
- Nonfat or low-fat milk (.5 cup)
- Skim milk (1 cup)
- Vanilla Greek yogurt - nonfat (5.5 oz. carton
- Sugar-free - low-fat yogurt - lemon flavored (6 oz.)
- Sour cream - f.f. (8 oz.)
- Light dairy sour cream (1 cup)
- Apple juice (4.5 cups)
- Orange juice (.33 cup)
- Prepared pesto (.33 cup)
- Purchased salsa (1 cup)

Meat

- Bacon (5 slices)
- Beef tenderloin steaks (2 @ 6 oz. each)
- Chicken breast (1 lb.)
- Chicken cutlets (4 @ 4-5 oz. each)
- Pork shoulder roast - boneless (2 lb.)
- Pork tenderloin - trimmed of fat (1 lb.)
- Cod fillets (4 @ 4 to 5 oz. each)
- Uncooked shrimp - 26-30 per pound (1 lb.)

Frozen

- Vanilla ice cream - f.f. (1 cup)
- Frozen banana (1 sliced)
- Frozen cantaloupe (2.5 cups)
- Fresh/frozen corn (2 cups) + Corn kernels (.5 cup)
- Frozen peas (2 cups)

Fruit

- Apples - ex. Granny Smith/Honeycrisp (3 medium
- Small Golden Delicious apples (1.75 lb./6)
- Apricots (1 lb. + 1 cup)
- Avocados (2)
- Mashed banana (2 cups) + (half of 1)
- Blueberries (1 cups)
- Cantaloupe or other melon chunks (3.5 cups)
- Fresh cranberries (1 cup)
- Kiwi (1)
- Lemon (2)
- Lime zest - grated (4.5 tsp.)
- Lime juice (3 tbsp.)
- Medium nectarines (2)
- Peaches (2 medium)
- Fresh pineapple chunks (1 cup) + (4 chunk @ .5-inch each)
- Red grapes (4)
- Fresh strawberries (4) + (4 cups)
- Juice (from 2 oranges)
- Watermelon (3 cups)

Veggies

- Fresh asparagus spears (4)
- Carrots (1 cup)
- Cucumber (1)
- Fresh green beans (1 lb.)
- Kale (1.5 cups)
- Mixed mushrooms (4 cups
- Fresh mixed wild mushrooms - ex. -button - shiitake - crimini or oyster mushrooms (8 oz.)
- Medium red onion (2) + (.5 cup)
- Yellow onion (2.5 cups)
- Onion (1 large) + (2 small) + (2/3 cup)
- Green onion (2)
- Sweet onions - ex. Vidalia (2.5 cups)
- Scallions (2 thinly sliced)
- Carrot (1 cup)
- Celery (1.5 cups)
- Iceberg lettuce (1 head)
- Romaine (1 bunch)
- Lettuce leaves (6)
- Raw spinach (4 cups)
- Mixed salad greens (8 cups - torn)
- Spaghetti squash (1 medium or 4-5 lb.)
- Sweet potatoes (1 lb.)
- Garlic (30 cloves)
- Fresh baby spinach (5 oz./about 8 cups)
- Large tomatoes (2)
- Diced fresh tomatoes (3 cups)
- Ripe tomatoes (approx. 4 cups/2 lb.
- Grape tomatoes (3 cups)
- Roma tomatoes (4)
- Leeks - whites parts only (2)
- Red pepper (1)
- Baby spinach (5 oz./about 6 cups)
- Yukon Gold potatoes (1 lb.)
- Freshly minced basil (8-10 torn leaves) + (.25 cup)
- Fresh cilantro (.25 cup)
- Fresh tarragon (1 tbsp.)
- Fresh thyme leaves (2 tbsp.) + (2 sprigs)
- Fresh parsley (.25 cup + 4 tbsp.)

Week Five - Meal Plan

Breakfasts	Snack time	Lunchtime	Snack time	Dinnertime
Day 1 Green Smoothies 15 mg	Mediterranean Layered Hummus Dip+ your favorite pita chips 275 mg	Potato Fennel Soup 104 mg	Blueberry Cheesecake** Sodium: 532 mg	Grilled Fish with Peperonata 461.5 mg
Day 2 White Cheddar - Black Bean Frittata 378 mg	Fruit & Nut Bar 4 mg	Strawberry-Blue Cheese Steak Salad 452 mg	Leftover Blueberry Cheesecake Sodium - 532 mg	Orange Rosemary Roasted Chicken - 95 mg
Day 3 Berry Muesli 45 mg	Buffalo Chicken Salad 367mg	Green Bean & Tomato Soup 535 mg	Creamy Fruit Dessert 241 mg	Low-Sodium Dash Meatloaf 55 mg
Day 4 Overnight Peanut Butter Oats 229 mg	Almond Chai Granola 130 mg	Apple Salad with Figs & Almonds 33 mg	Fruit Cake 117 mg	Skillet Lemon Chicken & Potatoes with Kale 377.9 mg
Day 5 High-Protein Strawberry Smoothie 141 mg	Apples & Dip 202 mg	Salmon Chowder 207 mg	Leftover Fruit Cake 117 mg	Pork & Cherry Tomatoes 517.7 mg
Day 6 Blueberry Low-Sodium Pancakes 150 mg	Leftover Almond Chai Granola 130 mg	Citrus Salad 11 mg	Grapefruit-Lime & Mint Yogurt Parfait 115 mg	Pineapple Chicken Stir-Fry 325 mg
Day 7 Baked Banana-Nut Oatmeal Cups 165.6 mg	Berries Marinated in Balsamic Vinegar 56 mg	Quick Creamy Tomato Cup-of-Soup 245	Leftover Day Grapefruit-Lime & Mint Yogurt Parfait 115 mg Or Fruit Cake 117 mg	Peppery Barbecue-Glazed Shrimp with Vegetables & Orzo 553.8 mg

Week Five - Ingredient Shopping List

The Pantry

- Chai tea bags (2)
- Crushed red pepper (1 pinch)
- Quick-cooking oats (3 cups) + Rolled oats (4.5 cups)
- Fennel seed (1 tbsp.)
- Fennel (.25 cup)
- Panko breadcrumbs (.75 cup)
- Dessert Shortbread biscuits (2)
- Baked pita chips
- Whole-grain tortillas (2 - 12-inch in diameter)
- Brown rice (.66 or 2/3 cup)
- Whole-grain orzo (1 cup)
- Almonds (2 cups)
- Unsalted peanuts (2 tbsp.)
- Toasted chopped pecans (.5 cup)
- Pine nuts (2 tbsp.)
- Toasted walnuts (.75 cup)
- Sweetened shredded coconut (1 cup) + Toasted shredded coconut (4 tbsp.)
- Greek olives (.5 cup)
- Assorted chopped dried fruit - currants, cherries, figs, or dates (2 cups)
  Dried fruit: Apricots - raisins or dates (.5 cup)
- Chicken/vegetable broth - reduced-sodium (6 cups)
- Chicken broth - l.s. (.5 cup)
- Canned black beans (1 cup)
- Unsweetened applesauce (.5 cup)
- Mandarin oranges (15 oz./430 g can)
- Water-packed sliced peaches (14.5 oz. can/410 g)
- Canned unsweetened pineapple chunks (1 cup)
- Crushed pineapple packed in juice (.5 cup)
- Water-packed pineapple chunks (8 oz./230 g can)
- Sugar- & fat-free cheesecake pudding mix (2 pkg.)

Optional Toppings:

- Sliced ripe olives
- Additional salsa

Refrigerated

- Large eggs (15)
- Butter (2 tsp.)
- 1% milk (.75 cup)
- Milk - l.f. (4.5 cups)
- Crumbled feta cheese (1 cup)
- Fat-free cream cheese (12 oz.)
- Low-fat cottage cheese -low-salt (.5 cup)
- Plain fat-free yogurt (4.5 cups)
- Fruit yogurt (1 cup)
- Fat-free whipped dessert topping (1 container)
- Salsa (.25 cup)
- Hummus (10 oz. carton)
- Apple juice - unsweetened (.5 cup)
- Orange juice (1 cup)
- Pineapple juice - unsweetened (3 tbsp.)

Meat

- Chicken breast (.5 lb.)

- Chicken breasts (3-4 oz.) breast halves (3 @ 8 oz. each)
- Chicken legs & thighs (3 @ 8 oz. each) + thighs (1 lb.)
- Lean ground beef (1.5 lb.)
- Pork tenderloin (1.25 lb.)
- Skinned banded rudderfish/swordfish/mahi-mahi (1.5 lb.)
- Jumbo shrimp - thawed if frozen (1 lb.)

Frozen

- Frozen blueberries (.5 cup)

Fruit

- Apple (.5 cup) + (4 medium or 8 small)
- Ripe bananas (2)
- Blueberries/favorite fruit (2 cups)
- Red grapefruit (5 large)
- Lime juice (2 tbsp.)
- Zest of lime (2 tsp.)
- Zest and juice (1 medium orange + 1 lemon)
- Lemon (2 large)
- Oranges (2)
- Fresh/frozen strawberries (1 cup) +Fresh sliced strawberries (3 cups)
- Raspberries - blueberries & strawberries (.5 cup each)
- Fresh mint leaves

Veggies

- Bok choy (1 cup)
- Garlic cloves (14)
- Bell pepper (1 cup)
- Carrots (2 large) + (4 medium)
- Celery (3 stalks)
- English cucumber (1 large)
- Sweet green bell peppers (.33 cup)
- Red bell pepper (1.33 cups)
- Any color bell peppers (8 cups)
- Fresh ginger (1.5 tsp.)
- Fresh green beans (1 lb.)
- Baby kale (6 cups)
- Whole chipotle peppers (2)
- Green onion (.5 cup)
- Onion (1.5 cup)
- Medium red onion (1) + (.25 cup)
- Green onions (3)
- Capers (.25 cup)
- Scallions (3)
- Snow peas (1 cup)
- Spinach (4 oz)
- Spring greens (4 cups)
- Medium tomatoes (2)
- Diced fresh tomatoes (3 cups)
- Cherry tomatoes (5 cups)
- Baby Yukon Gold potatoes (1 lb.)
- Rutabaga root vegetable - thinly sliced (1 lb.) + (.5 cup)
- Zucchini (2 cups)

Fresh Spices:
- Basil (.25 cup)
- Cilantro
- Rosemary (3 tsp.)
- Tarragon (1 tbsp.)
- Fresh thyme & oregano (1 tsp. each) + Fresh oregano (2 tbsp.)

- Parsley (1 tbsp.)
- Chopped mint (2 tbsp.)
- Mixed tender fresh herbs as desired - parsley, basil, or mint (.25 cup)

Week Six - Meal Plan

Breakfasts	Snack time	Lunchtime	Snack time	Dinnertime
Day 1 Orange-Lover's Smoothies 40 mg	Peanut Butter Energy Balls 47.7 mg	Greek Meatball Mezze Bowls 542.5 mg	Lemon Bread 80.3 mg	Balsamic Roasted Chicken 257 mg + Brown Rice Pilaf 139 mg
Day 2 Leftover Baked Banana-Nut Oatmeal Cups 165.6 mg	Cinnamon-Raisin Oatmeal Cookies 74.2 mg	Cucumber Salad with Tzatziki 169.2 mg	Easy Peach Cobbler Dump Cake 30.8mg	Swordfish with Roasted Lemons 287 mg +Brussels Sprouts & Shallots 191 mg
Day 3 Zucchini & Tomato Pie Breakfast Pie 223 mg	Strawberry-Chocolate Greek Yogurt Bark 7.6 mg	Curried Sweet Potato & Peanut Soup 593.7 mg	Leftover Lemon Bread 80.3 mg	Roasted Turkey 161 mg + Acorn Squash with Apples 46 mg
Day 4 Blueberry & Lemon Scones 35 mg	Leftover Peanut Butter Energy Balls 47.7 mg	Roasted Turkey Sandwiches 161 mg (turkey only)	Flourless Honey-Almond Cake 208.3 mg	Spicy Jerk Shrimp 411.3 mg
Day 5 Breakfast Scrambled Egg Burrito 116 mg	Leftover Strawberry-Chocolate Greek Yogurt Bark 7.6 mg	Creamy Pesto Chicken Salad with Greens 453.9mg	Leftover Easy Peach Cobbler Dump Cake 30.8mg	Thai Chicken & Pasta Skillet 432 mg
Day 6 German Apple Pancake 71 mg	Leftover Cinnamon-Raisin Oatmeal Cookies 74.2 mg	Grits & Shrimp 637 mg	Leftover Flourless Honey-Almond Cake 208.3 mg	Slow-Cooked Braised Beef with Carrots & Turnips 538.4 mg
Day 7 Overnight Peanut Butter Oats 229 mg	Air-Fried Crispy Chickpeas 85.8 mg	Greek Turkey Burgers with Spinach, Feta & Tzatziki 677.5 mg	Glazed Chocolate-Pumpkin Bundt Cake 237.2 mg	Spinach-Stuffed Sole 140 mg

Week Six - Ingredient Shopping List

Optional Toppings:
- Strawberries/raspberries/sliced banana
- Granola
- More chia seeds or flaxseed meal

The Pantry

- Small hamburger buns - preferably whole-wheat (4)
- 1 @ 6–8-inch tortilla
- Bouillon granules - chicken-flavored - l.s. (1 tsp.)
- Red curry paste (4 tsp.)
- Pesto (.25 cup)
- Chopped toasted almonds or walnuts (.5 cup)
- Whole almonds - toasted 1.5 cups) + Sliced almonds, toasted (.25 cup)
- Chia seeds (.75 tbsp.)
- Unsalted dry-roasted peanuts (1 cup)
- Organic - salted peanut/almond butter - crunchy or creamy (2 tbsp.)
- Organic peanut butter or favorite nut butter (1 cup)
- Maple syrup/organic brown sugar/coconut sugar/stevia (1 tbsp. or as desired)
- Rolled oats - gluten-free (2.5 cups)
- Whole-wheat spaghetti - uncooked (6 oz. pkg.)
- Brown rice - cooked (2.33 cups)
- Cooked quinoa (2 cups)
- Low-sodium baking mix (.66 or 2/3 cup)
- Whole tomatoes - preferably San Marzano (28 oz. can)
- Unsalted chickpeas (15 oz. can)
- White beans (15 oz. can)
- Tzatziki (.5 cup)
- Thai peanut sauce (1 cup)
- Unsweetened pumpkin puree (15-oz. can)
- Light corn syrup (.25 cup)
- Mini chocolate chips (.5 cup)
- Unsweetened shredded coconut (.25 cup)
- Cocoa powder - not Dutch-process - unsweetened (.75 cup)
- Organic yellow cake mix (1 box/15.85 to 18 oz.)
- Red wine (1 cup)

Refrigerated

- Soft/silken tofu (.33 cup)
- Chilled orange juice (1.5 cups)
- 1% milk (.75 cup)
- Fat-free milk (1 cup)
- Unsweetened plain almond/coconut/soy/hemp milk (.5 cup)
- Lite coconut milk (1 cup)
- Chilled light vanilla soy milk (2 cups)
- Half & Half (.5 cup)
- Whole milk (.75 cup)
- Nonfat buttermilk (1 cup)
- Eggs (13 large)
- Refrigerated/frozen egg product - thawed (.25 cup) or lightly beaten egg (1)
- Low-fat plain yogurt (.5 cup)
- Whole-milk plain Greek yogurt (3 cups)
- Unsalted butter (11 tbsp.)
- Margarine - trans-fat-free (2 tsp.)
- Feta cheese (1 cup)
- Swiss cheese (.33 or 1/3 cup) (2 tbsp.)
- Shredded Swiss & Gruyere cheese (1 tbsp.)
- Low/no sodium pasta sauce or salsa (1 tsp.)

Meat

- Swordfish (4 fillets @ 6 oz. each)
- Fresh/frozen large shrimp (1.5 lb.)

- Beef chuck roast - trimmed (3-3.5 lb.)
- 93% lean ground turkey (2 lb.)
- Turkey (12 lb. – whole)
- Whole chicken (4 lb.) + shredded & cooked (2 cups)

Frozen

- Frozen chopped spinach (2 cups)
- Frozen sliced peaches (16 oz. pkg./about 3 cups)

Fruit

- Granny Smith apple (1) + Gala cooking apples (2)
- Fresh blueberries (1 cup)
- Fresh pineapple - halves
- Orange zest (1 tsp.)
- Lemons (3)
- Lemon peel (2 tsp.) + Juice (10 tbsp.) +
- Lime (2 wedges) + (2 tbsp.)
- Chopped fresh mint (2 tbsp.)
- Sliced strawberries (1.5 cups)

Veggies

- Serrano chili (1 rib)
- Red sweet pepper (2 cups)
- Mini sweet pepper (1-2 tbsp.)
- Fresh jalapeño chili pepper (1)
- Shallot (about 2 tbsp./1 medium)
- Acorn squash (1 small - 6-inches in diameter)
- Asparagus tips - cut in 1-inch pieces (.5 lb./about 2 cups)
- Carrots (2 cups/about 8 ounces) + (5 medium) + (2 large)
- Celery (2 stalks)
- Cucumbers (1 large or 2 small) (1 medium) (2 cups) (12 slices)
- Fresh mushrooms (.5 lb./about 2 cups)
- Turnips - peeled & cut into 0.5-inch pieces (2 medium)
- Fresh sugar-snap peas (10 oz. pkg.)
- Sweet potatoes (1 lb. @ ½-inch pieces)
- Zucchini (1 cup)
- Cherry tomatoes (1 pint)
- Roma tomatoes (8)
- Tomato (1 cup)

- Onion (1 cup) + Yellow onions (2) (1.5 cups + Medium onion (1)
- Red onion (2 cups + 3 tbsp.) + (8 thick rings @ about .25-inches)
- Mixed salad greens (5 oz. pkg./about 8 cups)
- Grape or cherry tomatoes (1 pint)
- Garlic cloves (13)
- Fresh ginger (1 tbsp.)
- Fresh basil
- Fresh cilantro (.75 cup)
- Parsley (1.25 cup)
- Chopped mint (3 tbsp.)
- Fresh rosemary (8 sprigs + 1 tbsp.)

Chapter 5:
DASH-Approved Restaurant Dining

The sodium may be a little rich in some of these, so just save your daily sodium for a special treat or save half of it for the next day!

Favorite 1: Veggie Salad with Brown Rice - Black Beans & Guacamole
Chipotle will provide you with this dish for the following nutritional counts:
Statistics (Each Portion):
- Protein Counts: 14 grams
- Carbohydrates: 67 grams
- Fat Content: 29.5 grams
- Fiber: 16 grams
- Sugars: 3 grams
- Sodium: 770 mg
- Calories: 575

Favorite 2: Blackened Chicken Tenders
Popeyes will provide you with five chicken tenders with a regular side of green beans.
Statistics (Each Portion):
- Protein Counts: 46 grams
- Carbohydrates: 10 grams
- Fat Content: 5 grams
- Sugars: 2 grams
- Dietary Fiber: 2 grams
- Sodium: 1593 mg
- Calories: 338

Favorite 3: Tuna Rolla & Buddha's Feast -Steamed
PF Chang will offer you a delicious treat in this delightful portion.
Statistics (Each Portion):
- Protein Counts: 44 grams
- Carbohydrates: 75 grams
- Fat Content: 10 grams
- Sugars: 23 grams
- Dietary Fiber: 11 grams
- Sodium: 990 mg
- Calories: 560

Favorite 4: Live Maine Lobster
Red Lobster will provide you with 1¼ pounds of steamed lobster with a baked potato for a side dish.
Statistics (Each Portion):
- Protein Counts: 38 grams
- Carbohydrates: 45 grams
- Fat Content: 36 grams
- Sugars: 2 grams

- Dietary Fiber: 5 grams
- Sodium: 310 mg
- Calories: 650

Favorite 5: Herb-Grilled Salmon with Steamed Broccoli and Parmesan-Crusted Zucchini
Olive Garden steps up with a delicious salmon platter.
Statistics (Each Portion):
- Protein Counts: 52 grams
- Carbohydrates: 21 grams
- Fat Content: 34 grams
- Sugars: 7 grams
- Dietary Fiber: 9 grams
- Sodium: 1185 mg
- Calories: 575

Favorite 6: String Bean Chicken Breast with a Half-Side of Steamed Brown Rice & A Full Side of Super Greens
Panda Express loads your platter with healthier options!
Statistics (Each Portion):
- Protein Counts: 20 grams
- Carbohydrates: 23 grams
- Fat Content: 11.5 grams
- Sugars: 8 grams
- Dietary Fiber: 9 grams
- Sodium: 850 mg
- Calories: 280

Favorite 7: Banh Mi Bowl
California Pizza Kitchen will provide you with a dishful of goodies!
Statistics (Each Portion):
- Protein Counts: 28 grams
- Carbohydrates: 40 grams
- Fat Content: 33 grams
- Sugars: 10 grams
- Dietary Fiber: 9 grams
- Sodium: 770 mg
- Calories: 540

Favorite 8: Lemon Pepper Grilled Rainbow Trout with Freshly Steamed Broccoli & Brussels Sprouts & Kale Salad
Cracker Barrel offers a lightly seasoned boneless fillet.
Statistics (Each Portion):
- Protein Counts: 50 grams
- Carbohydrates: 43 grams
- Fat Content: 34 grams
- Sugars: 29 grams
- Dietary Fiber: 5 grams
- Sodium: 800 mg
- Calories: 650

Favorite 9: Fish Bowl & Pinto Beans - Diced Onions - Quinoa - Chopped Cilantro - Diced Tomatoes & Fresh Jalapenos

Moe's Southwest Grill in Georgia - USA, will load your plate with delicious Southern cuisine. The full platter is a bit much for a serving, so portion it into two meals if desired.

Statistics (Each Portion):

- Protein Counts: 41 grams
- Carbohydrates: 88 grams
- Fat Content: 17 grams
- Sugars: 18 grams
- Dietary Fiber: 25 grams
- Sodium: 1043 mg
- Calories: 605

Favorite 10: Grilled Chicken Sandwich

Chick-fil-A offers this flavorful lemon-herb marinated breast of chicken option!

Statistics (Each Portion):

- Protein Counts: 29 grams
- Carbohydrates: 41 grams
- Fat Content: 6 grams
- Sugars: 9 grams
- Dietary Fiber: 4 grams
- Sodium: 720 mg
- Calories: 330

Favorite 11: Parmesan Rotisserie Quarter Dark-Roasted Chicken (2 drumsticks & 1 thigh) with Steamed Vegetables & Garlic-Dill New Potatoes

Boston Market's flavorful chicken is packed full of nutrients and superb flavor.

Statistics (Each Portion):

- Protein Counts: 46 grams
- Carbohydrates: 41 grams
- Fat Content: 27 grams
- Fiber: 6 grams
- Sugars: 7 grams
- Sodium: 1470 mg
- Calories: 570

Favorite 12: Simply Grilled Salmon with Veggies & Jasmine Rice

TGI Fridays is a break away from the rest with this delicious dish!

Statistics (Each Portion):

- Protein Counts: 39 grams
- Carbohydrates: 86 grams
- Fat Content: 38 grams
- Sugars: 3 grams
- Dietary Fiber: 4 grams
- Sodium: 1000 mg
- Calories: 830

Favorite 13: Grilled Chicken Salad

Chili's is an atmosphere, not to be ignored!

Statistics (Each Portion):
- Protein Counts: 36 grams
- Carbohydrates: 22 grams
- Fat Content: 23 grams
- Sugars: 11 grams
- Dietary Fiber: 5 grams
- Sodium: 1130 mg
- Calories: 430

Favorite 14: Turkey Gyro

Arby's will please you with its delicious sandwich!

Statistics (Each Portion):
- Protein Counts: 25 grams
- Carbohydrates: 48 grams
- Fat Content: 20 grams
- Fiber: 3 grams
- Sugars: 5 grams
- Sodium: 1520 mg
- Calories: 470

Favorite 15: Charbroiled Chicken Club Sandwich in a Lettuce Wrap

Hardees will hit the DASH measure without the bacon.

Statistics (Each Portion):
- Protein Counts: 16 grams
- Carbohydrates: 12 grams
- Fat Content: 16 grams
- Sugars: 8 grams
- Dietary Fiber: 1 gram
- Sodium: 660 mg
- Calories: 250

Favorite 16: Cheese & Fruit Protein Box

Starbucks is a delightful option for your DASH healthy choices.

Statistics (Each Portion):
- Protein Counts: 20 grams
- Carbohydrates: 34 grams
- Fat Content: 27 grams
- Sugars: 15 grams
- Dietary Fiber: 4 grams
- Sodium: 620 mg
- Calories: 450

Favorite 17: Grilled Salmon with Sweet Potato & Grilled Zucchini

Ruby Tuesdays provide yet another delicious way to enjoy salmon.

Statistics (Each Portion):
- Protein Counts: 45 grams
- Carbohydrates: 31 grams
- Fat Content: 29 grams

- Sugars: 10 grams
- Dietary Fiber: 5 grams
- Sodium: 1491 mg
- Calories: 588

Favorite 18: Impossible Whopper

Burger King provides the Whopper for DASH - just - hold the mayo!

Statistics (Each Portion):

- Protein Counts: 25 grams
- Carbohydrates: 58 grams
- Fat Content: 16 grams
- Sugars: 12 grams
- Dietary Fiber: 4 grams
- Sodium: 940 mg
- Calories: 470

Chapter 6:
Big Changes to Your Diet Begin - Always from Small Changes

With your meal plan and shopping list in hand, begin your journey to making changes in preparing your meals. Meal prep is a great place to begin, but first, you must know what your body's craving. No matter which of the dieting methods you choose to use, if you're living a busy lifestyle, sometimes, you just don't know what you want. Your body will tell you what's necessary to keep it going. The message is sent to you as a craving. Here are a few cravings with what your body needs and a quick fix for the issue:

Your Craving	What You Need	Fix It
Carbs/Bread/Pasta	• Nitrogen	• High Protein Meat
Sugary Food	• Phosphorous • Tryptophan	• Chicken • Beef • Lamb • Liver • Cheese • Cauliflower • Broccoli
Chocolate	• Carbon • Magnesium • Chromium	• Spinach • Nuts • Seeds • Broccoli • Cheese
Salty Foods	• Silicon	• Nuts • Seeds
Fatty or Oily Foods	• Calcium • Chloride	• Spinach • Broccoli • Cheese • Fish

Consider Meal Preparation to Eliminate Sodium Intake

Now that you have a meal plan, let's consider meal prep and how you can stretch your budget further. Meal prep might seem a bit challenging at first but just remember – you don't need to prep all of your meals at one time. You can begin with the meats one evening and veggies the next; it's all up to you!

Decide How to Prep.
Do you want to prepare all of the chicken, pork, or other meal selections one night and the veggies the next night? Or: Do you want to cook each meal individually but in bulk?

Purchase the containers you want to use.
These are some guidelines for those:
- Mason Jars – Pint or quart size
- Ziploc-type freezer bags
- Rubbermaid Stackable - Glad Containers
- Microwavable
- Freezer Safe
- Stackable
- BPA Free
- Reusable

Label the containers.
There are some other things you have to consider when freezing your meals. You should always label your container with the date that you put it in the freezer. You also need to double-check that your bottles, jars, or bags are each sealed tightly. If your containers aren't air-tight, your food will become freezer burnt and need to be trashed.

Set aside quiet time for prep day.
Choose a time when you won't have any interruptions.

Inventory the kitchen.
Purchase your food items in bulk to save money. Saving money while on the DASH diet is vital. Purchasing your items in bulk can make a severe impact. Check your area for local farms that raise their animals on pasture feeding or a local market for fresh produce. After you find a good deal, stock up and purchase pantry items such as seasonings and flour. You can freeze many things and save a bundle of cash.

Follow your meal plan.
You will begin with your six-week meal plan and build from there. As you proceed with your daily selections, make notes of which ones you enjoyed the most and the ones you want to omit for your next month's planning.

Chop your veggies in advance.
Prepare and freeze plenty of healthy fruits and yogurt into a delicious smoothie for the entire week. Enjoy one for breakfast or any time you have the craving.

Purchase foods in bulk to be used for taco meats, breakfast burritos, fajita fillings, soups, egg muffins, and so much more.

As you prep, include lean proteins for the weekends in a container for a quick grab 'n' go snack or luncheon for a weekend journey.

Tips for Vegetable & Meat Selections

Select fresh meats and dairy when possible.

Try to find meat and dairy that has an expiration date for as far in the future as possible. These choices will tend to remain fresh and last longer, which also applies to the "sell by" dates. The further in the future, either of these dates is, the surer you can bet that the food will last the week.

Select whole - not chopped meats & veggies.

You can save big by chopping your meats and vegetables. You will pay for the person that is doing the cutting for your convenience.

Freeze & reheat your meals -the healthy way.

For meals scheduled to be eaten at least three days after cooking, freezing is a great option. Freezing food is safe and convenient, but it doesn't work for every type of meal. You can also freeze the ingredients for a slow cooker meal and then dump the container into the slow cooker and leave it there. Save a lot of time so you can pre-prep meals up to one to two months in advance. The last food safety consideration you need to make concerning meal prepping is how you reheat food. Most people opt to microwave their meals for warming, but you can use any other conventional heating source in your kitchen as well.

However, you have to be careful with microwaving because over-cooking can cause food to taste bad. To combat this, cook your food in one-minute intervals and check on it between each minute.

You can also help your food cook more evenly and quickly but keeping your meat cut into small pieces when you cook it. You should never put food directly from the freezer into the microwave. Let your frozen food thaw first.

Food reheating and prep safety will become second nature over time. Meal prep can be overwhelming and require a lot of thought and patience, but it becomes a lot easier once you get used to it. Many of the mistakes are easy to avoid.

However, mistakes do happen, and as such, it's best to cook for short periods rather than longer ones, so you have less of a risk of making a mistake and needing to scrap everything you have prepared for that substantial time. While it is a lot and seems complicated, meal prepping is the best way to set yourself up for success with the DASH diet.

Example of How Meal Prep Works - The Shopping List:

- ✓ **_Choose Healthy Produce_**
  Carrots, red bell peppers, cucumbers, baby spinach, and any other DASH-friendly veggies you prefer.
- ✓ **_Protein Options_**
  Two cans of tuna, one pound of lunch meat of your choice (turkey, ham, roast beef), and two pounds of skinless chicken thighs, or one pound of salmon (to be used for lunch and dinner).
- ✓ **_Dairy Options_**
  Cheese sticks (of your choice), heavy cream, sour cream, grass-fed butter, DASH-friendly salad dressing, mayo, mustard, and eggs.
- ✓ **_Options - Dry Goods_**
  Coffee, avocado oil, pecans, almonds, salt, pepper, and your seasonings of choice

Method of Preparation:

1. From there, you will do the following steps to prepare your lunch and dinner for the week:

2. Get ten plastic containers ready to fill with your meals.

3. Prepare perishable items first - this is an important step because you can save a ton of time and money by preparing several items simultaneously. For example, if you have many chicken items during the week, prepare all of the chicken needed and either place it into individual wrappers or in the bottom of the refrigerator to use within the next day or so.

4. Chop up vegetables and put them in five different plastic containers.

5. Combine baby spinach salad with vegetables of choice to make five salads.

6. Boil eggs and peel.

7. Mix the canned tuna with mayo, mustard, salt, and pepper. Put the tuna salad in two different plastic containers that already have a salad or mixed vegetables in them.

8. Bake four pieces of chicken and four pieces of salmon. Season it with your seasonings of choice and cook them in avocado oil.

9. Combine four pieces of salmon and four chicken pieces with the ten containers that are already filled with salad and chopped vegetables.

10. Finish the ten meals by adding your choice of pecans, almonds, hard-boiled eggs, and cheese sticks. These will be snacks to supplement your meals.

You are ready to go and prepare all of your breakfast, lunch, and dinner for the coming week. This process will take two to three hours, but it will be well worth it as all of your meals are now ready for the week.

Handle Snack Time

You never know when the hunger 'pains' will strike, so you have to be prepared with the right substance at just the right time. These are some excellent spaces to hide the 'emergency' stash until it is time for mealtime preparation.

The Handy Backpack - Briefcase & Handbag

Always be prepared and become known as the person with everything!

- Less than 200 calories - several whole-grain granola bars
- Snack-size Ziploc baggie of ¼ cup of dried fruit trail mix and seed. Add the same amount of whole-grain cereal
- A small box or can of 100% vegetable or fruit juice
- Whole grain breakfast bars
- Have some handy Ziploc baggies of crunchy broccoli, carrots, cucumbers, or bell peppers for a super healthy snack.

The Vending Machine

Modernized machines are one of the areas that have shown improvements with so many health issues in today's society. You need to stick to a single serving size of 1- to 1½-ounce portions.

These are some of the good choices to seek:

- Baked tortilla or potato chips
- Pretzels
- Whole-grain breakfast bars
- Trail mix
- Single-serve flavored milk (fat-free or low-fat)
- 12-ounce serving sizes of 100% fruit or vegetable juice

The Desk Drawer

Whether you are at home or in the office, you should always be prepared with fresh fruit or similar items for that 'hungry' moment. These are a few other ways:

- Stock up on whole-grain pretzels and crackers
- Plain nuts and seeds are good for a healthy, fiber-filled snack.
- Sardines or Tuna in a bag is a quick fix. Select the ones packed in water.
- Hot or cold cereals in individual packages are good whether you have milk—or not!

The Office Lunchroom Refrigerator

Most businesses, even the smaller ones, will have an area with a refrigerator where you can store some healthy goodies. If not, grab a lunch box or cooler, and you are set. Consider these choices to stay in line with your DASH plan:

- Low-fat/fat-free yogurt, milk, cottage cheese, cheese slices or sticks, and similar items.
- Tzatziki – a sauce that can be used as a dip
- Frozen berries or fruit
- Deli roast beef, chicken, or turkey
- Hummus, bean dip, or Nut butter

Tips to Reset Your Diet & Lifestyle

o You can begin with subtle changes, so you don't end up craving items that are not in your DASH plan. These are some of the ways:

o Use only fat-free or low-fat or condiments.

o It is essential to attempt to use only half of your typical serving of salad dressing, margarine, or butter.

o Add a serving of vegetables to your dinner and lunch menus. Make dry beans a part of your diet plan.

o Limit meat options to six ounces daily. Make some of the meals strictly vegetarian.

o Add a serving of fruit as a snack or with your meal. Dried and canned fruits are quick and easy to use. However, make sure they don't have added sugar.

o Read the food labels and make choices that are lower in sodium content.

o For a snack, have some frozen yogurt (fat-free or low-fat), nuts or unsalted pretzels, raw veggies, unsalted-plain popcorn. Leave the sweets and salty chips alone.

You have many resources online; you have the option to plan many of your meals before you leave home. You should continue with your pre-planning. It will become more evident as you can branch out to enjoy dining out at many different restaurants. You just need to follow a few simple guidelines, as shown in this segment.

How to Choose Beverages When You Go Out to Eat?

You will want to choose beverages that are low in sodium. Choose coffee, tea, diet soda, fruit juice, club soda, or a glass of the best option of water. According to Healthline, choose from juices including pomegranate, prune, beet, or tomatoes. Have a glass of skim milk to help fight hypertension and blood pressure issues.

Avoid Super-Sized Portions

Before you began your DASH diet plan, you probably enjoyed dining out, and restaurants always gave you heaping portions. Use some of these suggestions to avoid overheating:

- Instead of an entree, substitute with an appetizer.
- Even if you're having dinner, request a lunch portion.
- Enjoy and share a meal with a friend.
- Ask the waiter/waitress to provide you with the container to store half of your meal before you begin eating.

Lower Your Salt Intake

One of the key objectives of the DASH diet plan is to cut back on salt. Even though salt often enhances flavor, in many restaurants, it gets heavily overused. These are a few additional tips to use while dining out:

- Limit condiments such as ketchup, mustard, and pickles that may be high in salt content.
- Remove the salt shaker from the table - out of reach.
- Request that your meal is to be prepared without added salt.
- Remain aware of certain foods that may be suggestive of being cooked with salt. For example, avoid cured or smoked dishes or plates that have soy sauce or broth.
- Opt for veggies and fruits instead of salty appetizers.

Lower Unhealthy Fat Intake

Your DASH diet plan will promote foods that are low in cholesterol and saturated fat. Lower the fat using the following techniques:

- Trim away any visible fat from poultry and meat products ordered. One portion should be about the size of a folded wallet. Even lean meats contain fat.
- Ask the chef to prepare your food using olive oil versus butter.
- Select foods that have been prepared with cooking techniques such as stir-frying, poaching, roasting, baking, broiling, grilling, or steaming.
- Avoid salad dressing and request it to be served on the side. Choose oil and vinegar.
- Choose from broiled or steamed fish and ask for fresh herbs or lemon on the side.
- Order steamed veggies and fruits without sauce or butter.

Use Caution Dining at Fast Food Establishments

With a little planning and these tips, you can enjoy your fast-food outing:

- Choose children's meals or regular size meals while on your dash diet plan.
- Choose a healthier option such as a single hamburger or a fish sandwich: Select yogurt, low-fat milk, or whole wheat bread.
- Make yourself familiar with the restaurant's nutritional information before you leave home.
- Ask for no added salt in your food preparation.
- Use caution when ordering fast-food salads. They may contain many extras, including salt and dressing.
- Select from healthier side dishes, including fresh fruit or a baked potato.
- Select food that has been steamed, broiled, or grilled. It's best to avoid battered and fried foods.
-

Try not to become obsessed with the results or focus on quick fixes, or you will lose sight that the diet is about regaining your health and developing a new way of eating. Set your goals on creating a lifestyle change that you can continue for the rest of your life.

Once you have your meal plan favorites charted, plan another one using your new food items, using caution to how much sodium is included. Here is a general list of how you accomplish all of your goals:

- *Step One:* Make the menu.

- *Step Two*: Plan the meals focusing on foods at your local market on sale.

- *Step Three*: Check your stock in the pantry, freezer, and fridge to know what items are needed.

- *Step Four*: Slowly build your pantry and spice supplies to provide various flavors to your diet plan.

- *Step Five*: Plan on using leftovers or freeze them for another time.

- *Step Six*: Stop for items using a seasonal chart, for instance, consider these: It's important to understand which foods you can and cannot eat, but it is equally important to obtain the freshest items available in your area.

Depending on where you live, some fruits and vegetables are fresh and available year-round. The following dates are a general guideline based on the United States' growing seasons. Use these veggies and fruits to enjoy the most delicious and healthy options:

Spring - March 1 to May 31:
- Fava Beans
- Fennel
- Artichokes
- Avocados
- Carrots
- Asparagus
- Chives
- Apricots

Summer - June 1 to August 31:
- Arugula
- Cucumber
- Beets
- Bell Peppers
- Carrots
- Radishes
- Zucchini
- Garlic

Autumn - September 1 to November 30:
- Fennel
- Apples
- Winter Greens
- Pomegranate
- Figs
- Pears
- Sweet Potatoes
- Winter Squash

Winter - December 1 to February 28:
- Apples
- Cabbage
- Cauliflower
- Carrots
- Broccoli & Broccoli Rabe
- Brussels Sprouts
- Beets

That is all it is to it!

Conclusion

I hope you have enjoyed each segment of the *Dash Diet Cookbook*; let's hope it was informative and provided you with all of the tools you need to achieve your goals, whatever they may be. The next step is to consider which delicious meal to prepare first. You have the first few weeks already mapped out and ready to go!

As a reminder, you will want to stay on track with your new methods used for the DASH approach to dieting.

The guidelines will help you stay in line with your goals:
- Switch refined grains for whole grains.
- Serve and enjoy an abundance of vegetables and fruits.
- Choose lean protein sources, including poultry, fish, and beans.
- Choose low-fat or fat-free dairy products.
- Cook with vegetable oils.
- Limit your intake of foods high in saturated fats such as full-fat dairy, fatty meats, and oils - including - coconut or palm oil.
- Limit your intake of foods high in added sugars, including candy and soda.

Other than the measured fresh fruit juice portions, this diet recommends you stick to low-calorie drinks such as water, tea, and coffee.
Here are very more simple tricks to help you reduce your salt intake:
- Use other citrus options, herbs, and seasonings when cooking to flavor your food instead of salt.
- Be sure to check the nutritional facts and ingredients labels for hidden sources of sodium.
- Use a phone app to keep track of your daily food intake.
- Watch out for anything packaged in advance, including pickled, cured, barbecued, smoked, or seasoned with broth, miso, soy sauce, tomato sauce, or Asian sauces. You can use them in moderation when included in your special recipe options.

The DASH diet is even more effective at lowering blood pressure when paired with physical activity. The pros suggest you perform at least ½ hour of moderate activity most days. Do something you enjoy or make daily tasks a more pleasurable event.

Ways to Get Walking:
- Walk instead of driving, whenever you can.
- If you take a bus, make an early stop, and walk part of the way.
- If you have a choice of an elevator or the stairs, you know the answer.
- Start making Saturday morning a family walking event.
- Take a Sunday walk instead of taking a Sunday drive.
- When you go shopping, park a few aisles further away and take a walk.
- While you are window shopping, go for a brisk walk in the mall.
- Leave the television off and take a leisurely half-hour walk to remove the stress of the day.
- Quit avoiding the hills, and go climbing.

Additional examples of moderate activity

- Housework (60 minutes) can invigorate you if you turn on a few tunes while you work.
- Go for a brisk walk (9 minutes per kilometer or 15 minutes per mile), popping in your music to get the rhythm flowing.
- Running is another wonderful way to eliminate some unwanted pounds (6 minutes per kilometer or 10 minutes per mile).
- Cycling can be a lot of fun if you have a partner who can also indulge (4 minutes per kilometer or 6 minutes per mile).
- Swimming laps is a very enjoyable event that will help you stay fit (20 minutes).

As you see, there is more to a new way of eating than just pushing your plate away at the table and cutting back on your sodium intake. It just takes a bit of adjusting to your current lifestyle.

You can do it!

Finally, if you found this book useful in any way, a review on Amazon is always appreciated!

Printed in Great Britain
by Amazon